Helicopter Gunship

4	Introduction
6	Helicopters Go to War
8	The Attack Helicopter
10	Bell UH-1 Huey
12	Bell AH-1 Cobra
14	Mil Mi-24
16	McDonnell Douglas AH-64A Apache
18	McDonnell Douglas AH-64D Apache Longbow
20	AgustaWestland Apache AH1
22	Boeing AH-64E Guardian
24	Aérospatiale SA341/342 Gazelle
25	Eurocopter EC665 Tiger
26	Kamov Ka-52 Alligator
27	Mil Mi-28
28	America's Helicopter War in Vietnam
42	Moscow's First Helicopter War
44	Apache Dawn 1991
60	Whiskey Cobra Action
64	Into Afghanistan 2001
68	Apache Strike in Afghanistan 2002
74	Destroying the Republican Guard
82	Operation Telic 2003
88	Britain's Apache over Helmand
94	Operation Panther's Claw
98	Strike from the Sea
104	Gunships Against 'ISIS'
110	Seize Kiev
112	Air Cav for the 21st Century

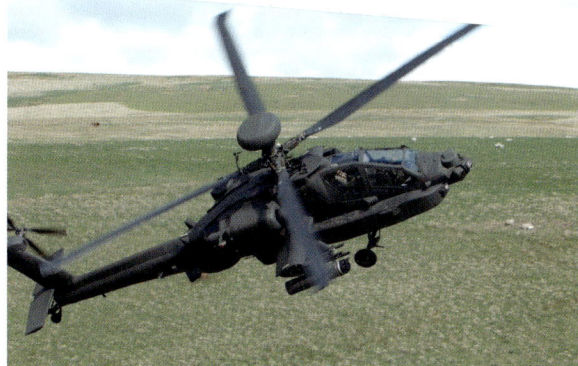

The iconic Apache is the world's ultimate attack helicopter. (UK MOD/CROWN COPYRIGHT)

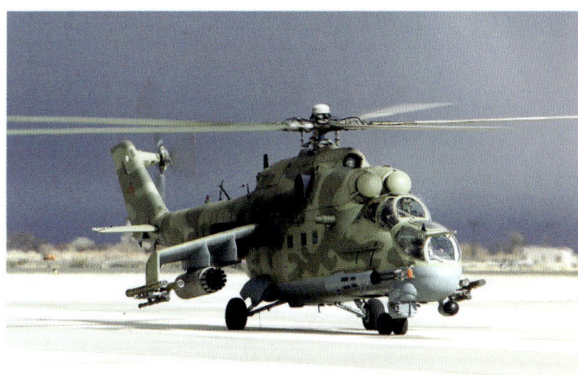

The Soviet-era Mi-24 is still on duty with more than 20 air arms. (US DOD/COMBAT CAMERA)

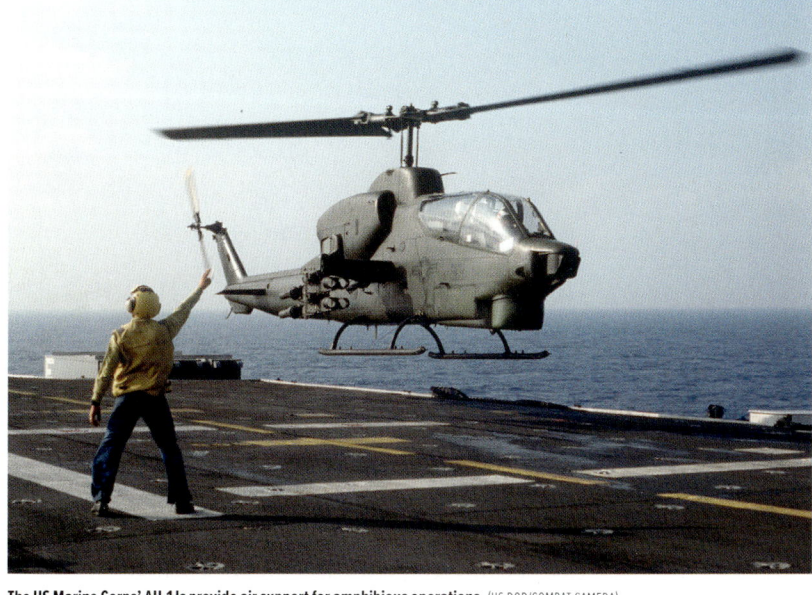

The US Marine Corps' AH-1Js provide air support for amphibious operations. (US DOD/COMBAT CAMERA)

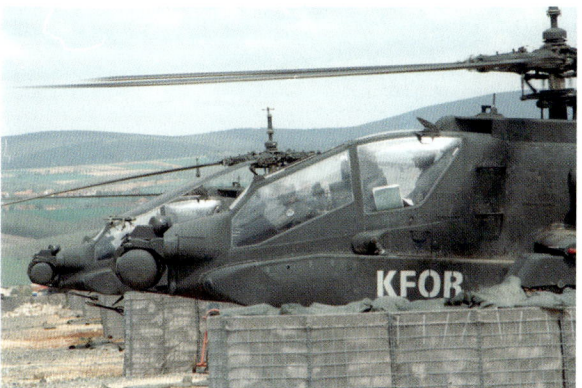

UAE AH-64E poised for a peacekeeping patrol over Kosovo. (TIM RIPLEY)

ISBN: 978 1 80282 329 5

Editor: Tim Ripley

Senior editor, specials: Roger Mortimer

Email: roger.mortimer@keypublishing.com
Design: SJmagic DESIGN SERVICES, India
Cover: Dan Hilliard
Advertising Sales Manager: Brodie Baxter
Email: brodie.baxter@keypublishing.com

Tel: 01780 755131
Advertising Production: Debi McGowan
Email: debi.mcgowan@keypublishing.com

Subscription/Mail Order
Key Publishing Ltd, PO Box 300,
Stamford, Lincs, PE9 1NA
Tel: 01780 480404
Fax: 01780 757812
Subscriptions email: subs@
keypublishing.com

Mail Order email: orders@keypublishing.com
Website: www.keypublishing.com/shop

Publishing
Group CEO: Adrian Cox
Publisher: Jonathan Jackson
Head of Publishing: Finbarr O'Reilly
Head of Marketing: Shaun Binnington
Key Publishing Ltd, PO Box 100,
Stamford, Lincs, PE9 1XP
Tel: 01780 755131

Website: www.keypublishing.com

Printing
Precision Colour Printing Ltd, Haldane,
Halesfield 1, Telford, Shropshire.
TF7 4QQ

Distribution
Seymour Distribution Ltd, 2 Poultry
Avenue, London, EC1A 9PU
Enquiries Line: 02074 294000.

Photo Credits: Tim Ripley, UK Ministry of Defence, US Department of Defense, US Navy, US Air Force, US Marine Corps, US Army, US National Archives, US Central Intelligence Agency, British Army, Royal Air Force, Royal Navy, UK Ministry of Defence, NATO, , Russian Ministry of Defence, Russian Aerospace Force, Israel Defence Force Spokesman, French Ministry of Defence, German Bundeswehr, Eurocopter, Westland Helicopters, Bell Helicopte4s Boeing, Lockheed Martin, BAE Systems, Thales, Sikorsky, RuthAS, Filip Vidinovski, Paramount Pictures, Maxar Technologies, Alan Radecki, Nicky Boogaard, Greg Goebel, Hunini, Peter Ellis, Radomil, Oren Rozen, Przemyslaw Idzkiewicz, JC Perrin, Dmitriy Pichugin, Oleg V. Belyakov, Vitaly V. Kuzmin, Allocer, Icemanwcs, Mikhail Evstafiev, Mke1024.

The author has attempted, where possible, to credit the originators of all the images used in this publication. Any errors will be corrected in future editions.

Gunship

Attack Helicopters at War

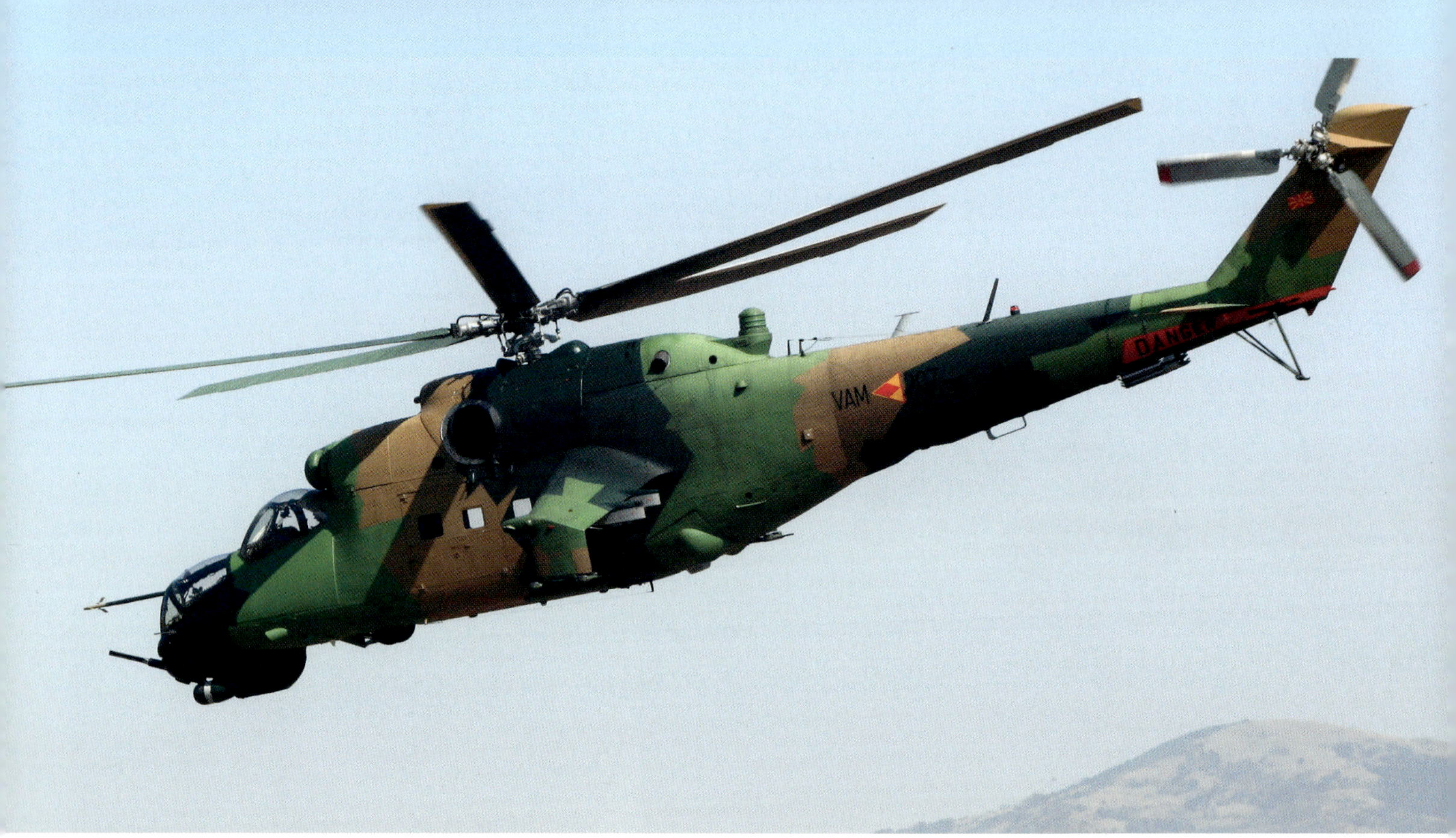

ABOVE: A Mi-24 on patrol over Macedonia. The iconic gunship is still used by more than 30 air arms. (FILIP VIDINOVSKI)

In an iconic 12-minute long sequence in the 1979 Hollywood movie, *Apocalypse Now*, US Army helicopter gunships take part in a dramatic air assault operation to capture a Viet Cong-held village.

Huey gunships 'prep' the objective with rockets and cannons before troop transport helicopters deliver the assault force onto its objective. This all takes place to a backing track of Wagner's *Ride of the Valkyries*.

There was plenty of artistic licence on display in the film but beneath the Hollywood treatment it captured the essence of going to war in helicopters in Vietnam in the 1960s and early 1970s.

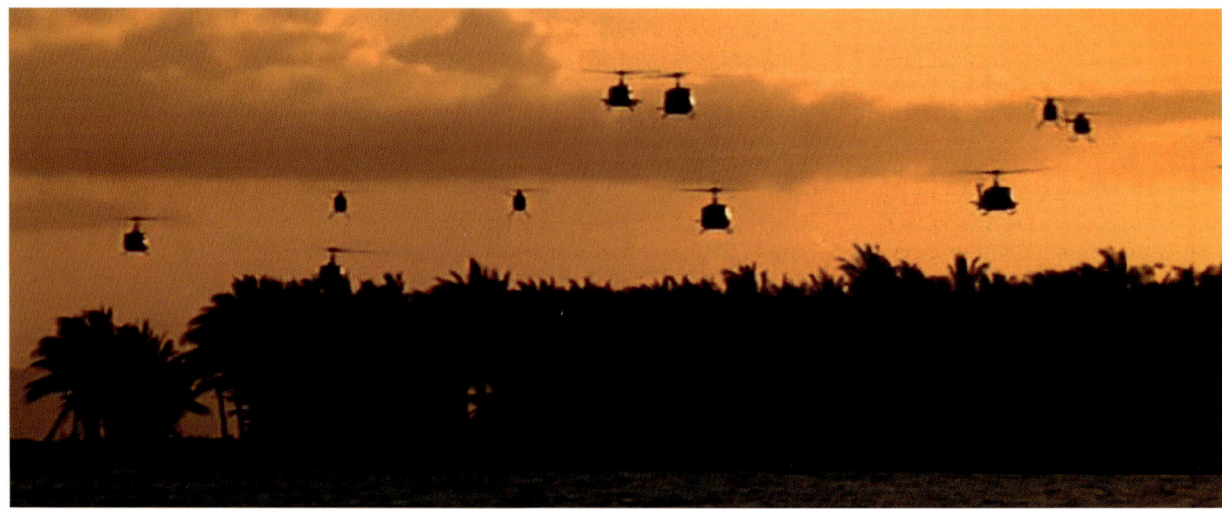

RIGHT: The movie *Apocalypse Now* gave the US Army helicopters' operations in Vietnam the full Hollywood treatment. (PARAMOUNT PICTURES)

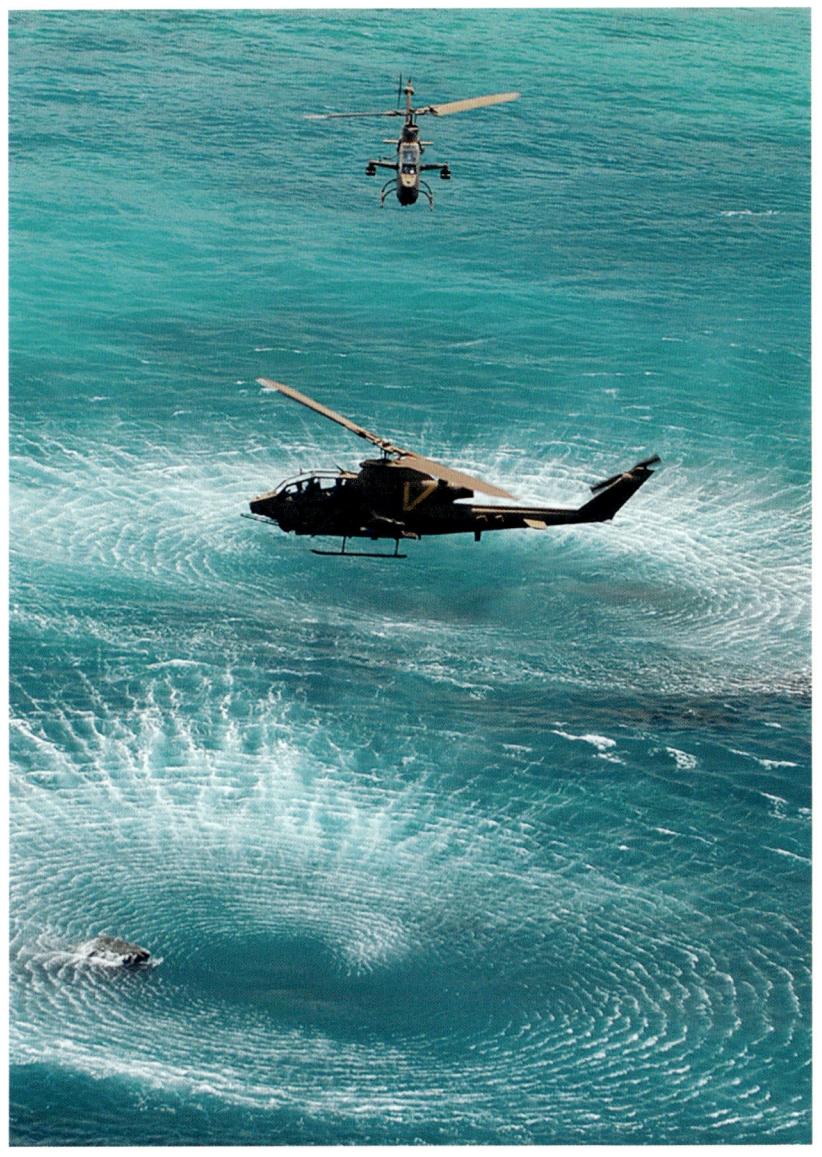

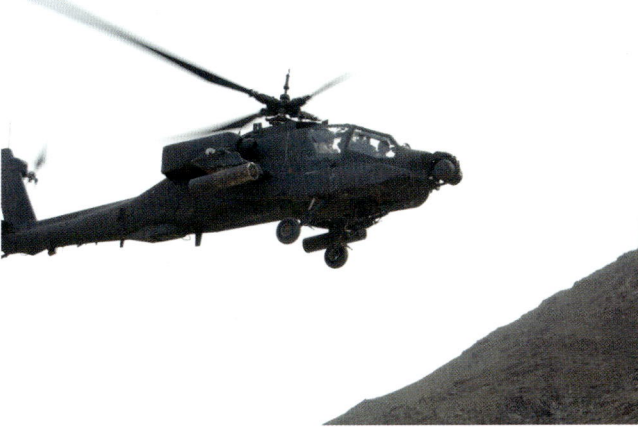

summer of 2001, the paralysing fear caused by the approach of helicopters rapidly became apparent. Within seconds of hearing the sound of Macedonian Mi-24 gunships, experienced and confident insurgents were transformed into hunted prey. They rapidly abandoned their vehicles and ran for cover in roadside ditches, forests, and buildings.

Overhead we could fleetingly see the Mi-24s loaded with missiles and rockets, but they were moving so fast the insurgents were never able to bring their weapons to bear against them. All they could do was remain hidden from view until the gunships were low on fuel and returned to base.

In the 50 years since the end of the Vietnam War, attack helicopters have been in service with armies and air forces around the world. In *Helicopter Gunships at War* we tell the story of how warfare has been changed by these devastating weapons.

Tim Ripley
Editor

The lead character, Captain Willard, played by Martin Sheen, produced a famous quote about the 'Air Cav' unit portrayed in the film, saying: "The First of the Ninth was an old cavalry division that traded in their horses for helicopters and went tear-assing around 'Nam looking for the s**t."

The 1st Squadron, 9th Cavalry was a real unit. It was part of the 1st Cavalry Division during the Vietnam War. It even had a flamboyant, commanding officer, Colonel John B Stockton, who was reputed to be the basis for the Colonel Kilgore character in *Apocalypse Now*. Just like the fictional commander of the Air Cav, Colonel Stockton had a strong line in motivational speaking and later commented, "You wanted every member of the unit to start believing that he's in the best unit in the United States Army. We're different. We're different because we're better."

During the Vietnam War gunships, or attack helicopters, were a new type of weapon. They revolutionised warfare. They could deliver devastating firepower with pin-point accuracy. Unlike US Air Force fast jets or heavy bombers they were under the direct control of US Army ground commanders so they could be rapidly co-ordinated with infantry or tank assaults. Their vertical take-off and landing capability meant that helicopter gunships could be based close to the front line in remote forward bases, so they were ready for action at a few minutes notice.

Helicopter gunships flew at low level so their crews were better able to spot targets that the pilots of high flying strike jets couldn't see. While this allowed them to accurately strike the enemy, it also meant that they were far more vulnerable to enemy fire than air force jets. Helicopter pilots had to employ their wits and skill to shield their machines from enemy fire by using speed and terrain – woods, hills, and large buildings – to mask their approach.

The impact on enemy soldiers of being stalked by attack helicopters cannot be underestimated. During a visit by your editor to Albanian insurgents in Macedonia in the

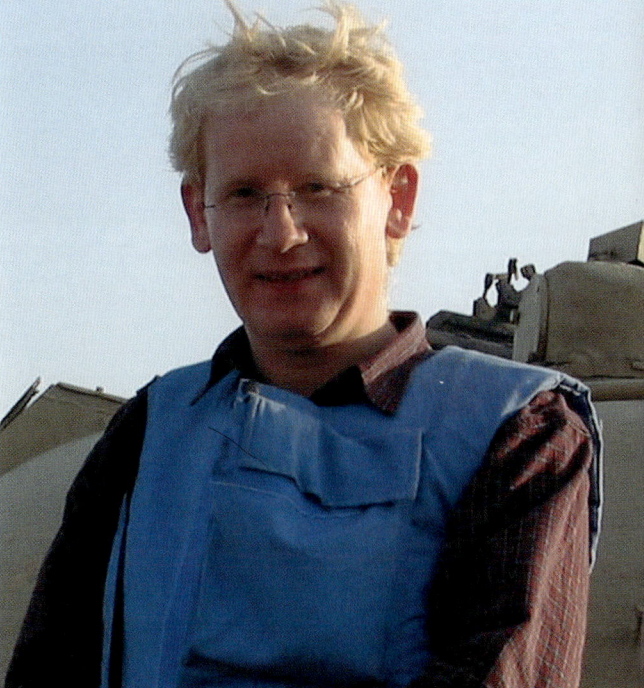

Helicopters Go To War

RIGHT: US Marine Corps HRS-2/S-55 helicopters conducted the first combat movement of troops during the Korean War in 1951. (USMC)

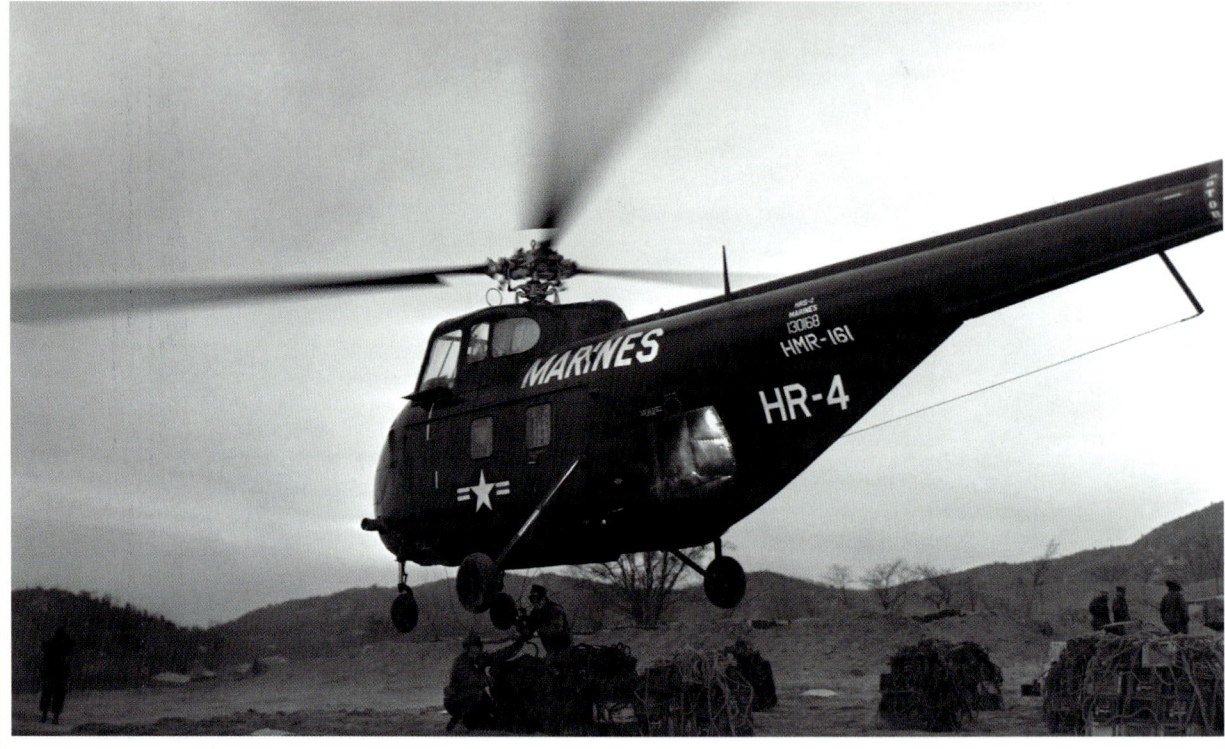

Aviation pioneer, Igor Sikorsky, is credited with designing the first mass-produced military helicopter, the Sikorsky R-4. The idea of using rotating blades to generate a 'disc' that could be used to create lift had been around for many years, but Sikorsky was able to turn the concept into a functioning helicopter that could be built in numbers economically.

The Germans had used basic auto-gyros in small numbers during the early years of World War Two but only a handful ever saw service. Sikorsky flew his prototype R-4 in January 1942 and the following year the US Army Air Force placed its first order. Both the US and British military recognised the battle-winning potential and urged Sikorsky to accelerate testing and production of the helicopter.

By January 1944, the first R-4s were in Southeast Asia, serving with the US contingent fighting the Japanese in the jungles of Burma. One made history by rescuing the downed pilot of a crashed Allied aircraft.

Helicopter technology moved rapidly after World War Two and all the branches of the US military had operational helicopter units by the start of the Korean war in 1950. They were quickly deployed to help the United Nations' forces fight off the Communist invasion. US Army and US Air Force helicopters were used extensively to rescue downed airmen or recover battlefield casualties using the iconic Bell H-13 Sioux. This

BELOW LEFT: Igor Sikorsky's R-4 was the first mass-produced military helicopter. (RUTHAS)

BELOW RIGHT: US Marine Corps' HUS-1/UH-34D Seahorse helicopters in flight over the Mekong Delta in Vietnam in 1962 during the early days of US intervention in that war. (US NAVY)

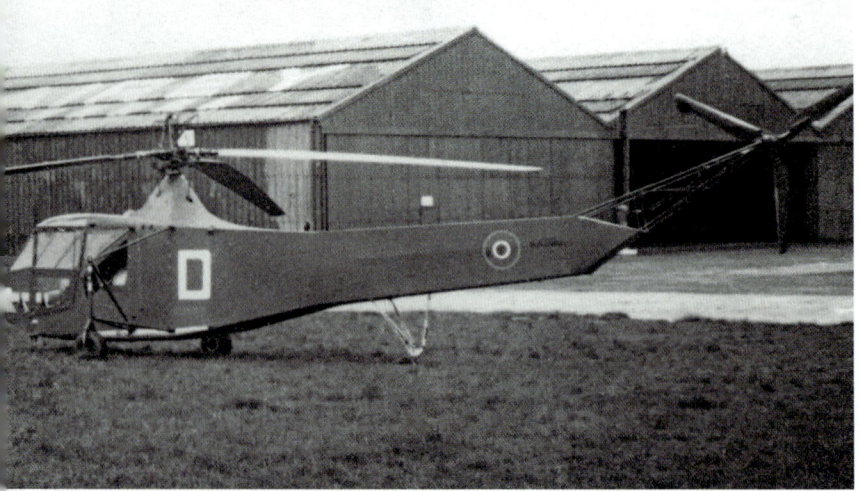

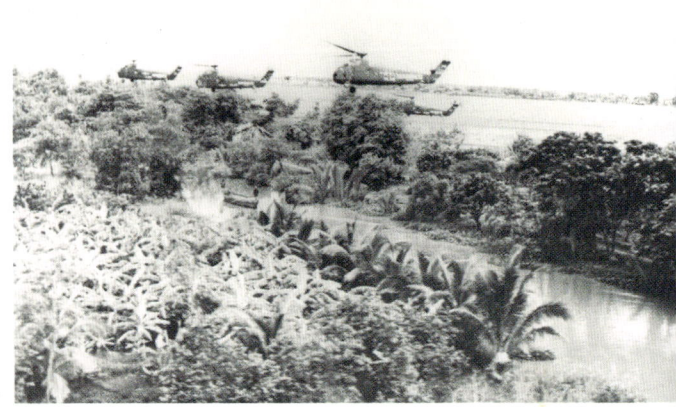

helicopter, with it distinctive glass bubble cockpit, was immortalised in the opening sequence of the film *MASH*, which featured a fictional US Mobile Army Surgical Hospital during the Korean war.

The first recorded instances of helicopters moving troops into battle in Korea took place in September 1951 during Operation Windmill I and involved the US Marine Corps' Sikorsky S-55 Chickasaw, or as the service called it, the HRS-1. The USAF and US Army designated this helicopter the H-19 and in British service it was known as the Whirlwind. This was the first US military helicopter that could lift a useful load of troops or cargo.

Operation Windmill I, saw the USMC helicopters move eight tons of cargo and 74 Marines close to the frontline. A week later more than 200 US Marines were also flown forward to the same area. They were landed just outside the combat zone and then walked into battle.

The distinction of conducting the first-ever combat air assault operation into enemy-held territory in helicopters fell to the British Royal Marines and Fleet Air Arm during the 1956 Suez conflict. British Whirlwinds and Bristol Sycamore helicopters flew 425 troops from 42 Commando ashore from the carriers HMS *Ocean* and HMS *Theseus*.

French forces had used a handful of helicopters, including S-55s, to evacuate casualties from the besieged garrison at Dien Bien Phu in Vietnam in 1953 and they soon saw the potential of these aircraft. When Algerian insurgents rose in revolt in 1954 the French military launched a large campaign in what proved to be a doomed attempt to keep control of the North African country. Its vast desert and mountainous terrain proved ideal for helicopter operations

and the French conducted several air mobile operations to move troops by this means.

France is also credited with using armed helicopters or gunships in action for the first time, although the exact date and location was

not recorded. In 1956, the French Air Force, Armée de l'Air, and the French Army Light Aviation, Aviation Légère de l'Armée de Terre or ALAT, experimented with arming the troop-carrying S-55s with machine guns and small rockets to provide fire support as they landed troops. Bigger and more powerful Piasecki/Vertol H-21s and French-built Sikorsky H-34 Choctaw helicopters were then armed with forward-firing machine guns, cannons, and rockets to create the world's first dedicated gunships. These new gunships flew escort missions for troop transports during large air assault operations. In 1961, ALAT dispatched Sud Aviation Alouette III light helicopters, armed with Nord SS.11 wire-guided antitank missiles, to Algeria to provide precision aerial firepower.

Just as the French war in Algeria was winding down, the US military was being sucked into a new conflict in Southeast Asia and very soon the helicopter would be the defining weapon of that war.

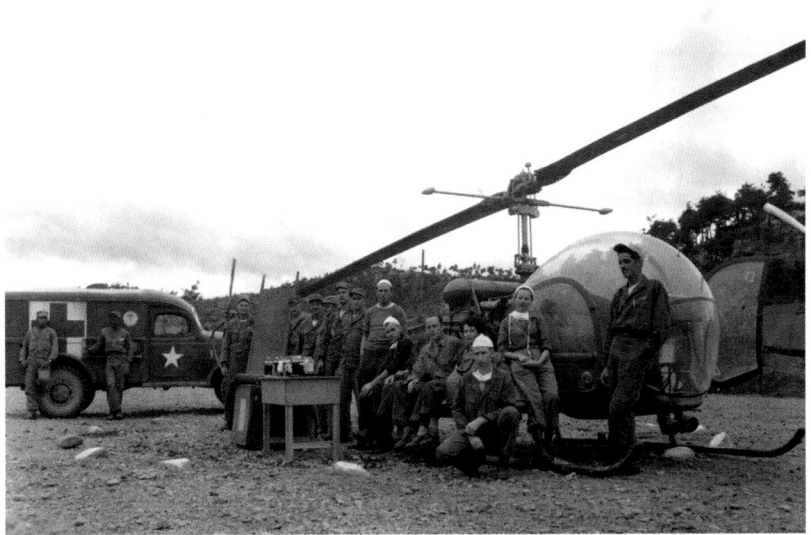

LEFT: The iconic H-13 Sioux's role in evacuating casualties from the battlefields of Korea was made famous in the Hollywood movie, *MASH*. (US ARMY)

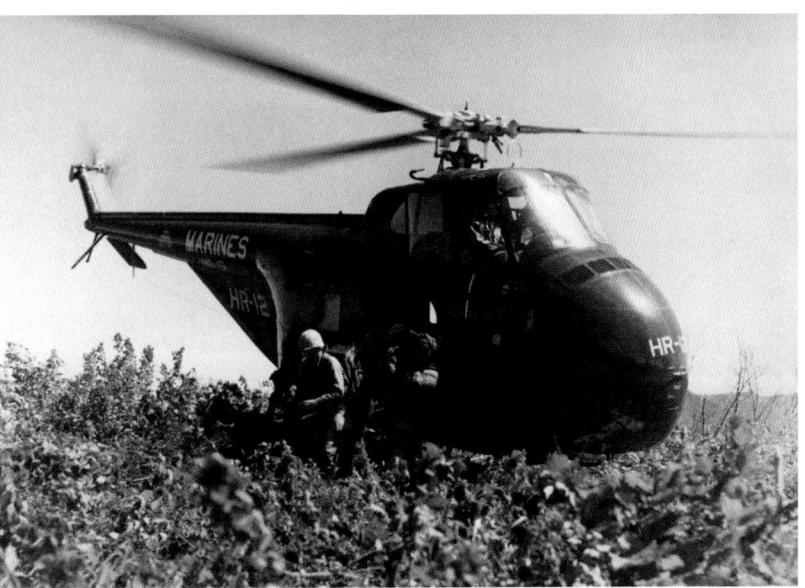

LEFT: The HRS-2/S-55 was the first US military helicopter that could lift a worthwhile load of personnel and cargo. (USMC)

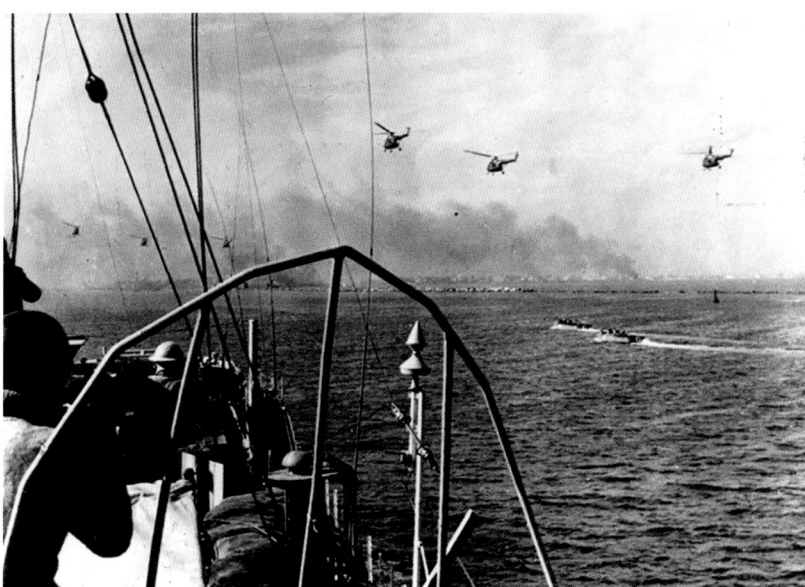

LEFT: Royal Navy Whirlwind and Sycamore helicopters conducted the first-ever air assault operation from a warship during the 1956 Suez Crisis. (ROYAL NAVY)

The Attack Helicopter

What Makes a Good Gunship?

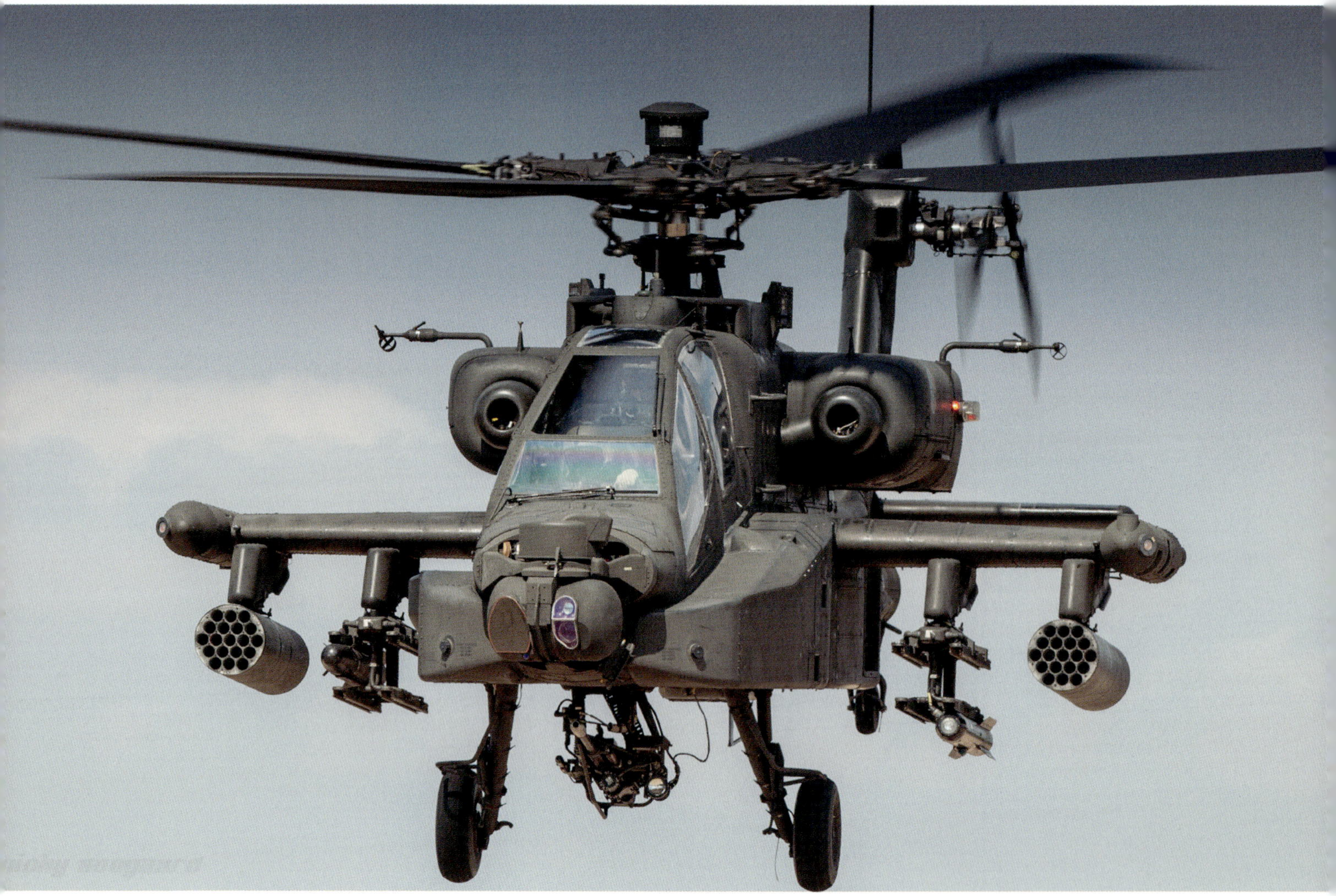

ABOVE: The business end of an AH-64D of the Royal Netherlands Air Force (NICKY BOOGAARD)

There are several essential ingredients in a successful attack helicopter that differentiate them from other military rotorcraft. First of all, they are designed and built around their weapons system. They are all about firepower, so attack helicopters are optimised to carry an array of weapons such as forward-firing guns, rockets, and guided missiles. They need to have effective sensors to allow their crew to find targets and guide their weapons to those targets. Speed and manoeuvrability are also essential requirements to allow crews to dodge enemy fire and approach their targets from unexpected directions.

The first generation of armed helicopters, developed in the 1950s and 1960s, were simple transport or observation helicopters that had

RIGHT: A US Marine Corps AH-1W heads into action during a training exercise in the California desert. (ALAN RADECKI)

weapons strapped on their fuselage. This was a quick and easy way to field aerial firepower but these first gunships were far from ideal.

It was not until the famous Bell AH-1 Cobra took to the skies in the late 1960s that purpose-built attack helicopters saw action. The Cobra used the engine, transmission and tail section of the classic UH-1 Huey but did away with its troop-carrying compartment, which reduced weight

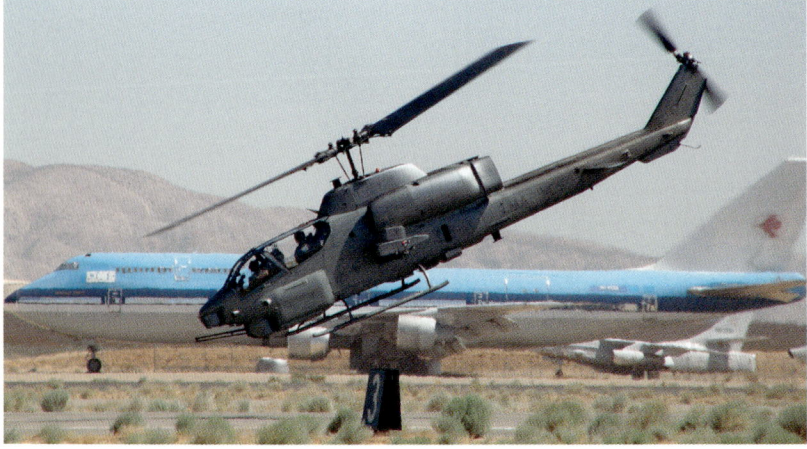

and enhanced manoeuvrability. Its pilot and gunner sat in a tandem configuration at the front of the helicopter to give them a superb view of the battlefield. Small stub wings were stacked with rockets and guns. A rotating turret under the nose contained a mini-gun or grenade launchers.

The instant success of the Cobra in Vietnam saw other nations move to field their own dedicated attack helicopters and the US Army soon set to work improving the Cobra. This coincided with rapid developments in anti-tank guided weapons in the 1960s and it soon become possible to employ those from helicopters, creating flying tank killers.

In the United States the Hughes Aircraft Company (now Raytheon) developed the BGM-71 TOW (Tube-launched, Optically tracked, Wire-guided) missile and this was soon used in action in Vietnam on specially modified UH-1Bs.

In the Soviet Union the adaptation of the Cobra was watched with interest and in 1968 the development of what became known as the Mil Mi-24, or Hind as it was code-named by NATO, got underway.

The Mi-24 featured the tandem cockpit and stub weapon carrier wings of the Cobra but retained a troop-carrying compartment, leading some Western observers to believe it would be used in the air assault or air mobile role to deliver troops to the battlefield. This belief proved to be mistaken and the Soviets used the Mi-24 almost exclusively in the attack role. The troop-carrying

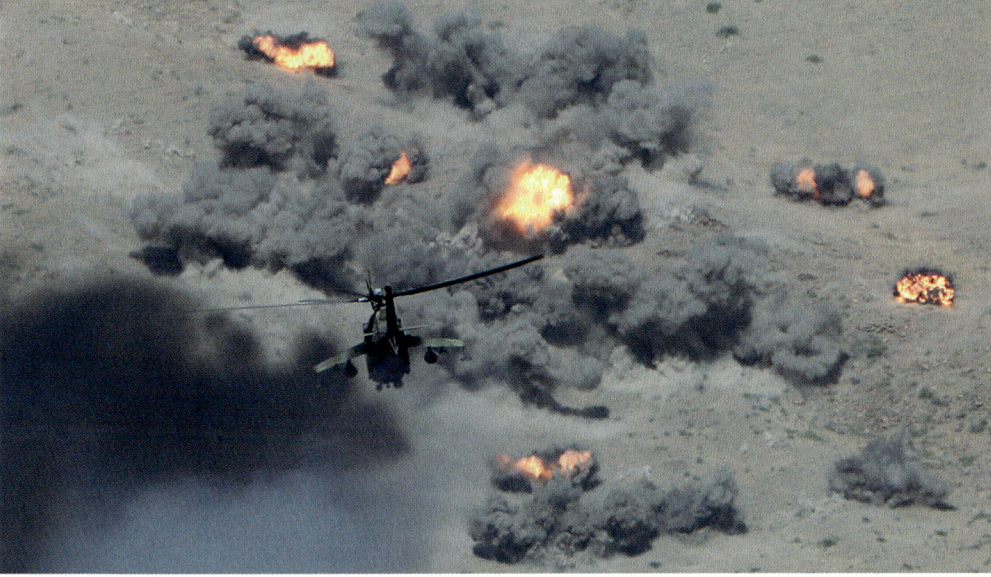

compartment was meant to carry cargo and maintenance personnel during long- distance deployments. Mi-24s were the first attack helicopters to feature extensive use of armour to enhance survivability, leading to their nickname, the 'flying tank'.

The 1980s and 1990s saw rapid advances in the development of sensor technology and this was soon incorporated on attack helicopters. Thermal imaging sensors allowed the helicopter crew to spot targets at long range at night, with computer technology being used to 'slave' sensors to weapon sights to allow rapid and accurate target engagement.

Battlefield radars were also installed on attack helicopters, most famously the Longbow radar mounted on a disc above the rotor hub of the McDonnell Douglas AH-64D Apache Longbow variant. This allowed the crew to identify and target the enemy in fog and rain that would normally impact the performance of thermal imaging sensors.

The 1980s also saw the widespread fielding of defensive aid suites to better protect attack helicopters from shoulder-launched man-portable surface-to-air missiles, known as MANPADs, or radar guided anti-aircraft guns.

Attack helicopters of the 21st century are purpose-designed killing machines, bristling with weapons, advanced sensors, and defensive systems. Armed helicopters have come a long way from the days of strapping a couple machine guns in the open door of a Huey over Vietnam.

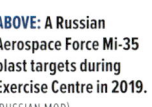

ABOVE: A Russian Aerospace Force Mi-35 blast targets during Exercise Centre in 2019. (RUSSIAN MOD)

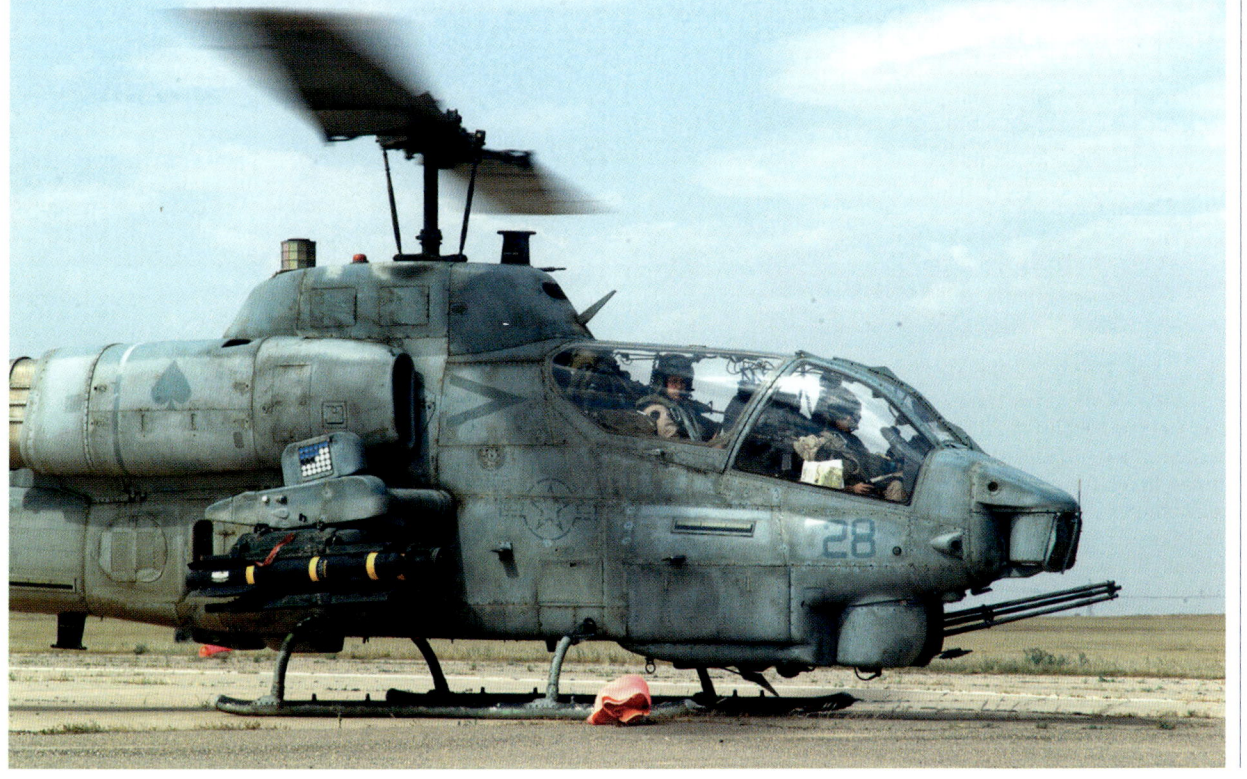

LEFT: Cannons in nose-mounted turrets and guided weapons on stub-wing weapon pylons give modern gunships awesome fire power. (US DOD/COMBAT CAMERA)

Bell UH-1 Huey

America's First Gunship

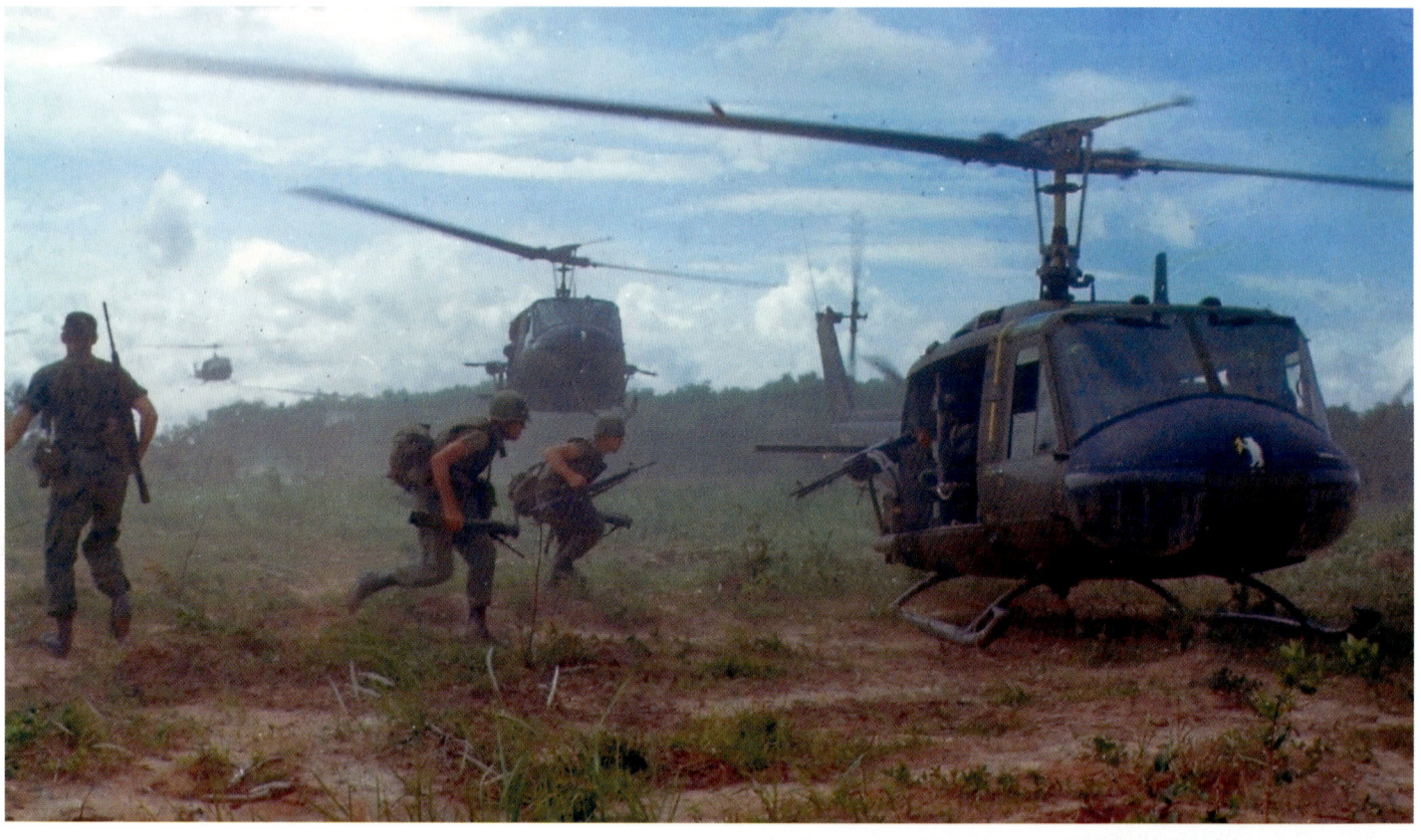

The Huey was the iconic helicopter of the Vietnam War in the 1960s and 1970s. It served in a wide range of roles including troop transport, cargo carrier, reconnaissance, casualty evacuation and attack. Until the arrival of the dedicated AH-1 Cobra in 1967, the Huey gunship, or Hog, was the US Army and US Marine Corps primary armed helicopter.

Huey was the nickname of the basic Bell 204, or HU-1 Iroquois, as it was first designated by the US military. The name Huey is forever linked to the Vietnam War. Out of around 12,000 US Army helicopters sent to the wars in Southeast Asia up to 1973, just over 7,000 were Hueys. Nearly half of them were lost in combat or accidents but several hundreds were recovered, repaired, and sent back into action.

The Huey went through many evolutions as the US Army learned lessons on the battlefields of Vietnam. The first version used in large numbers by the US Army was the UH-1B, which could carry seven passengers. It was followed by the

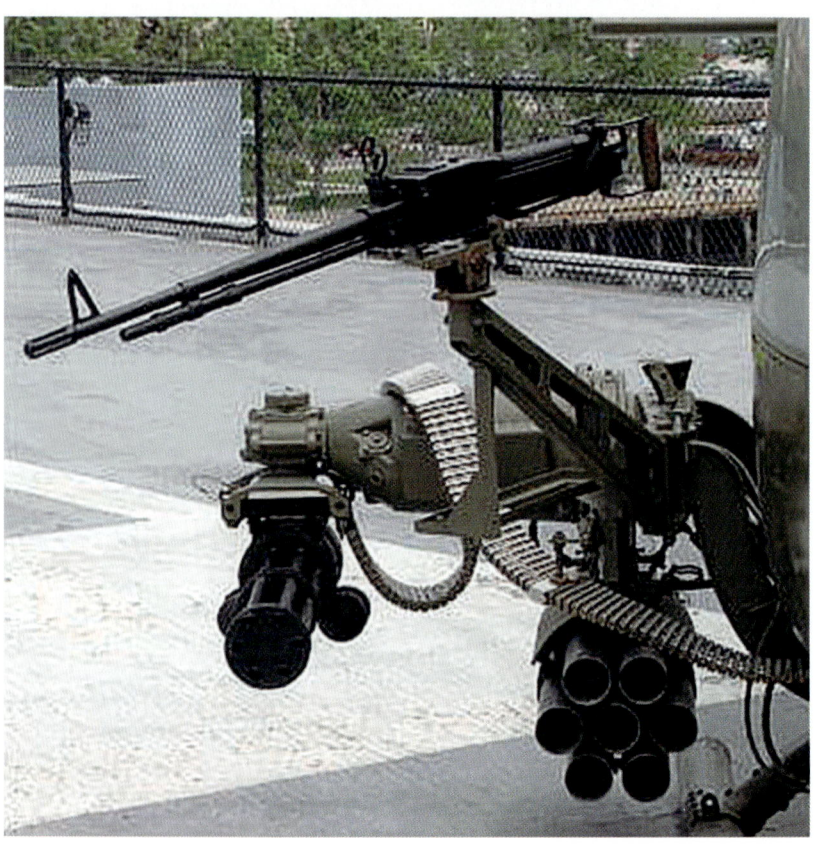

Bell UH-1 Iroquois (Huey)	
In service:	From 1963
Used by:	US Army, US Marine Corps and 70+ other air arms
Manufacturer:	Bell Helicopter
Produced:	from 1956 to 1987 (all variants)
Number built:	16,000 (all variants)
Specifications for UH-1B	
Powerplant:	Lycoming T-53 free-turbine
Fuselage Length:	12.1m (39ft 7.5in)
Height:	4.3m (14ft 7in)
Rotor Diameter:	13.4m (44ft)
Gross Weight:	3,855kg (8,500lb)
Range km:	480km (260nm)
Max Speed:	236km/h (147mph)
Armament:	4 x M-60 7.62mm machine guns, 2 x M157 2.75 rocket pods, M75 40mm grenade launcher

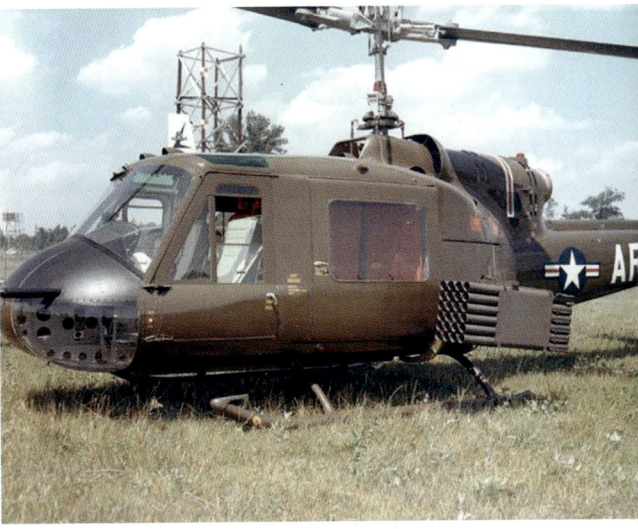

ABOVE: US Army Aerial Rocket Artillery units used UH-1 Hueys equipped with 48 rocket tubes to put down devastating firepower. (US ARMY)

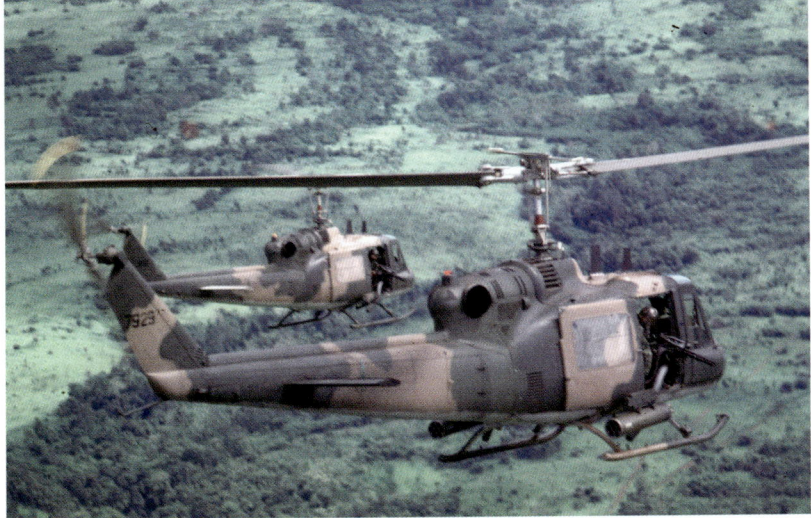

LEFT: Vietnam-era UH-1 Huey gunships usually hunted for their targets in pairs. (USAF)

UH-1C that had a more powerful engine. The US Marine Corps operated their own version, the UH-1E.

To enhance the troop-carrying capacity of the basic Huey, the US Army ordered the UH-1D, or Bell 205, which featured an improved engine as well as a stretched and enlarged cabin to enable it to carry 11 personnel. It first entered service in 1963 and was in widespread use with US Army air mobile units in the air assault, or troop-carrying, role when American ground troops entered the Vietnam war two years later. These troop-carrying Hueys were known as 'Slicks' by their crews. Medical evacuation Hueys were called 'Dusters' after the radio call sign, Dust Off, for an evacuation mission. In 1967 the improved UH-1H entered service in Vietnam to augment the UH-1Ds.

Every Huey could, in theory, sport door machine guns for self-defence, but the US Army wanted to give the helicopter an offensive capability as well, by adding forward-firing rocket pods, cannons and machine guns. These were directed by the pilots using sighting systems similar to those used by fighter jets. The first

gunships were converted UH-1Bs that sported two M157 2.75in rocket pods and two forward-firing M60 7.62mm machine guns. In 1965 a dedicated gunship variant of the UH-1C entered service that had weapons pylons or stub wings for forward-firing rockets, machine guns, M134 Gatling mini-guns and rockets. A version of the UH-1B armed with the first BGM-71 TOW wire-guided anti-tank missiles arrived in Vietnam in early

1972. These were the first US Army helicopters to use this new type of weapon in combat.

Huey gunships served in a variety of roles and with a number of helicopter units in Vietnam. Each air assault company had gunships attached, to fly escort for their troop-carrying Slicks. To provide fire support the US Army created Aerial Rocket Artillery units, equipped only with a Huey variant fitted with 24-tube rocket pods. The classic gunship role was with Air Cavalry, or Air Cav, units, whose job it was to hunt the Viet Cong in combination with smaller scout helicopters. Huey gunships in Air Cav units were the first to be replaced by new Cobras when they arrived.

When the US Army began pulling out of Vietnam in 1970 many of its Huey gunships were handed over to the South Vietnamese military and saw combat service until the end of the war in 1975.

Since the 1960s more than 16,000 UH-1 variants have been built by Bell and its overseas industrial partners. The iconic Huey remains in service with the US military in a variety of roles and has been used by dozens of foreign armed forces.

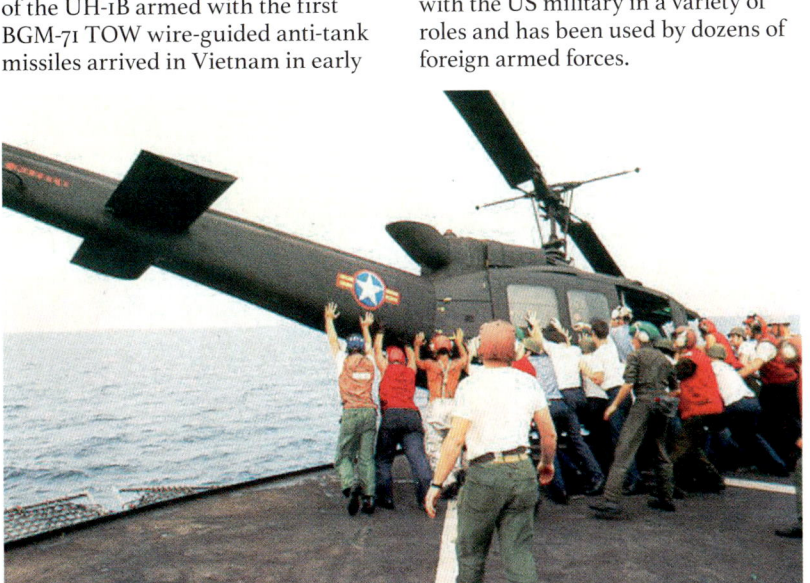

LEFT: The end of the Vietnam War in 1975 was fittingly marked by a helicopter-borne evacuation of the last Americans and South Vietnamese allies from Saigon. This ended with Vietnamese Hueys being pushed over the side of US Navy amphibious ships. (USMC)

Bell AH-1 Cobra

The Classic Gunship

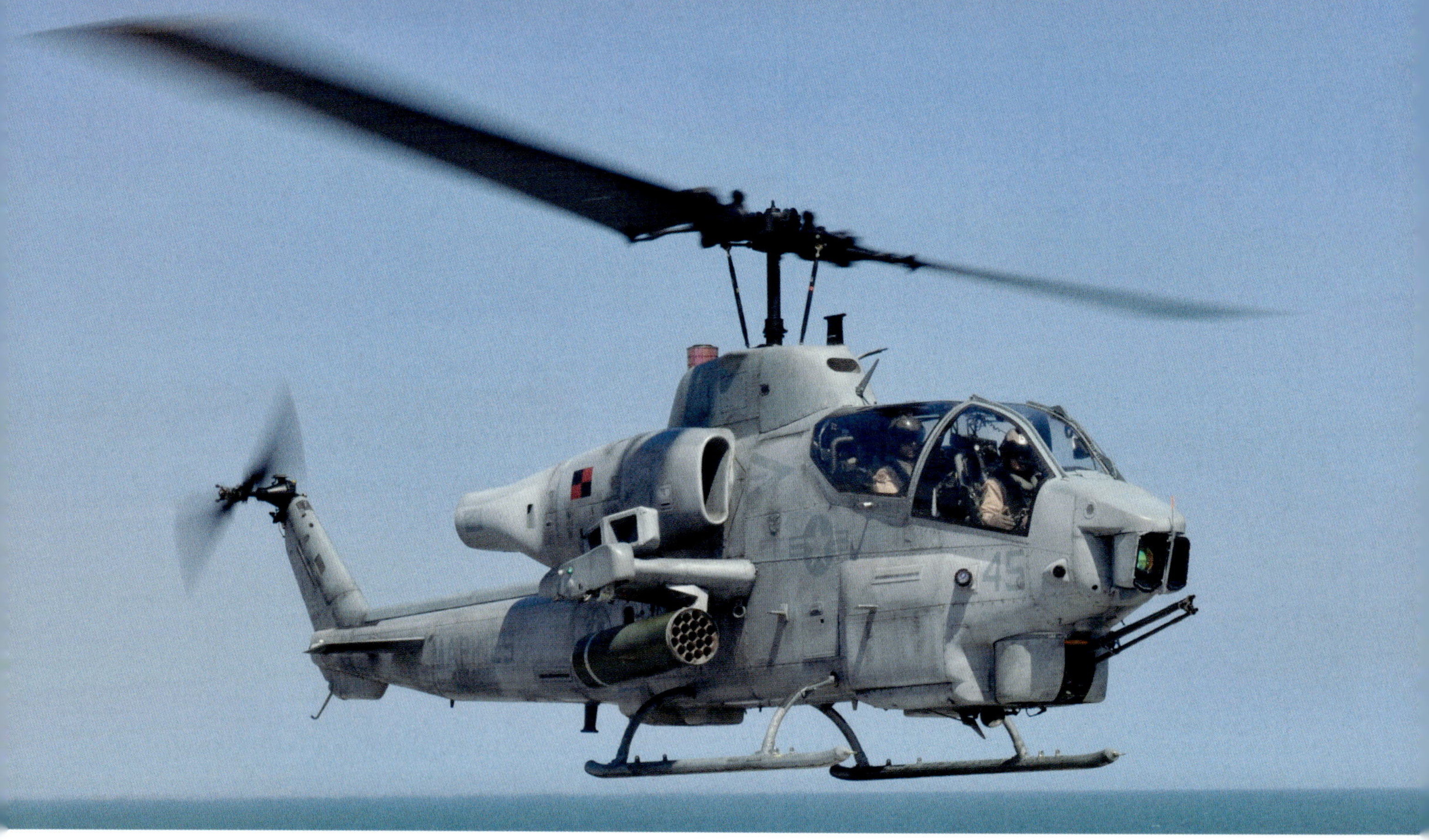

ABOVE: The US Marine Corps' twin engine AH-1s were the ultimate versions of the classic Cobra gunship. (US DOD/COMBAT CAMERA)

Bell's classic attack machine was the first helicopter that was purpose-designed to employ weapons. It entered US Army service almost by accident after Bell was knocked out of the competition for the next generation attack helicopter in 1964 by Sikorsky and Lockheed. The AH-56 Cheyenne was selected by the US Army but when Lockheed ran into technical problems and the programme slipped, Bell was well placed to offer up a solution to meet the urgent need for dedicated attack helicopters in Vietnam.

Using its own funds, Bell hired aircraft designer Richard Ten Eyck to start work in February 1965 on adapting their established UH-1 design to become an attack helicopter.

By September 1965 the first prototype was flying and by April 1966 Bell was under contract to build its first 100 AH-1Gs.

The classic Cobra with its tandem cockpit design and stub wing weapon pylons was an instant success after the first helicopters arrived in Vietnam in August 1967.

US Army Air Cav units were the first to receive the AH-1G and the aircraft were used aggressively to hunt Viet Cong guerrillas in the jungles of South Vietnam, Cambodia, and Laos. AH-1Gs were teamed with Hughes OH-6 Cayuse, or Loaches as they were soon nicknamed, which were scout helicopters that flew at low level looking for signs of enemy activity. Once the enemy had been found – usually after they opened fire on the Loach – the AH-6Gs would start their attack runs.

After its intense service in Vietnam from 1968 to 1972, the US Army decided to drop the AH-56 but keep its AH-1s in service. An aggressive

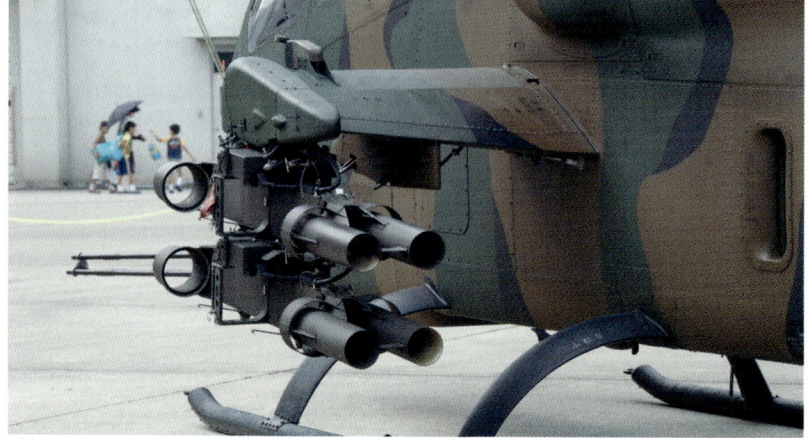

RIGHT: By adding TOW missiles the US Army turned the Cobra into a highly effective tank killer. (HUNINI)

Bell AH-1 Cobra

In service:	1967 to date
Used by:	Bahrain, Japan, Jordan, Kenya, Pakistan, Philippines, Spain, South Korea, Thailand, Turkey, US Army, US Marine Corps
Manufacturer:	Bell Helicopters
Produced:	1966 to 2019 (all variants)
Number built:	1,116 (all variants)

Specifications for AH-1G Cobra

Powerplant:	1 × Lycoming T53-L-13 turboshaft
Length:	53ft (16m)
Main rotor diameter:	44ft 0in (13.4m)
Height:	13ft 6in (4.11m)
Max take-off weight:	9,500lb (4,309kg)
Maximum speed:	149kts (171mph, 276kmph)
Range:	310nm (360 miles, 570km)
Crew:	one pilot, one co-pilot/gunner

Armament

2 × 7.62mm (0.308in) multi-barrel Miniguns, or 2 × M129 40mm grenade launchers, or one of each, in the M28 turret. (When one of each is mounted, the minigun is mounted on the right side of the turret, due to feed requirements.)

2.75in (70mm) rockets – 7 rockets mounted in the M158 launcher or 19 rockets in the M200 launcher

M18 7.62mm Minigun pod or XM35 armament subsystem with XM195 20mm cannon

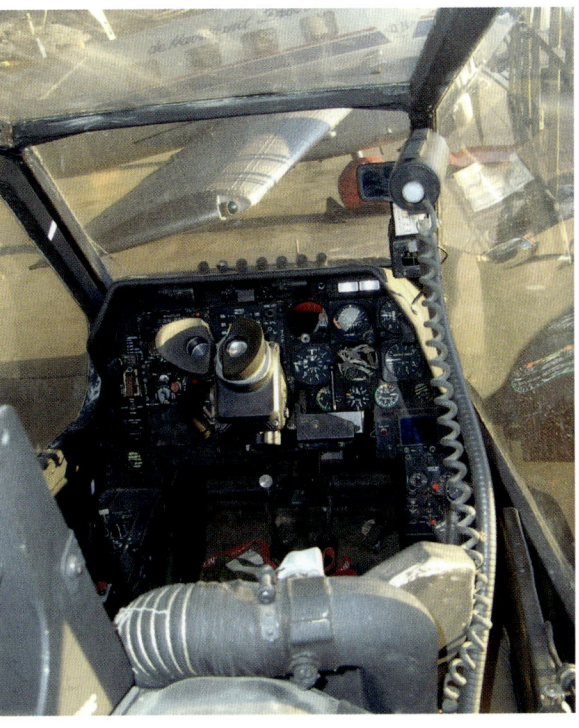

ABOVE: The front cockpit of a Cobra housing the gunship's weapon sights. (PETER ELLIS)

programme of upgrades took place in the 1970s, including the fitting of new engines, sensors and the BGM-71 TOW missile as standard. The ultimate US Army version was the AH-1F, which saw service in the 1991 Gulf War.

The US Marine Corps was late to the attack helicopter game in Vietnam, but soon became enthusiastic users of the Cobra. Once the Vietnam war had ended the USMC started to modify the Cobra to support its global amphibious operations, including fielding the two-engine AH-1T variant. This feature enhanced the helicopter's safety when operating over water.

During the 1980s the USMC ordered the replacement AH-1W, or Whiskey Cobra, which could fire the laser AGM-114 Hellfire missile. This was the same weapon used on the US Army AH-64A Apache. The AH-1W received its combat début in the 1991 Gulf War and subsequently saw action in Afghanistan in 2001 and Iraq in 2003. Cobras are routinely embarked on US Navy amphibious ships and have been used to fly protective missions during non-combatant evacuation and combat search and rescue missions from Saigon in 1975 and Grenada in 1983, as well as intervention missions in Somalia in 1992-93, Bosnia in 1995 and Libya in 2011 and 2016.

By 2010 the USMC had begun to field its replacement, the AH-1Z Viper. This featured many improvements including a bearingless and hingeless rotor system that has 75% fewer parts than the AH-W's four-bladed articulated systems. Its rotor blades are made of composite materials to give them increased ballistic survivability, and it has a semi-automatic folding system for storage aboard amphibious assault ships. New and larger weapons pylons allow a combination of AIM-9 Sidewinder heat-seeking air-to-air missiles, 2.75in Hydra 70 rocket pods or quad AGM-114 Hellfire missile launchers to be carried. The AN/APG-78 Longbow fire-control radar can also be mounted on a wingtip station to allow for target detection in bad weather or at night.

The Cobra has been used extensively by the US Army and Marine Corps. More than a dozen other armed forces have the operated versions of the AH-1 and orders continue to be received for the AH-1Z.

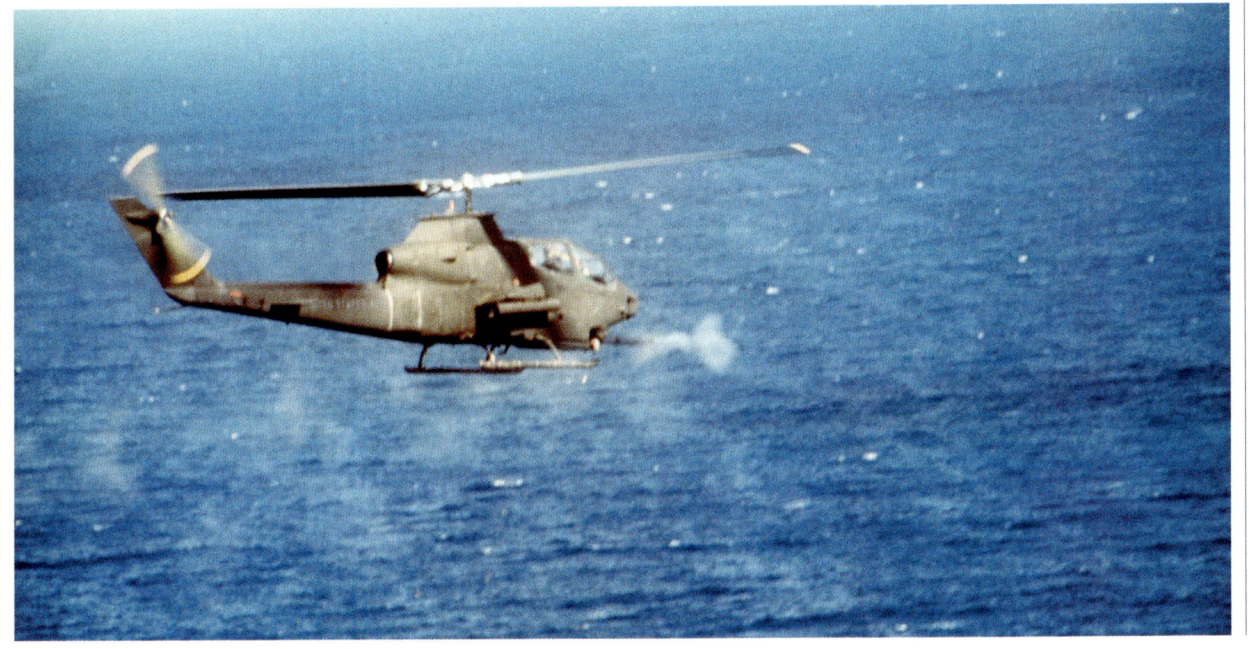

LEFT: AH-1s have seen action in all of America's wars since Vietnam. This AH-1S is blasting targets during the 1983 US invasion of Grenada. (US DOD/COMBAT CAMERA)

Mil Mi-24

The Flying Tank

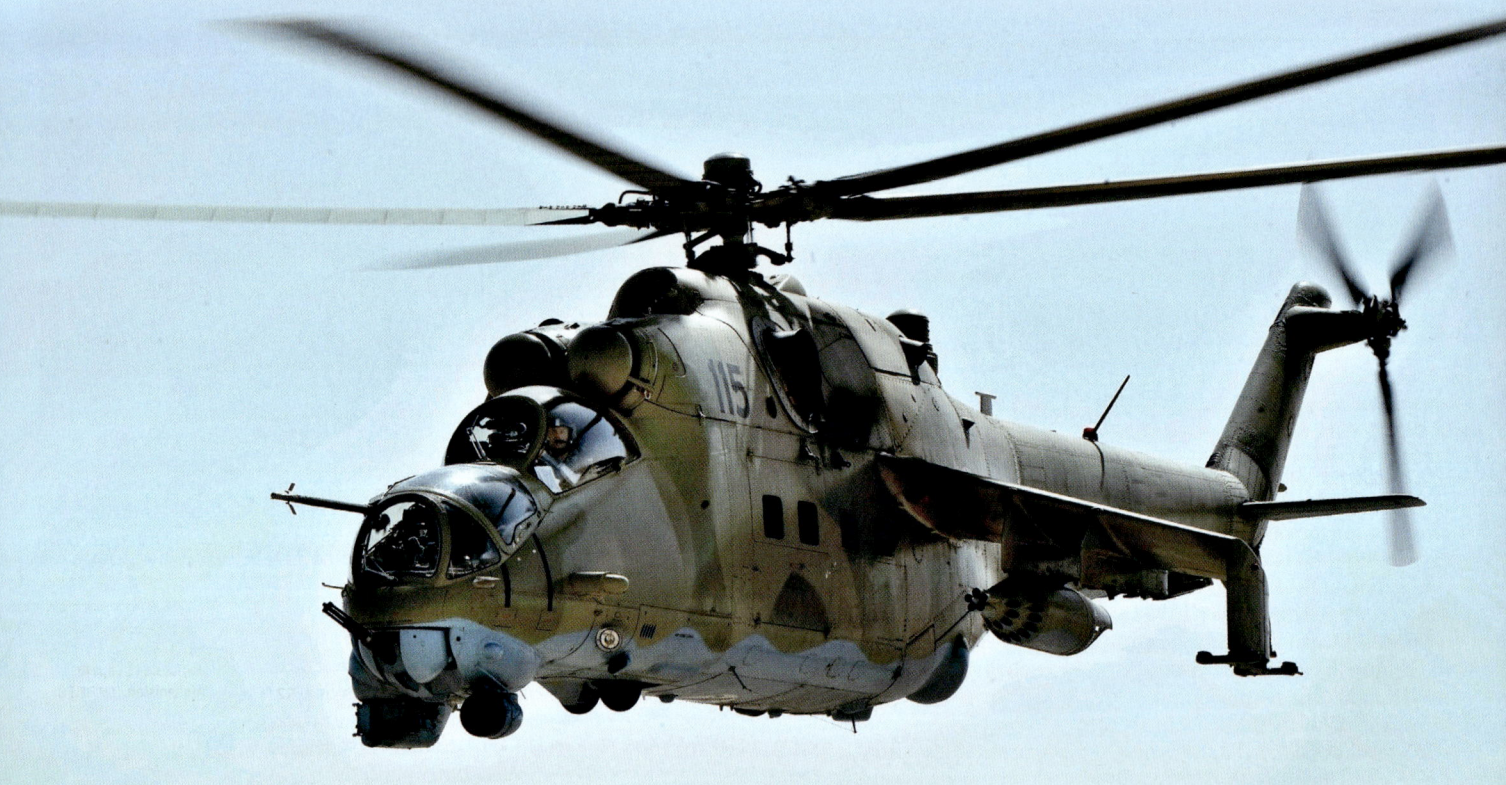

ABOVE: The distinctive silhouette of an Afghan National Air Force Mi-24 over Kabul. (US DOD/COMBAT CAMERA)

Russia's classic Mil Mi-24 attack helicopter was developed in the late 1960s in response to the deployment of US armed helicopters in Vietnam. The appearance of the Bell AH-1 Cobra impressed the Soviet military and it wanted to equip the Red Army with its own attack helicopter.

Like Bell, the Mil OKB design bureau took a proven helicopter and

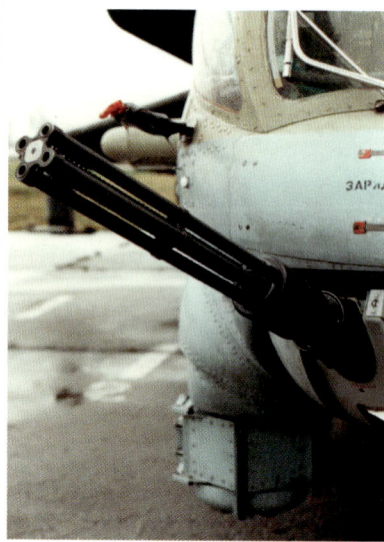

RIGHT: p.14-2 Mi-24Vs sporting a 12.7mm Gatling gun in its nose turret. (TIM RIPLEY)

adapted it to become a dedicated attack machine. They took the rear fuselage, engines and transmission from the existing Mi-8 transport helicopter and optimised its front fuselage section to operate weapons. The first prototype flew in the 1970s but that early version boasted a 'green house' glass cockpit rather than the tandem design of later variants. By 1974 the first Mi-24s were serving with the Group of Soviet Forces in Germany and had been given the code-name 'Hind' by NATO.

The Soviet designers introduced some innovative features to the Mi-24, including armoured protection for the crews and critical components. It was also the first dedicated attack helicopter to enter service armed with guided anti-tank weapons. From the start, Western intelligence agencies were keen to gain insights into the Mi-24. In the 1970s and early 1980s, because its cargo cabin could carry up to eight passengers, it was presumed that the Mi-24 was a hybrid attack/assault helicopter. It later emerged that the Soviets never used it in the air assault role, only to move support personnel and equipment during long distance deployments.

Early versions were equipped with the 9M117 Fleyta (NATO AT-2 Swatter) radio-controlled anti-tank missile mounted under the helicopter's stub wings. The Mi-24 D (NATO Hind-D) entered production in 1973 and was the first version that featured the under-nose turret with a single 12.7mm four-barrel Yak-B machine-gun.

By 1976 the definitive Cold War-era variant, the Mi-24V (NATO Hind-E) was in production and this used the longer range 9M114 Shturm (NATO AT-6 Spiral) missile. This variant was also known as the Mi-24W.

The Soviets were always looking to enhance the fire power of the Mi-24 and soon fielded the P variant (NATO Hind-F) which had two fixed side-mounted 30mm GSh-30-2K twin-barrel cannons.

After it had seen initial service with the Soviet army in Eastern Europe in the 1970s, it was not long before Moscow's Warsaw Pact allies began receiving the Mi-24. The Soviet Union also began exporting a modified version of the Mi-24-D to Third World allies, which was designated the Mi-25. Later it began exporting the Mi-24E under the designation Mi-35.

Mil Mi-24

In service:	1972 to date
Used by:	Russian Aerospace Forces and 30+ other air arms
Manufacturer:	Mil OKB design bureau. Final assembly Rostvertol and Mil Moscow Helicopter Factory
Produced:	1968 to date
Number built:	2,648

Specifications for Mi-24V

Powerplant:	2 × Isotov TV3-117 turboshafts
Length:	17.5m (57ft 5in)
Main rotor diameter:	17.3m (56ft 9in)
Height:	6.5m (21ft 4in)
Max take-off weight:	12,000kg (26,455lb)
Maximum speed:	335km/h (181kts)
Range:	450km (280 miles, 240nm)
Crew:	pilot, weapons system officer and technician (optional)
Capacity:	8 troops / 4 stretchers

Armament

Internal guns

12.7mm Yakushev-Borzov Yak-B Gatling gun or GSh-23L 23mm twin cannon in nose turret

Fixed twin-barrel GSh-30K cannon on the Mi-24P

External stores

9M17 *Fleyta* (in the Mi-24A-D)

9K114 *Shturm* complex (in the Mi-24V-F)4 × FAB-100 bombs

KGMU2V submunition/mine dispenser pods

UB-16 S-5 rocket pods

UB-32 S-5 rocket podsS-8 rocket pods

S-24 240mm rocket pods

UPK-23-250 gun pod carrying the GSh-23L 23mm cannon

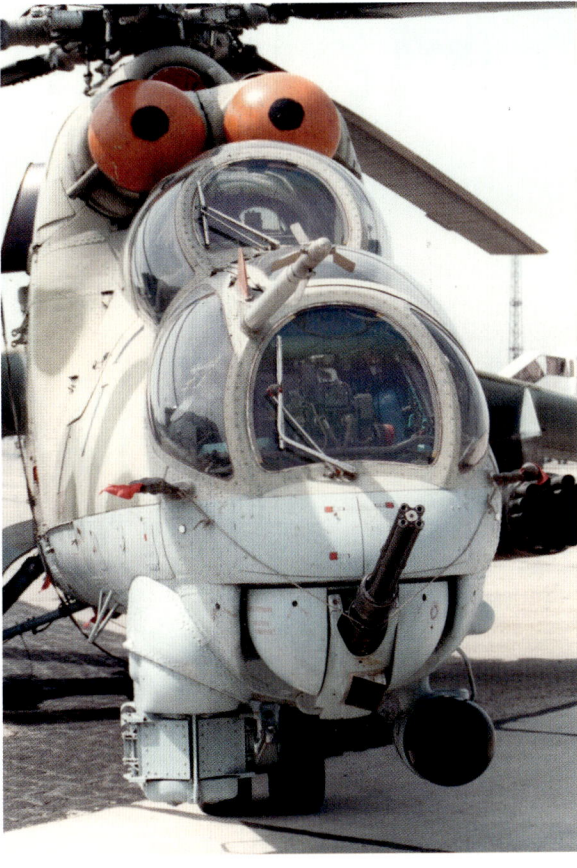

ABOVE: The stepped turret of the Mi-24 led it be nicknamed the 'Crocodile' by Russian troops in Afghanistan. (TIM RIPLEY)

BELOW LEFT:
A combination of gun pods, rockets and guided weapons are usually carried by Mi-24s. (RADOMIL)

BELOW RIGHT: 1970s-era Mi-24Ds sported an array of dials in their cockpits. Modern era Mi-35s have digital avionics. (MKE1024)

Hundreds of Mi-24s were sent to Afghanistan in the 1980s and proved highly effective in the central Asian country's extreme climate.

With the collapse of the Berlin Wall in 1989, and the dissolution of the Warsaw Pact and the collapse of the Soviet Union in 1991, several former Soviet republics gained their independence and claimed ownership of the former Red Army Mi-24s that were present on their territories. By the mid-1990s, over 2,000 Mi-24s were in use by more than 30 air arms around the world.

The newly established Russian Federation continued to use the Mi-24 extensively and invested in developing an advanced version optimised for night operations. This included night vision systems, a GLONASS/GPS navigation system and jam-proof communications equipment.

The Russian Aerospace Forces continue to have large numbers of Mi-24 variants in service and they have seen action in Chechnya, Georgia, Syria, and Ukraine. Plans to replace it with the Kamov Ka-52 or Mil Mi-28N have continuously been delayed for technical and financial reasons, so the Mi-24/35 is set to continue in Russian service for many years to come.

During its career the Mi-24 was initially dubbed the 'Flying Tank' by the Soviets because of its heavy armour and armaments. In Afghanistan, Soviet soldiers started to call it the 'Hunchback' or 'Crocodile' on account of its distinctive silhouette created by the stepped cockpit.

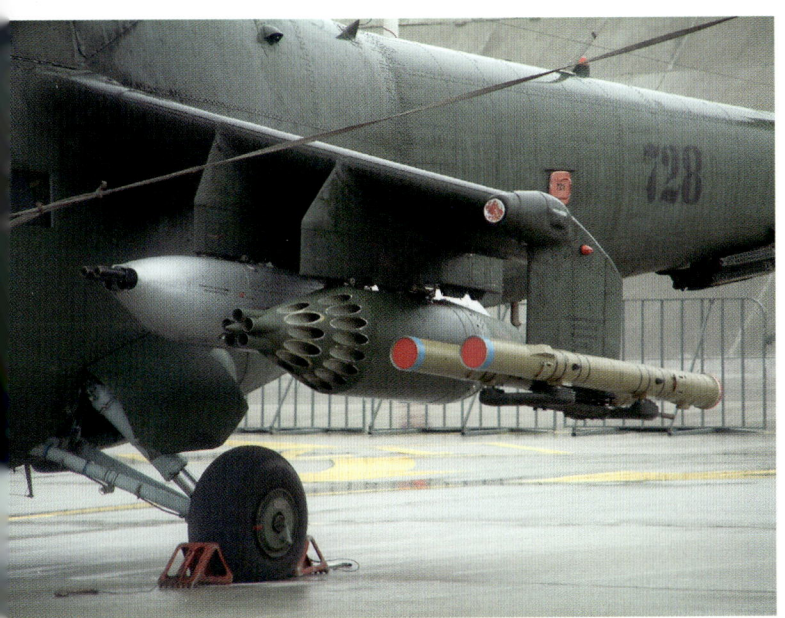

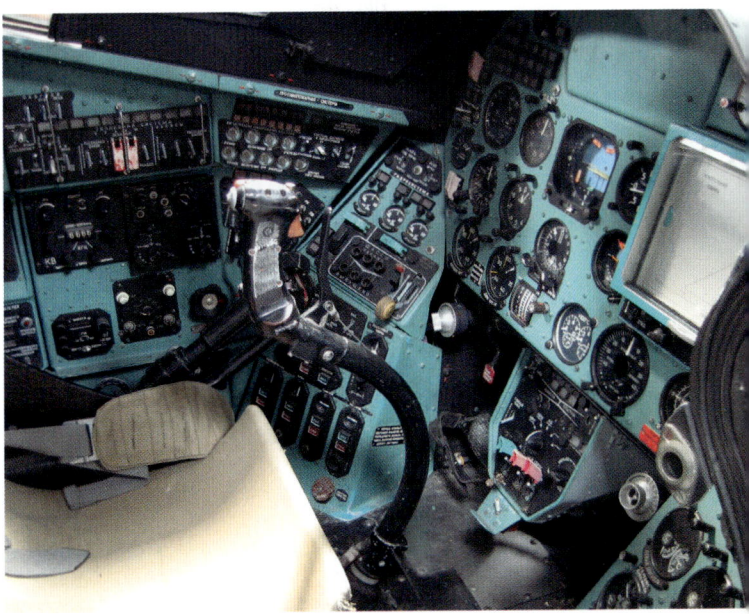

McDonnell Douglas AH-64A Apache

America's Tank Killer

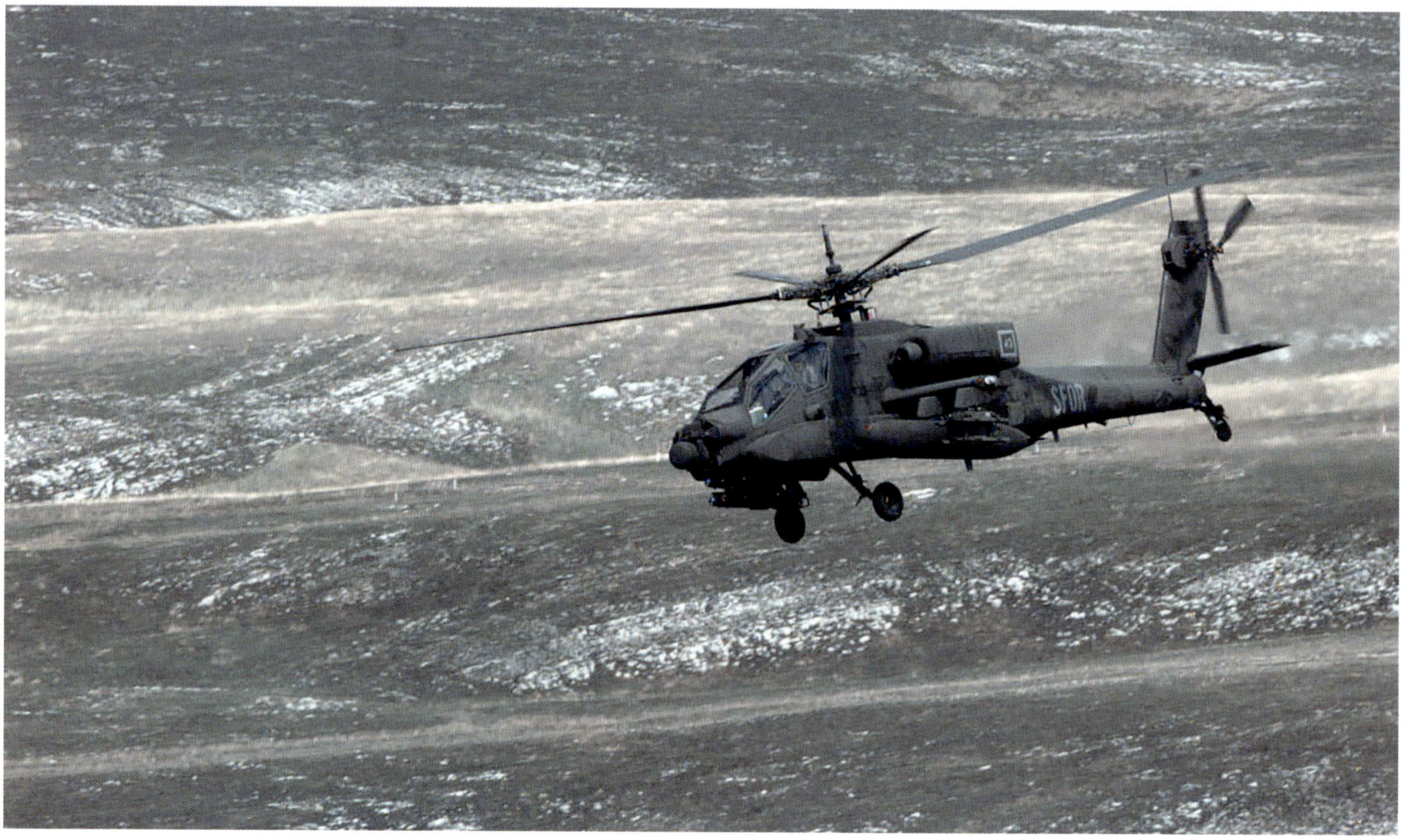

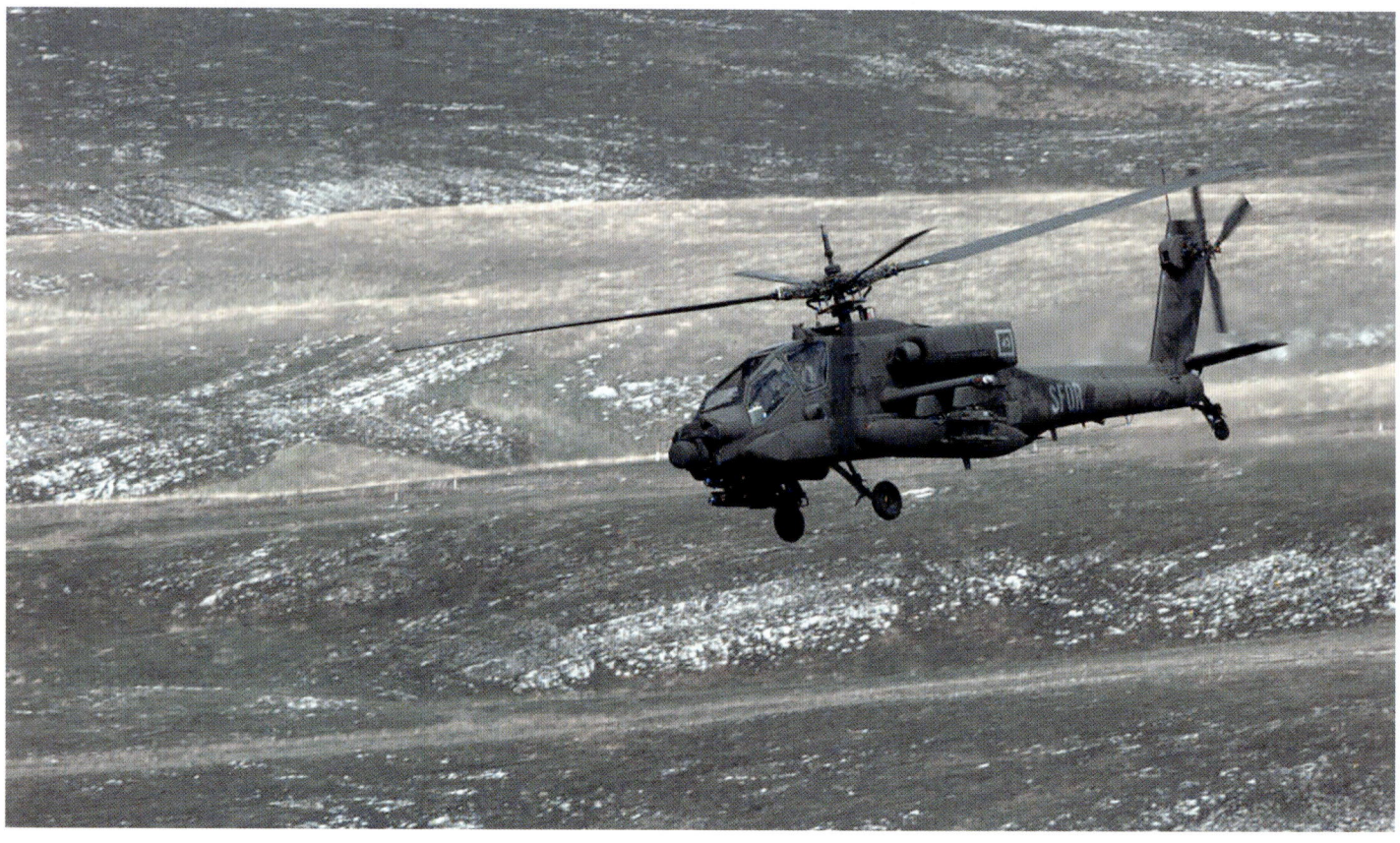

The success of the Bell AH-1G Cobra in the Vietnam War prompted the US Army to look for an attack helicopter that could help it counter the build-up of Soviet tanks in Central Europe.

In 1972 the Army had cancelled the Lockheed AH-56 Cheyenne after it ran over budget and failed to perform in tests. The Pentagon then launched the Advanced Attack Helicopter, or AAH, competition and this came to fruition in 1976 with the Hughes Model 77 (YAH-64) being selected as the winner against the Bell 409 (YAH-63).

The AH-64 adopted the tandem cockpit arrangement that had proved so successful on the Cobra, but the Apache featured modern night vision sensors to allow it to operate around the clock. It had two engines that gave it more power to allow it to carry up to 16 of the new AGM-114 Hellfire missiles. This was a generation ahead of the old wire-guided TOW missiles carried by the Cobras. The Hellfire could be guided by either a laser or radar homing that allowed it to find and kill tanks even when they were hidden in forests or under camouflage netting.

The Apache's Target Acquisition Designation Sight/Pilot Night Vision System (TADS/PNVS) gave a huge

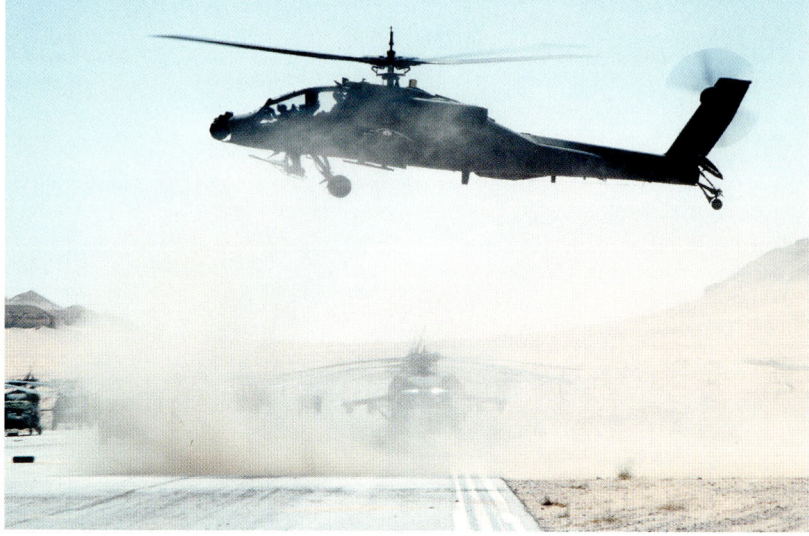

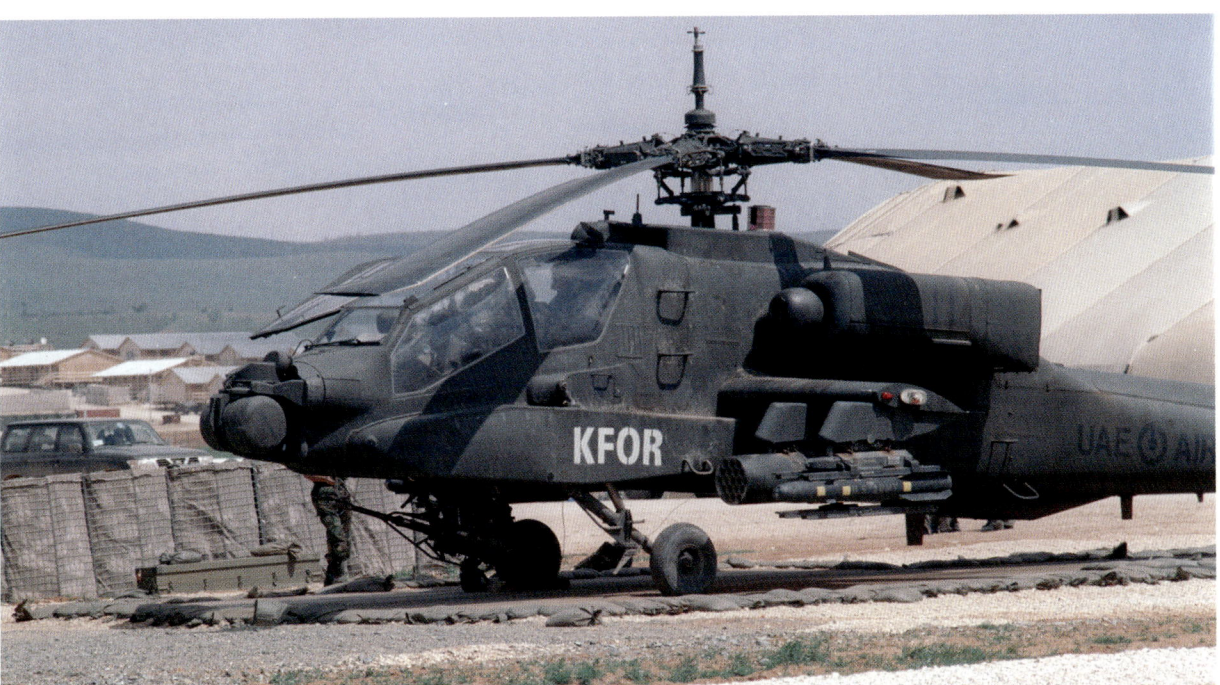

leap in performance over the Vietnam War-era sensors that were in service in the 1970s. In a new innovation, the TADS/PNVS imagery could be projected into the eyepiece of the Apache crews' helmets. This in turn was slaved to the helicopter's 30mm cannon so the gunner could look at a target and almost instantly train the cannon on it without looking down at his controls. This was a revolutionary development that allowed Apache crews to bring down fire on the enemy in a few seconds. The technology has since been adopted by other attack helicopters.

Battlefield survivability was enhanced by the incorporation as standard of defensive systems to detect and decoy heat-seeking missiles aimed at the helicopter. The crew also sat in tandem in an armoured compartment for added protection. The US Army eventually bought 821 AH-64A models and 116 were sold to international customers including Egypt, Greece, Israel, Saudi Arabia, and the United Arab Emirates. The Army then began converting its A model helicopters into enhanced AH-64Ds. The service's last AH-64A was taken out of service in July 2012 for conversion at Boeing's facility in Mesa, Arizona.

US Army Apaches first saw service in the 1989 US invasion of Panama and 278 were dispatched to the Middle East in 1990 for Operation Desert Storm. Over the next two decades AH-64As were deployed on peace-keeping duties in Bosnia and Kosovo. Israel used its AH-64As in action in Gaza and Lebanon. UAE AH-64As were deployed on peacekeeping duty in Kosovo and Saudi Apaches have seen action in Yemen.

McDonnell Douglas AH-64A Apache	
In service:	1997 to date
Used by:	US Army, Egypt, Greece, Israel, United Arab Emirates, Saudi Arabia
Manufacturer:	Hughes/McDonnell Douglas
Produced:	1981-1996
Number built:	1,000+
Specifications	
Powerplant:	2 x T700-GE-701
Length:	17.73m (58ft)
Height:	3.87m (12.8ft)
Rotor Diameter:	14.63m (48ft)
Maximum Operating Weight:	15,075lb (6,838kg)
Maximum Level Flight Speed:	284km/h (153kts)
Range :	400km (215nm)
Crew:	2
Armament	
Guns:	M230 Chain Gun, 1200 rounds
Missiles:	AGM-114 Hellfire
Rockets:	Hydra 70

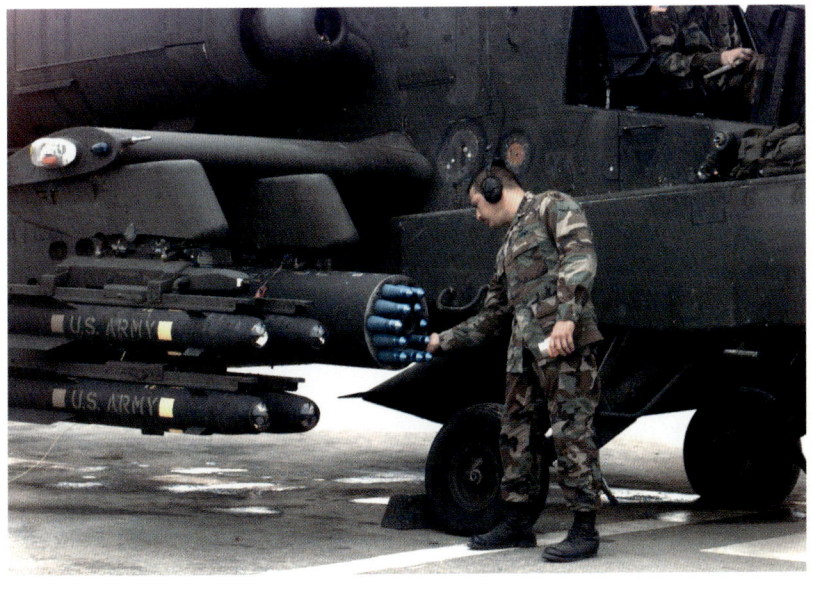

McDonnell Douglas AH-64D Apache Longbow

A New Generation Attack Helicopter

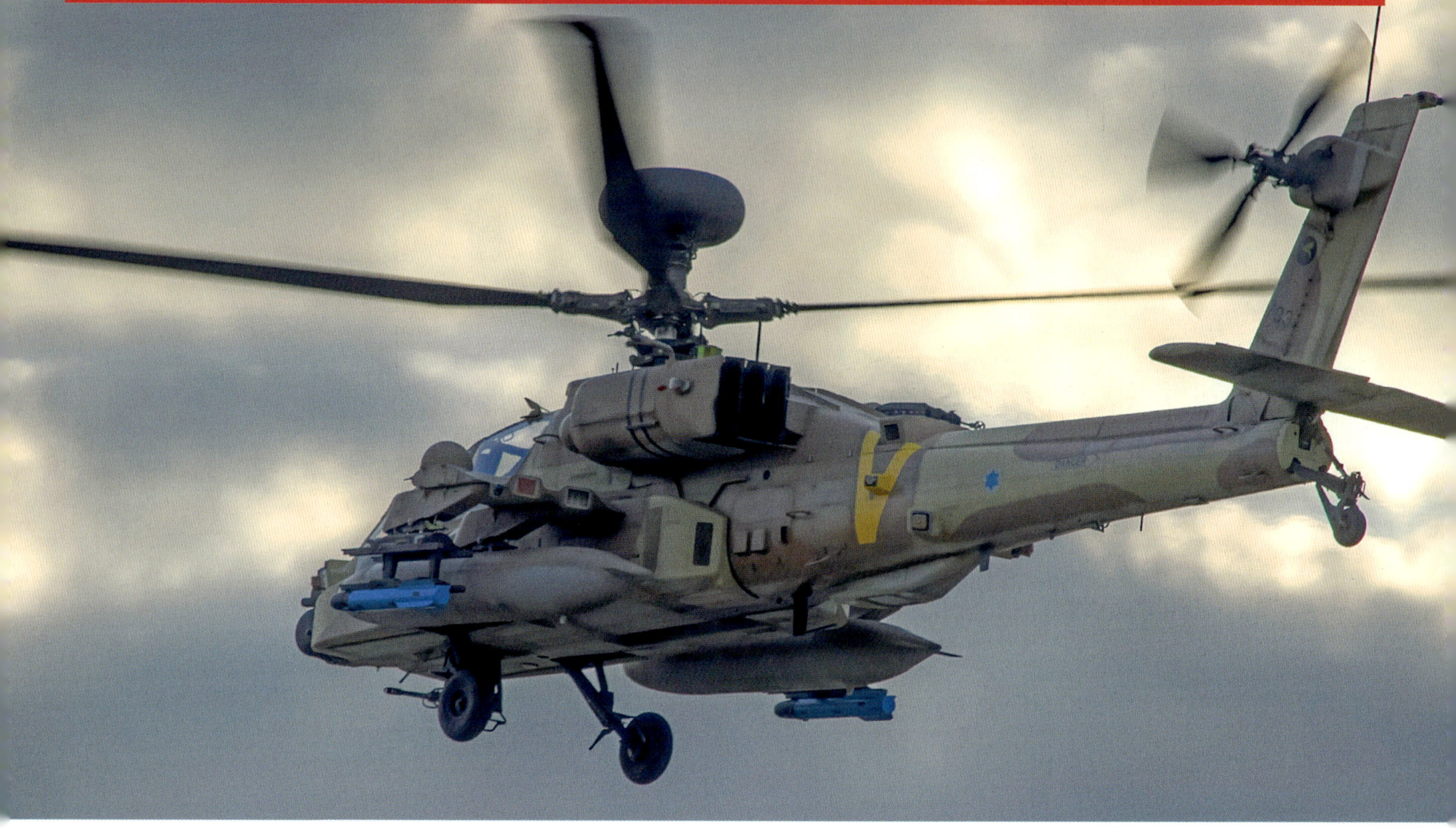

ABOVE: The distinctive Longbow radar transformed the AH-64D into an all-weather tank killer. (OREN ROZEN)

BELOW: The US Army teamed its AH-64D with OH-58D Kiowa Warriors to scout out for targets. (US DOD/COMBAT CAMERA)

Even before the classic McDonnell Douglas AH-64A Apache demonstrated its capabilities during the 1991 Gulf War, the US Army had been investigating how to improve its performance.

During the 1980s McDonnell Douglas studied an AH-64B, featuring an updated cockpit, a new fire control system and other upgrades. In 1988 funding was approved for a multi-stage upgrade programme to improve sensor and weapon systems.

During US Army AH-64A deployments to Europe in the late 1980s commanders had requested systems that would allow the helicopter to find and then engage targets at night and in bad weather. The Target Acquisition Designation Sight/Pilot Night Vision System (TADS/PNVS) used on the AH-64A were found to have serious limitations in the European climate, the thermal images from the sensors being significantly degraded in cold and damp conditions. Although the TADS/PNVS was very effective in the Iraqi deserts during Operation Desert Storm, the US Army realised that a more ambitious upgrade was needed to keep the Apache fighting at peak efficiency over the coming decades.

The result was the AH-64D Apache Longbow. This was designed around the Longbow millimetric radar that could identify large metal targets such as tanks, trucks, and artillery pieces at ranges up to 50km in rain, fog, or snow storms. The helicopter's targeting systems allowed its crew to match radar contacts to weapons at the click of a few switches. In theory, AH-64D could use this technology

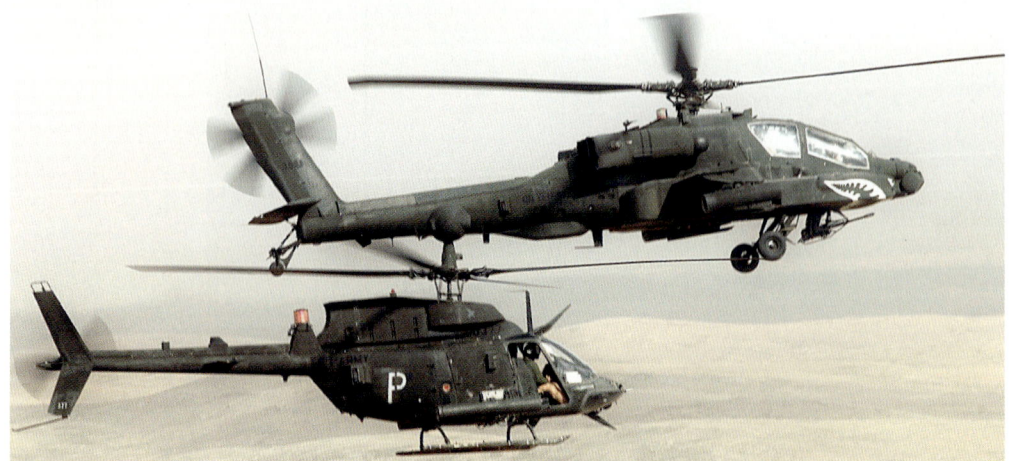

McDonnell Douglas AH-64D Apache Longbow

In service:	1997 to date
Used by:	US Army, Egypt, Greece, Indonesia, Israel, Japan, Kuwait, Netherlands, Saudi Arabia, Singapore, United Arab Emirates, United Kingdom
Manufacturer:	McDonnell Douglas/Boeing
Produced:	1995 to 2008
Number built/converted:	1,100+

Specifications

Powerplant 2 x T700-GE-701C engines

Length:	17.73m (58ft)
Height:	4.72m (15.6ft)
Rotor Diameter:	14.63m (48ft)
Maximum Operating Weight:	7270kg (16,027lb)
Maximum Level Flight Speed:	149kts (276km/h)
Range:	476km (257nm)
Crew:	2

Armament

Guns: M230 Chain Gun, 1,200 rounds

Missiles: AGM-114 Hellfire, Stinger, Spike

Rockets: Hydra 70

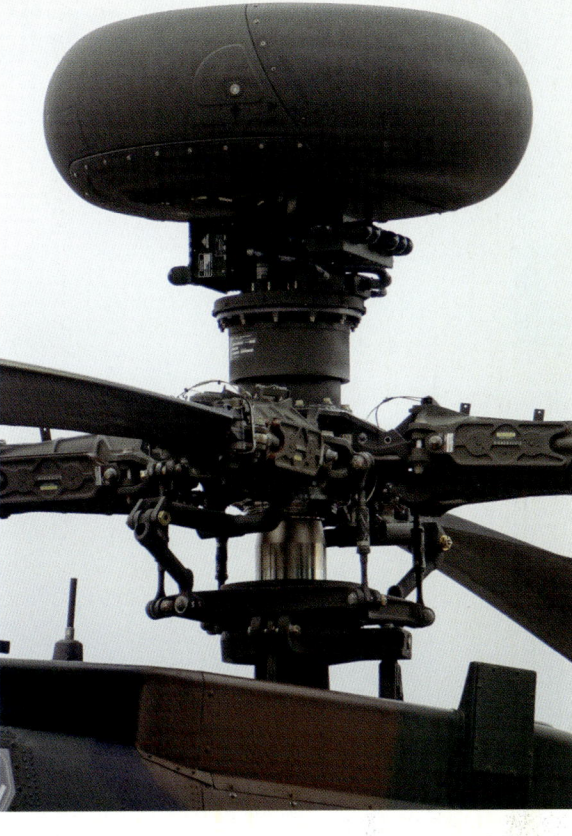

ABOVE: The Longbow millimetric radar was mounted above the AH-64D's rotor head to improve its detection performance.
(US DOD/COMBAT CAMERA)

BELOW: Often AH-64D operators did not fly with the Longbow radar in scenarios where they did not expect to face enemy tanks and there was a need to improve their helicopter's performance.
(US DOD/COMBAT CAMERA)

to find and engage up to 256 targets simultaneously. This turned the AH-64D into a true all-weather weapon system.

In August 1990 development of the AH-64D Apache Longbow was approved by the Pentagon's Defense Acquisition Board. The first AH-64D prototype flew on 15 April 1992.

During testing, six AH-64D helicopters were pitted against a larger group of AH-64As. The results demonstrated the AH-64D to have a sevenfold increase in survivability and a fourfold increase in lethality compared to the AH-64A.

On 13 October 1995 full-scale production was approved. A $1.9-billion five-year contract was signed in August 1996 to upgrade 232 of the US Army's AH-64As into the new AH-64D variants. The first production AH-64D flew in March 1997. The AH-64D programme cost more than $11 billion through to 2007.

The US Army then began a rolling programme to convert its AH-64As to the AH-64D configuration. Other improvements have been progressively incorporated in the helicopter including a major project to replace the legacy TADS/PNVS with a more modern system. In 2021 the US Army still operated some 440 AH-64Ds but were in the process of re-manufacturing them in AH-64E models. More than 300 AH-64Ds were in service with overseas air arms.

Starting in 2005, the US Army began fitting the Modernized-TADS/PNVS (M-TADS/PNVS), or Arrowhead sensor system, to its AH-64Ds. This sensor has enhanced thermal imagers that improve the ranges and clarity of the images that Apache crews see in the cockpit displays. Lockheed Martin, which makes the Arrowhead, says it gives a 150% performance and reliability improvement, while reducing costs through lower maintenance requirements. Egypt, Netherlands, Saudi Arabia, and the United Kingdom all opted to upgrade their AH-64Ds and new customers had it fitted as standard.

Several foreign Apache users have followed the US Army's lead and upgraded their legacy air frames. This was accelerated by Boeing and the US Army terminating logistical support for the older A-model air frames.

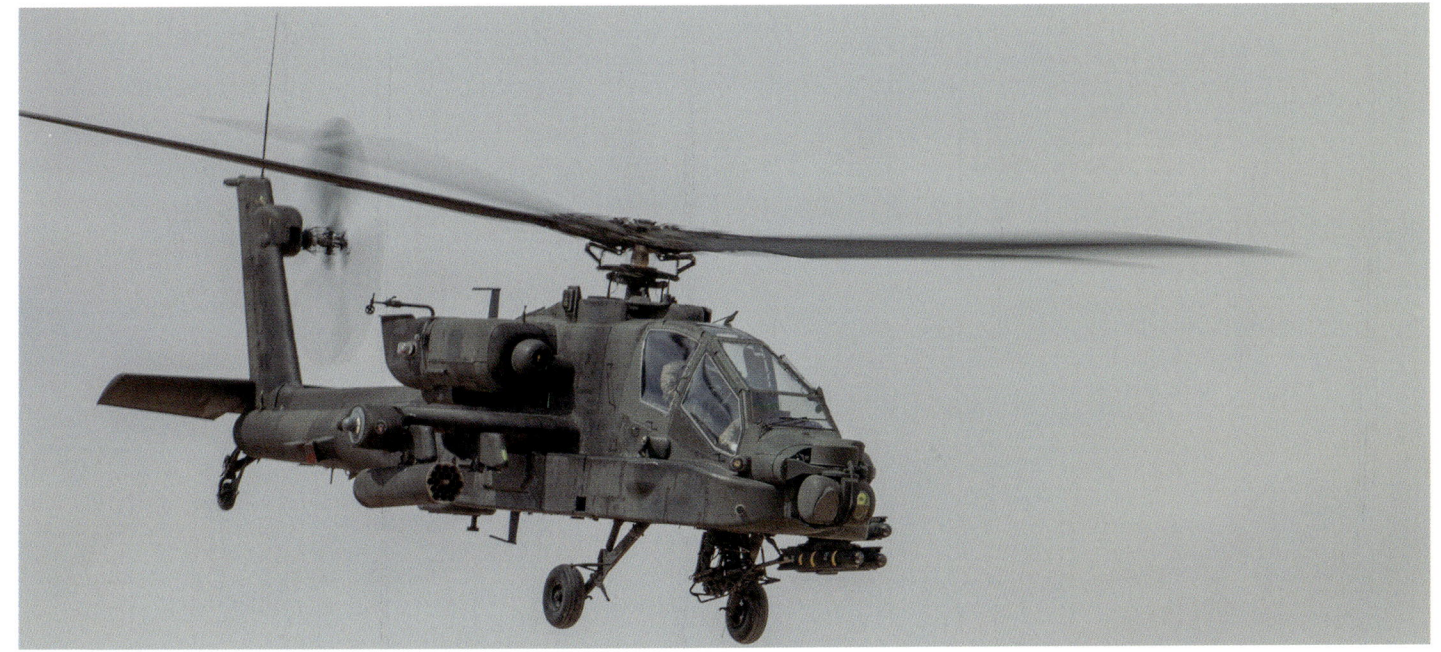

AgustaWestland Apache AH1

The Queen's Apache

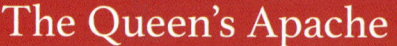

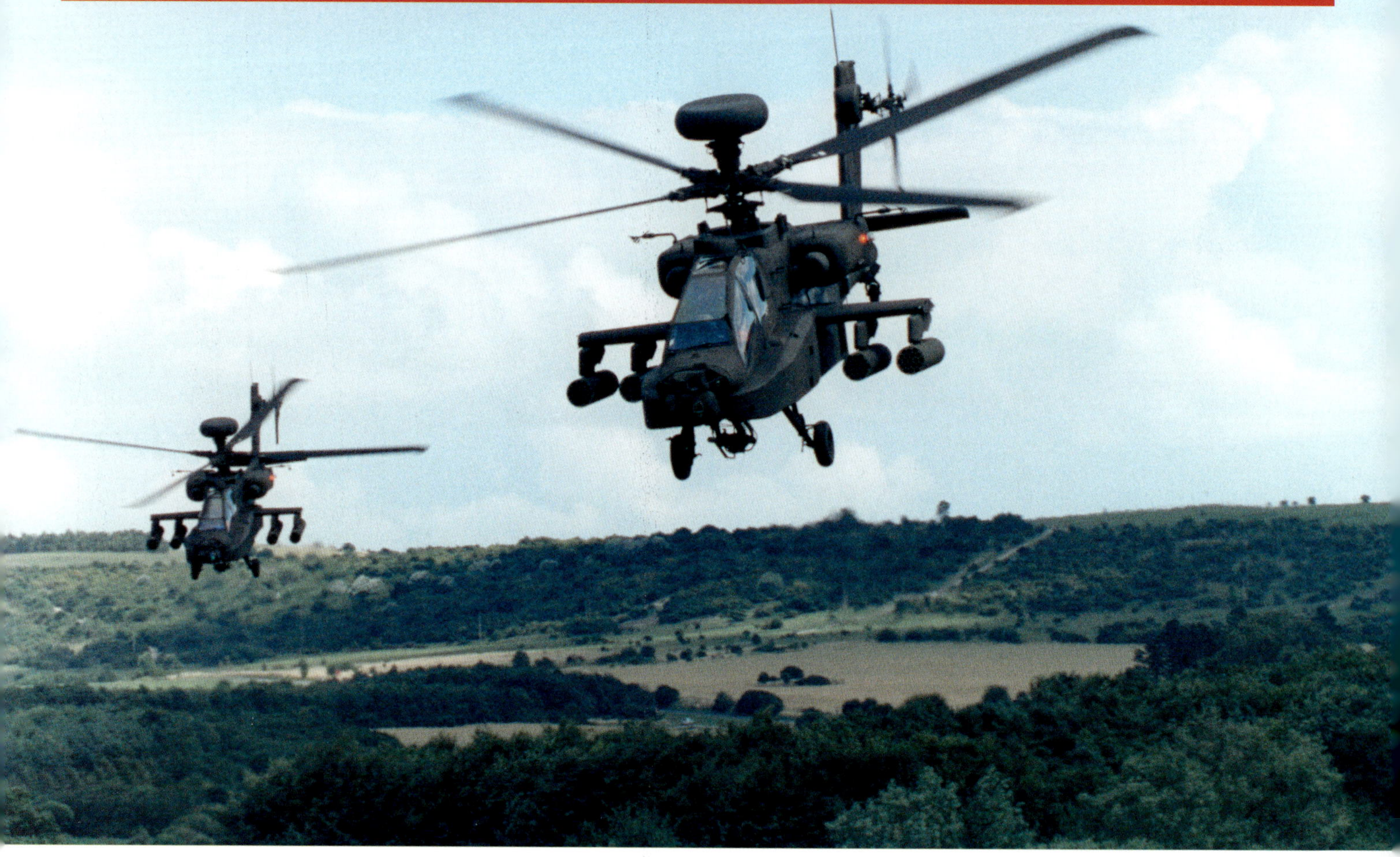

ABOVE: The Army Air Corps trained hard ahead of the Apache AH1s first operational deployment to Afghanistan in 2006. (MOD/CROWN COPYRIGHT)

RIGHT: Ground crew at forward arming and refuelling points act like Formula 1 pitstop crews to replenish the weapons and fuel of Apaches between missions. (MOD/CROWN COPYRIGHT)

Britain's Apaches are unique and feature a large element of 'UK-specific' technology, which makes them very different from the McDonnell Douglas AH-64D Apache Longbows of the US Army and a number of other air arms. In several respects the British Apaches are more capable than their American counterparts. Westland Helicopters – which became AgustaWestland and is now owned by the Italian company Leonardo – assembled the helicopters at its Yeovil plant. It was initially dubbed the Westland Attack Helicopter (WAH-64) Apache Longbow but the British Army subsequently designated them Apache AH1. To the McDonnell technicians who worked on the helicopters at the Mesa plant in Arizona they were known as 'the Queen's Apaches'.

The biggest difference between the UK Apache AH1 and its US counterpart is the integration of the Rolls-Royce Turbomeca RTM322 turboshafts, which were more powerful than the engines used on US Army Apaches.

A whole array of weapons and other systems were sourced from UK companies or locally assembled in the UK.

While the AAC's Apaches use standard RF and laser-guided Hellfire missiles alongside standard 30mm cannon ammunition, the UK decided to adopt as its area effects munition the CRV7 unguided rockets made by the Canadian company Bristol Aerospace. The initial batch of Hellfires for the Army Air Corps were built by Shorts (now Thales) in Belfast.

The British also opted for a home-grown solution to protect their Apaches from surface-to-air missile

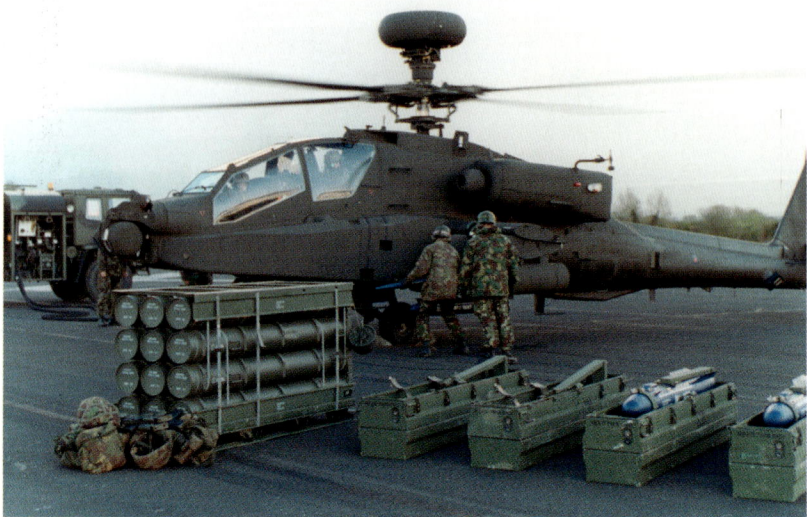

AgustaWestland Apache AH1	
In service:	2001 to present
Used by:	British Army
Manufacturer:	Westland Helicopters, then AgustaWestland via McDonnell Douglas/Boeing
Produced:	1995 to 2004
Number built:	67 were built for the Army Air Corps, 30 were in use by the British Army in 2022
Specifications	
Powerplant:	2× Rolls-Royce/Turbomeca RTM322 turboshaft
Length:	17.57m (57ft 7in)
Rotor diameter:	17.63m (57ft 10in)
Height:	4.9m (16ft)
Max take-off weight:	7,746kg (17,076lb)
Maximum speed:	293km/h (158kts)
Range:	296km (160nm)
Crew:	2
Armament	
Guns:	M230 Chain Gun, 1200 rounds
Missiles:	Hellfire
Rockets:	CRV7 with Flechette (Tungsten dart) or High-Explosive Incendiary Semi-Armour Piercing (HEISAP) warheads

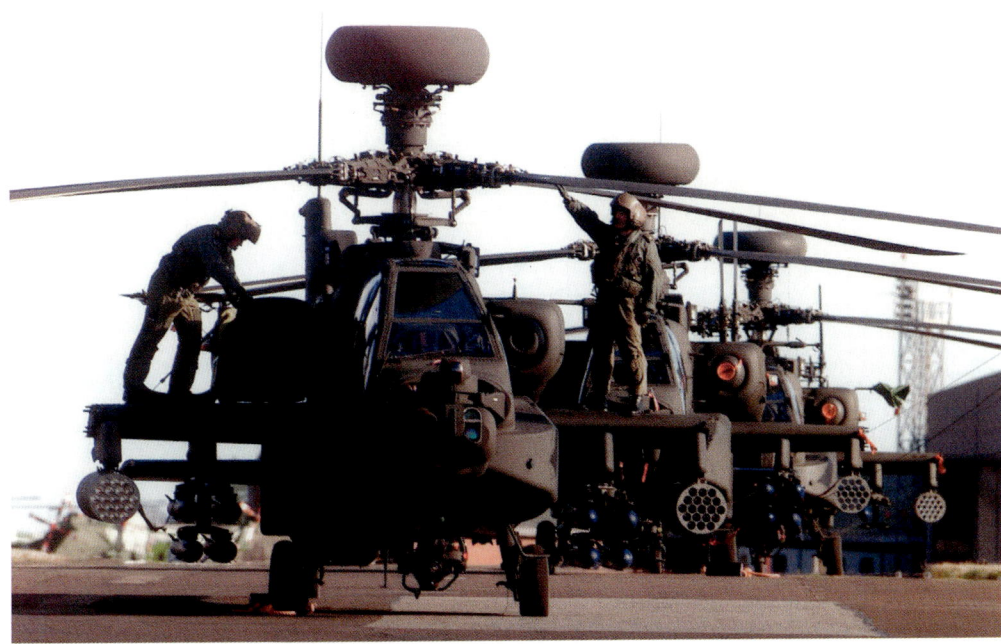

ABOVE: Apache AH1s feature many UK-specific components and weapons that distinguish the type from its US-counter-part.
(AGUSTAWESTLAND)

threats and selected GEC-Marconi (now BAE Systems Avionics) to supply the Helicopter Integrated Defensive Aids Suite (HIDAS). This features warning sensors to detect missile launches and automatic systems to employ counter-measures and decoys, including a British-made Sky Guardian 2000 Radar Warning Receiver and Type 1223 laser-warning system, linked for automatic control to W Vinten Vicon 78 Series 455 chaff-flare dispensers.

A UK specific communications suite was also purchased, based on Thomson (now Thales) SATURN AM/FM Have Quick II secure air-to-air radios, contracted in November 1999. British Army standard Bowman tactical radios were also installed.

After technical and training glitches delayed entry to service, the first Apache squadron was declared operational in 2004. Two years later the first Apache was deployed to Afghanistan to support the arrival of British troops in Helmand province. This was the first time the British Army had used its attack helicopters in action.

Over the next eight years Apaches were in almost daily action, providing close air support for British and allied troops in combat with Taliban insurgents.

In another first, Apaches embarked on the helicopter carrier, HMS *Ocean*, in May 2011 to fly attack missions against targets in Libya. The missions from the ship in the Mediterranean were flown as part of combined strike packages with French Gazelle helicopter gunships and RAF Typhoon strike jets.

The remaining Apaches are now a core part of the British Army's 1 Aviation Brigade and regularly deploy to the Baltic States as part of NATO's enhanced forward presence.

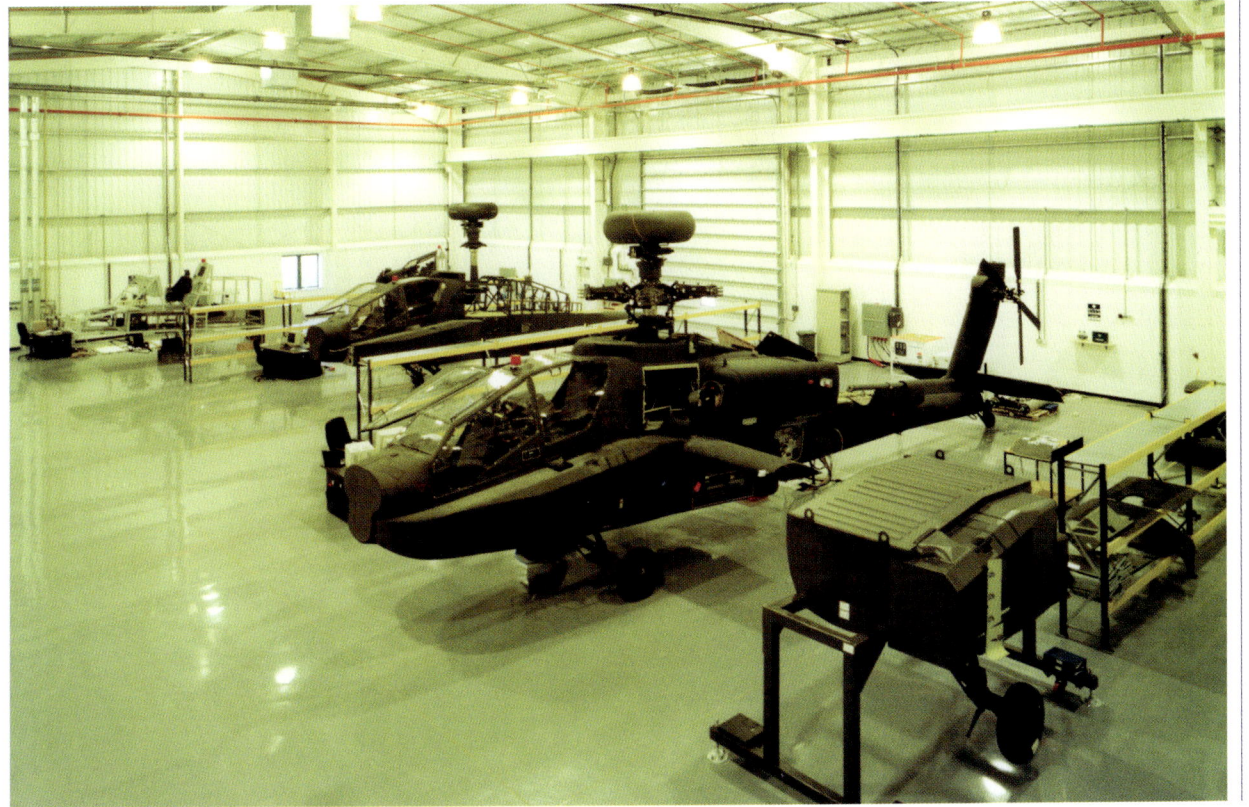

LEFT: The British Apache AH1s were assembled at the Yeovil plant of Westland Helicopters, later AgustaWestland.
(AGUSTAWESTLAND)

Boeing AH-64E Guardian

Improving the Apache

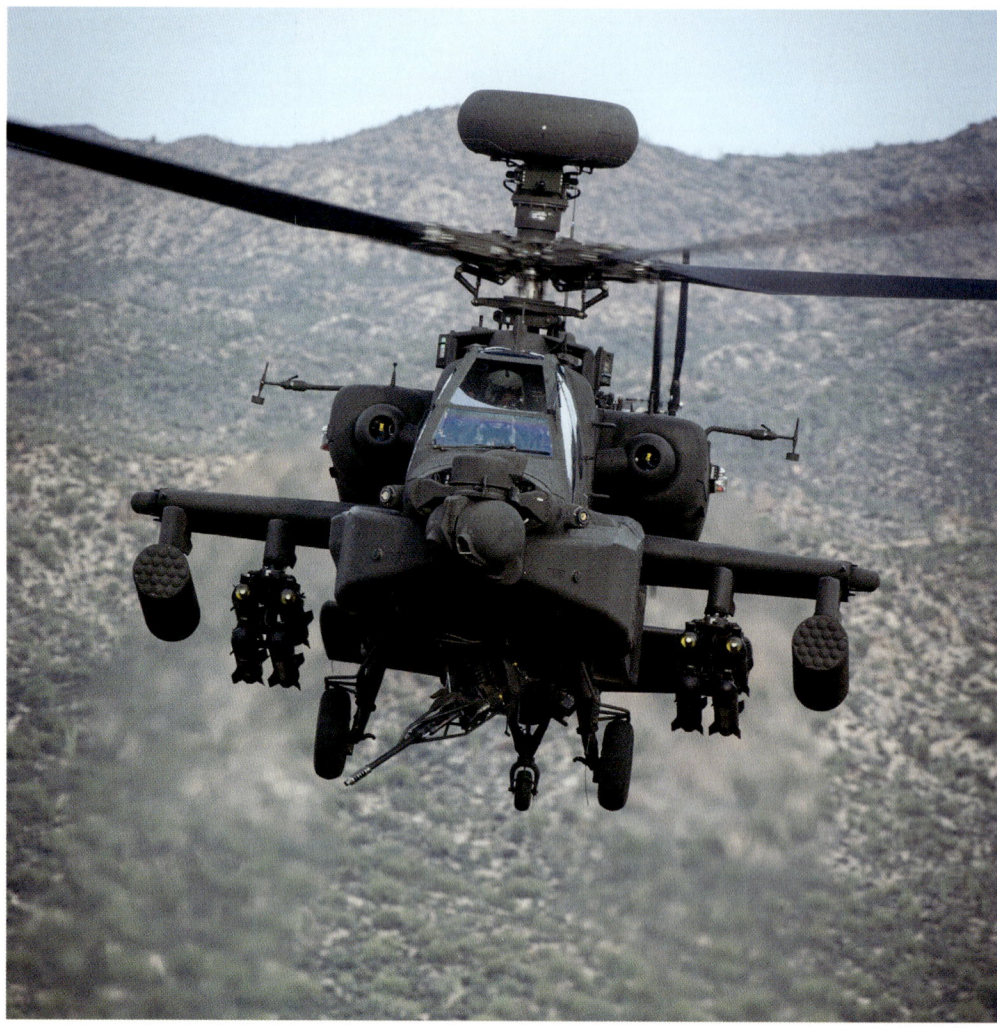

The latest variant of the iconic Apache features improved weapons, sensors, and engines to make it more lethal and survivable on the battlefields of the future. The US Army officially knows it as the AH-64E Version 6.0 but it is nicknamed by its crews the "64 Echo".

US Army Aviation commanders wanted to enhance their Apache's combat performance by giving it new and more powerful engines and making it easier for crews to share battlefield information with fixed-wing strike aircraft, helicopters, and ground forces.

This new helicopter features more powerful General Electric T700-GE-701D engines, new transmissions, new composite rotor blades and improved landing gear. The heart of the enhancements are new avionics and digital communications via a Joint Tactical Information Distribution System. This allows the crew to access and share information rapidly with ground forces and other aircraft, including the facility for the AH-64E crew to control unmanned aerial vehicles flying as part of joint missions. A maritime mode is provided to enhance the performance of the Longbow radar when operating over water. Embedded system-level diagnostics are also incorporated in the new helicopter to allow ground

ABOVE: Externally the AH-64E looks very similar to the AH-64D but it features many internal improvements to its engines, systems, and weapons. (BOEING)

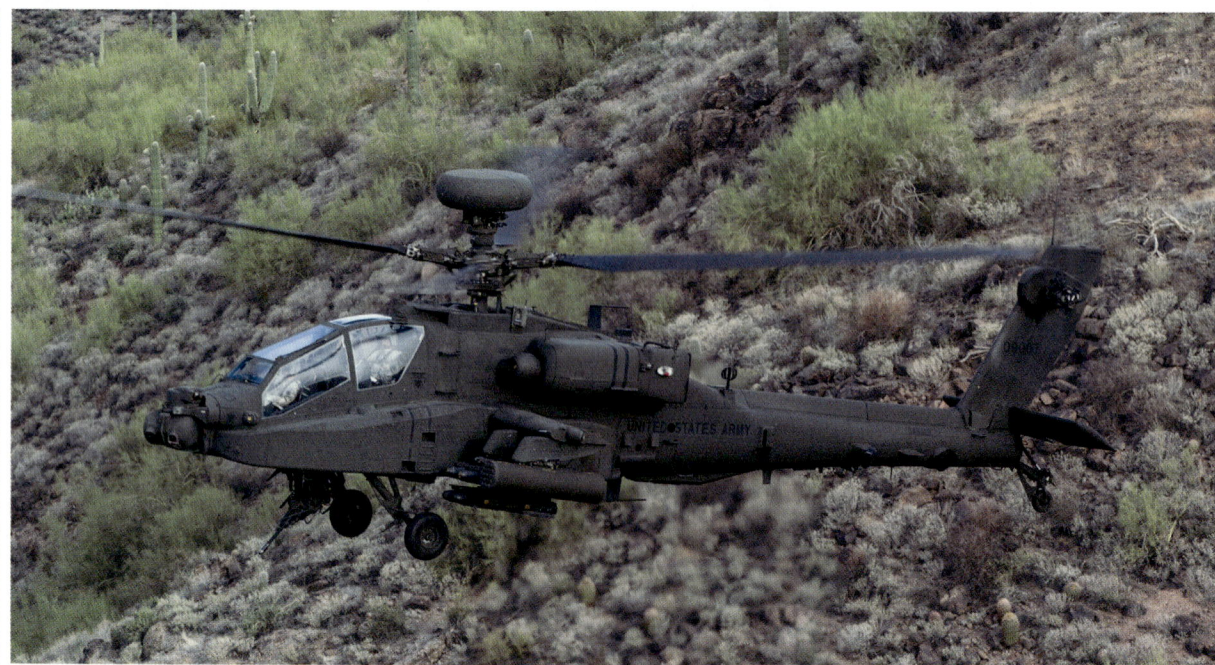

RIGHT: The US Army is in the process of upgrading all its AH-64Ds to the new 64 Echo standard. (BOEING)

Boeing AH-64E Guardian	
In service:	2012 onwards
Used by:	US Army, India, Indonesia, Morocco, Qatar, Saudi Arabia, South Korea, Taiwan, and the United Kingdom
Manufacturer:	Boeing
Produced:	2011 to date
Number built:	600 new-build and re-manufactured airframes
Specifications	
Powerplant:	2 x T700-GE-701D engines
Length:	17.7m (58ft)
Height:	5m (16ft 4in)
Rotor Diameter:	14.63m (48ft)
Maximum Operating Weight:	10,432kg (23,000 lb)
Maximum Level Flight Speed:	276+ km/h (149+ kts)
Range:	476km (257nm)
Crew:	2
Armament	
Guns:	M230 Chain Gun, 1200 rounds
Missiles:	AGM-114 Hellfire, Joint Air-to-Ground Missile (JAGM)
Rockets:	Hydra 70

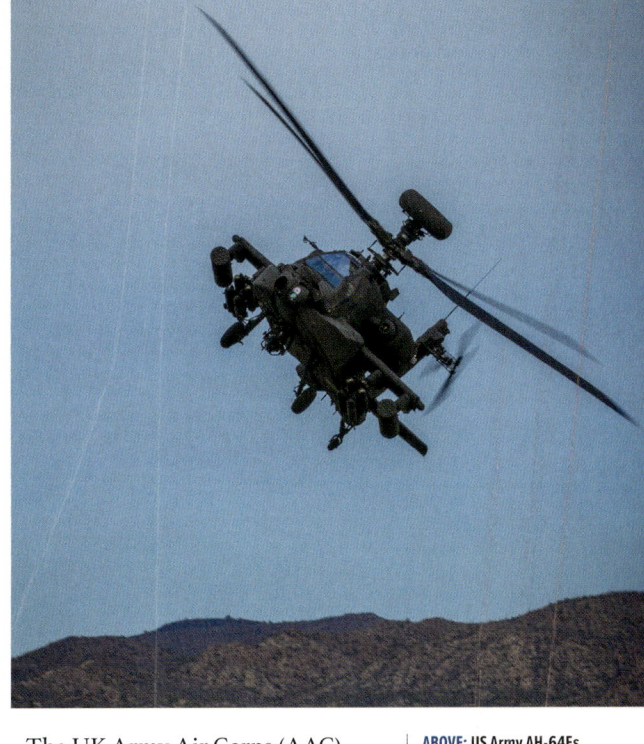

ABOVE: US Army AH-64Es have seen action in Afghanistan, Iraq, and Syria. (BOEING)

crews to rapidly assess maintenance requirements between missions.

The first deliveries of pre-production helicopters began in November 2011. They were initially designed as AH-64D Block III but, in a sign of the importance of the project, in 2012 the helicopter was re-designated as AH-64E Guardian. Test flights went well, and full-rate production was approved by the US Army in October 2012, with plans for the service's 634 AH-64Ds to be upgraded to AH-64E standard. In November 2013, the AH-64E achieved initial operating capability and five months later the 1st Battalion, 229th Attack Reconnaissance Battalion deployed with its 24 AH-64Es to Afghanistan in the type's first combat deployment. The AH-64E has gone through several iterations and Version 6.0 is the model currently in production for US and overseas customers.

Boeing has since moved production fully to the AH-64E and secured several export orders including to India, Indonesia, Morocco, Qatar, Saudi Arabia, South Korea, Taiwan, and the United Kingdom. Most of these are new-build aircraft but the UAE and UK are re-cycling some components from their legacy AH-64Ds.

The UK Army Air Corps (AAC) has designated the AH-64E Apache AH2 in UK service. Contracts were placed for the first 50 of the improved versions in July 2016. These helicopters involve the use of fuselages and other components donated from old UK Apache AH1 airframes, including their Longbow radars.

Unlike the original British variant of the Apache, which was assembled by Westland Helicopters in Yeovil, the majority of the work on the new variant is being conducted at the Boeing plant at Mesa in Arizona.

BELOW: The first UK AH-64Es were airlifted to Wattisham Flying Station in Suffolk in November 2020. (MOD/CROWN COPYRIGHT)

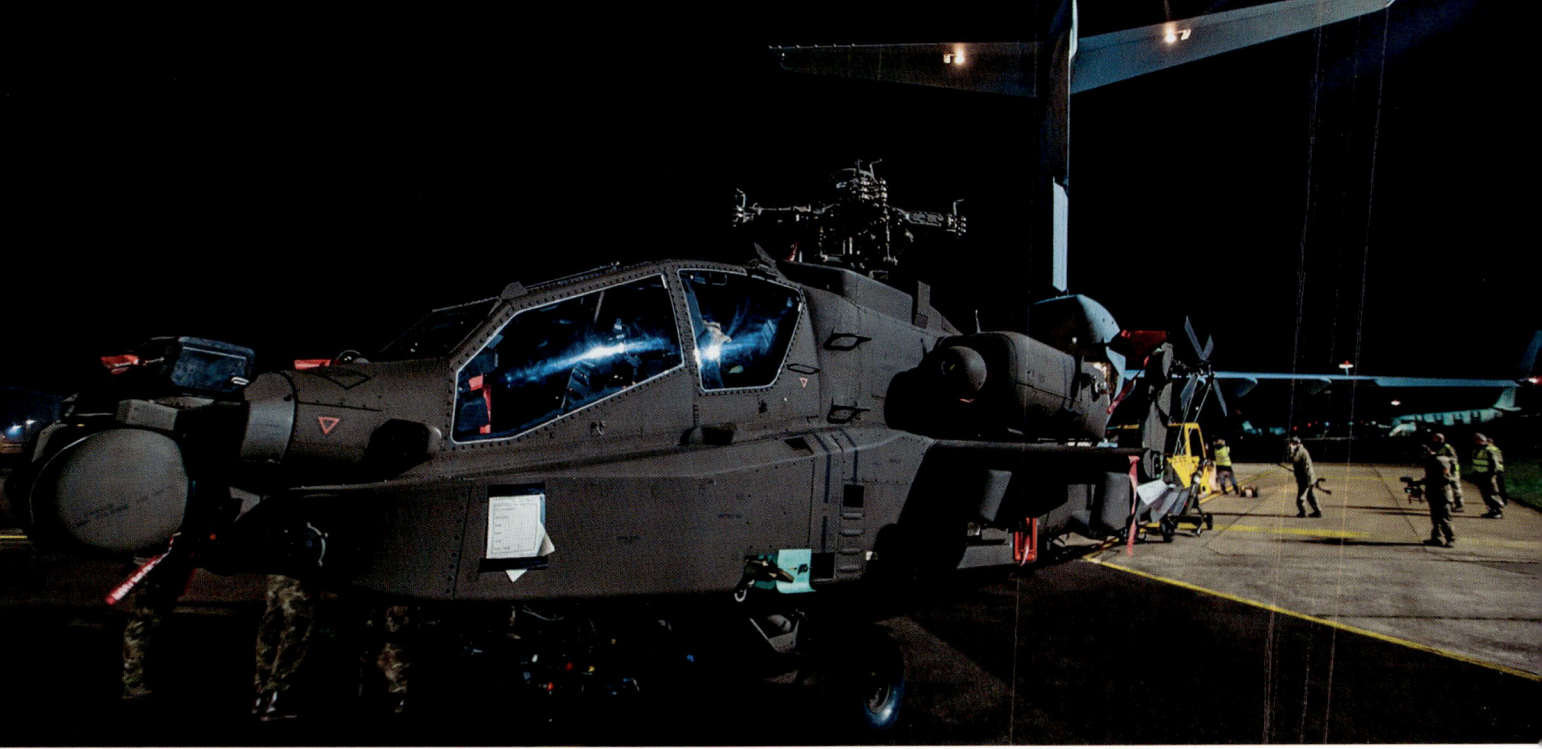

Aerospatiale SA341/342 Gazelle

France's Fast Mover

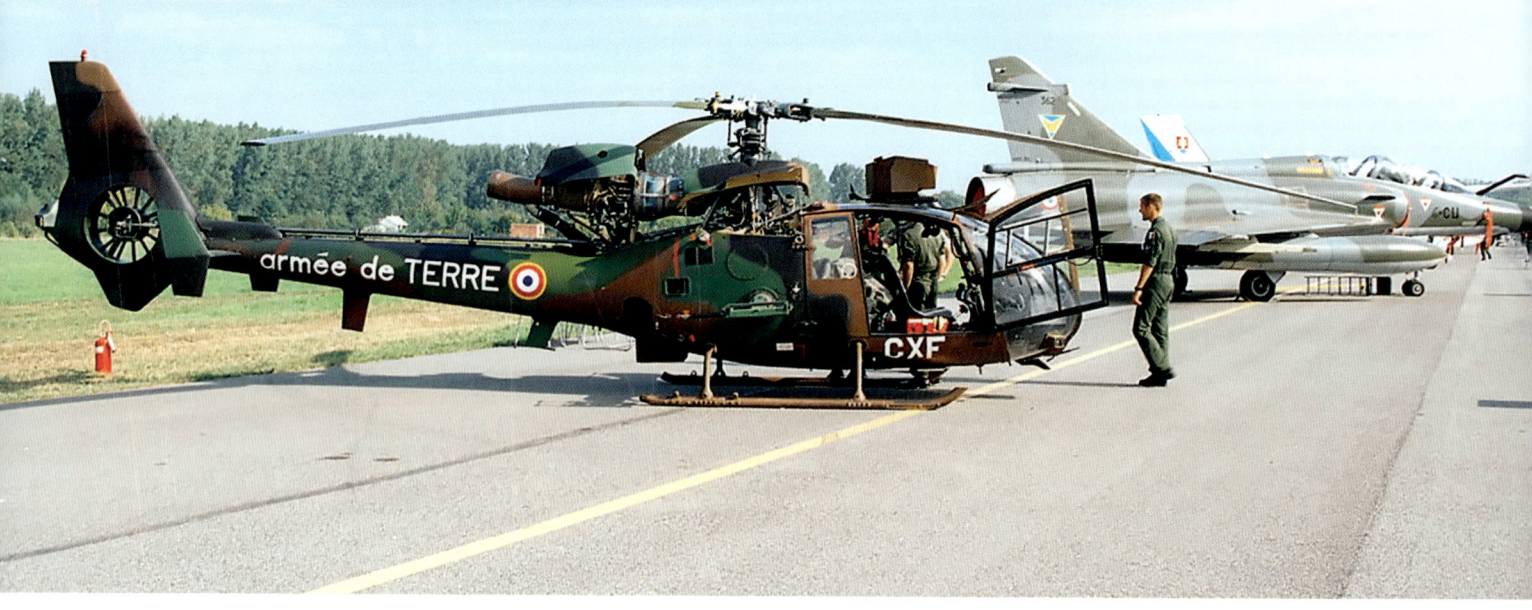

ABOVE: ALAT SA-341s spearheaded the French advance in Iraq in February 1991. (US DOD/ COMBAT CAMERA)

BELOW: Upgraded SA-342s continue to be in service in the ALAT. (PRZEMYSLAW IDZKIEWICZ)

The iconic Gazelle had its origins in an Anglo-French co-operation deal in the 1960s to field a family of helicopters. This resulted in the Puma medium transport helicopter, the Lynx armed army and naval helicopter, as well as the Gazelle attack, utility, and observation helicopter.

In France the project was led by Sud Aviation, which subsequently became Aerospatiale. The prototype Gazelle made its maiden flight on the April 7, 1967 and entered service with the French Army's Light Aviation branch, Aviation Légère de l'Armée de Terre (ALAT), in 1971. By the time production had ended in 1996, more than 1,775 had been built in France, the United Kingdom and Yugoslavia.

A total of 340 Gazelles were procured for the Aviation Légère de l'Armée de Terre (ALAT) – 171 SA 341Fs with the Turboméca Astazou IIIC turboshaft, and 161 SA 342M dedicated anti-tank variants with the more powerful Turboméca Astazou XIVH engine.

The ALAT used the Gazelle primarily as an anti-tank gunship (SA 342M) armed with Euromissile HOT missiles. A light support version (SA 341F) equipped with a M621 20mm cannon was used, as well as anti-air variants carrying the Mistral air-to-air missile. The latter anti-tank and reconnaissance versions also carried the Viviane thermal imagery system, so were known as the Gazelle Viviane. The Gazelle has been replaced in frontline duties by the Eurocopter Tiger but continues to be used for light transport and liaison roles.

Aerospatiale SA341/342 Gazelle	
In service:	1974 to present
Used by:	French ALAT
Manufacturer:	Sud Aviation, Aerospatiale
Produced:	1967 to 1996
Number built:	109 in use with French ALAT in 2022
Specifications	
Powerplant:	1 × Turbomeca Astazou IIIA turboshaft
Length:	11.97m (39ft 3in)
Rotor diameter:	10.5m (34ft 5in)
Height:	3.15m (10ft 4in) overall
Maximum speed:	310km/h (190mph, 170kts) at sea level
Range:	361km (224 miles, 195nm)
Crew:	1 or 2
Capacity:	up to 3 or 4 passengers
Armament:	6 x HOT missiles, 2 x forward-firing 7.62mm machine guns (optional)

Eurocopter EC665 Tiger

Europe's Gunship

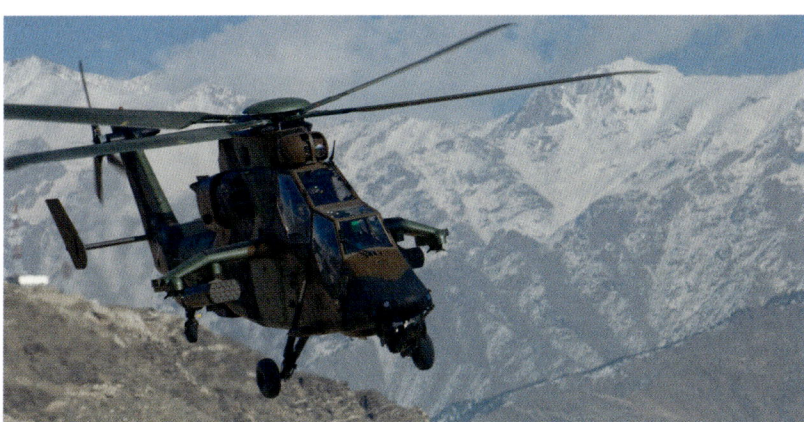

F rance and Germany joined forces in 1984 to launch a project to replace the anti-tank missile-armed Aerospatiale Gazelle and MBB Bo 105 light battlefield helicopters.

The project was beset by funding delays so it was not until 1999 that the first production contract was placed with Eurocopter, which became Airbus Helicopters. Now formally named the Tiger, the attack helicopter's crew sit in a tandem cockpit. It has an under-nose turret for a 30mm cannon and stub-wing weapon pylons. There are three basic variants:

- UHT (Unterstützungshubschrauber Tiger or Support Helicopter Tiger). A medium-weight multi-role fire support helicopter built for the German Armed Forces. It has a night vision sight mounted above the rotor hub.
- Tiger HAP/HCP (Hélicoptère d'Appui Protection or Support and Escort Helicopter/ Hélicoptère de Combat Polyvalent or Multipurpose Combat Helicopter). It features the under-nose 30mm cannon turret but does not have a mast-mounted sight.
- Tiger HAD (Hélicoptère d'Appui Destruction or Support and Destruction Helicopter). Essentially identical to the HAP version but better suited for operations in hot environments, with 14% more engine power available due to the upgraded enhanced MTR390 engine.

The first French and German Tigers entered service in 2005 and export orders were secured in Australia and Spain.

France, Germany, and Spain all deployed their Tigers to Afghanistan, with the French helicopters seeing action first in 2009. French Tigers operated from an amphibious landing ship in the 2011 Libyan war. They were subsequently deployed to Mali in 2013, while German Tigers were sent to the North African country in 2017.

In 2022, France and Spain announced that they would upgrade their Tigers to the new Mk III configuration, including a new helmet-mounted sight system, the enhanced vision system, radios, datalinks for manned-unmanned teaming, new air-to-surface and air-to-air missiles, guns and rockets, improved countermeasures, a new navigation system synchronised to the Galileo global positioning system and an updated avionics suite that includes new tactical data and battlefield management systems.

LEFT: The Tiger is the attack helicopter of the French, German, Spanish and Australian armed forces.
(US DOD/COMBAT CAMERA)

Eurocopter EC665 Tiger	
In service:	2005 to date
Used by:	Australia, France, Germany, Spain
Manufacturer:	Eurocopter/Airbus
Produced:	1999 to 2011
Number built:	180
Specifications for Tiger HAP/HCP	
Powerplant:	2 × MTR MTR390 turboshaft engines
Length:	14.08m (46ft 2in)
Rotor diameter:	13m (42ft 8in)
Height:	3.83m (12ft 7in)
Max take-off weight:	6,000kg (13,228lb)
Maximum speed:	315km/h (196mph, 170kts)
Crew:	2 (pilot and weapon systems officer)
Armament	
1× 30 mm (1.18 in) GIAT 30 cannon in chin turret	
Inner hardpoints:	
20mm (0.787in) cannon pod	
68mm (2.68in) SNEB unguided rocket pod	
70mm (2.75in) Hydra 70 unguided rocket pod	
AGM-114 Hellfire missiles	
Spike-ER missiles	
PARS 3 LR missiles	
HOT3 missiles	
Outer hardpoints:	
Mistral air-to-air missiles	
Air-to-Air Stinger missiles	
68mm (2.68in) SNEB unguided rocket pod	
70mm (2.75in) Hydra 70 unguided pod	

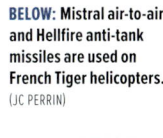

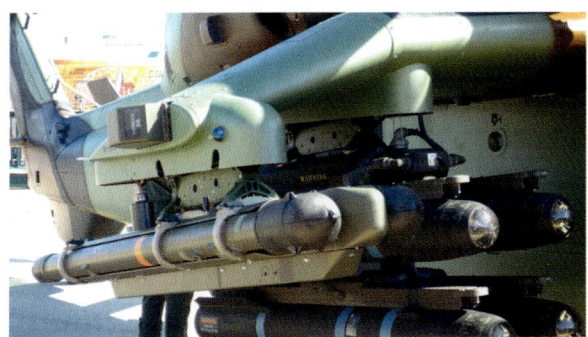

BELOW: Mistral air-to-air and Hellfire anti-tank missiles are used on French Tiger helicopters.
(JC PERRIN)

Kamov Ka-52 Alligator

Russia's Predator

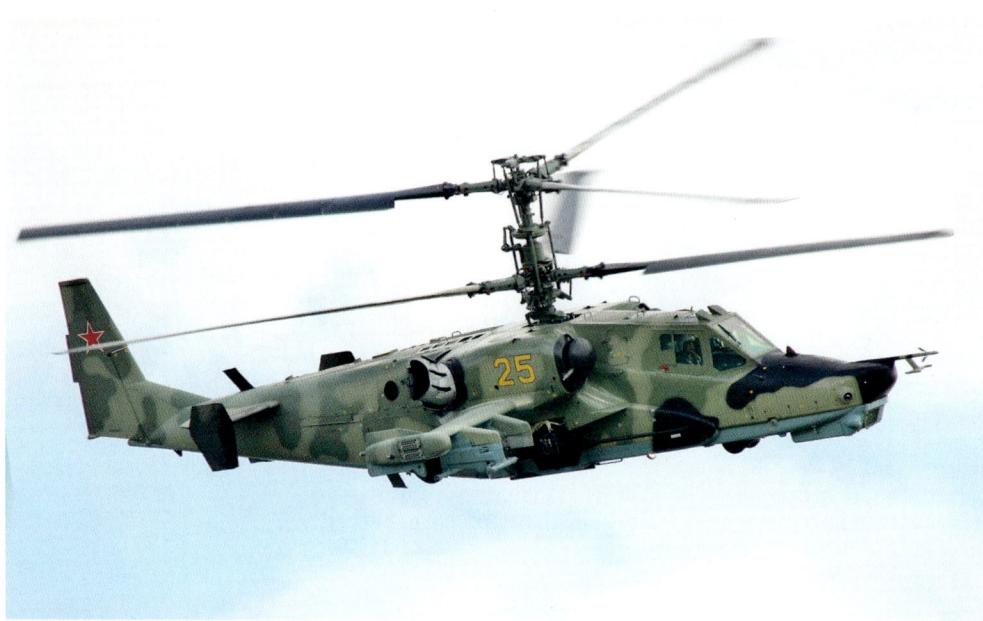

ABOVE: The twin-seat Ka-52 is now in frontline service with the Russian Aerospace Forces. (DMITRIY PICHUGIN)

The Kamov OKB design bureau began work in the 1980s on an attack helicopter that featured its distinctive coaxial rotor system. This allowed the helicopter to do away with the antitorque rotor, or tail rotor that counteracts the main rotor torque and controls the fuselage rotation. As a result of not requiring a tail rotor, coaxial rotor-equipped helicopters can use all their power for forward flight, so they are faster and more manoeuvrable than traditional helicopters.

Kamov proved the concept worked on the Ka-25/27 naval helicopter and the design bureau was keen to use it on battlefield helicopters.

The original Ka-50 Night Shark variant was a single-seat machine, but as more complex sensors and weapons were added in the 1990s it was decided to incorporate a second crew member sitting beside the pilot. This Ka-52 Alligator has since entered Russian Aerospace Forces' service.

Throughout its life the Ka-50/52 has been locked in competition with the rival Mi-28, both having similar roles, weapon systems and sensor fits.

In the 1980s the first Ka-50 design gained the seal of approval of the Soviet military which selected it over the Mi-28 as the replacement for the classic Mi-24. The demise of the Soviet Union meant serial production was never given the go-ahead but a handful of prototypes had been built and handed over to the military for testing. In the early 1990s approval was given for Kamov to begin working on the two-seat Ka-52 and this new variant included ground surveillance radars, night vision equipment and six hard points for multiple weapons.

Production of the Ka-52 began in 1996 and the first frontline units took delivery of the helicopters in 2011. More than 100 were in service in 2022. The Russian Aerospace Forces first used the helicopter in combat in Syria in 2016 and they have since been in action in Ukraine in 2022.

Egypt is the only export customer, and it took the Ka-52K Katran variant, which has folding rotor blades, for use on ships.

BELOW: Ka-52s have seen action in Syria and Ukraine. The large pod is a ground surveillance radar. (OLEG V. BELYAKOV)

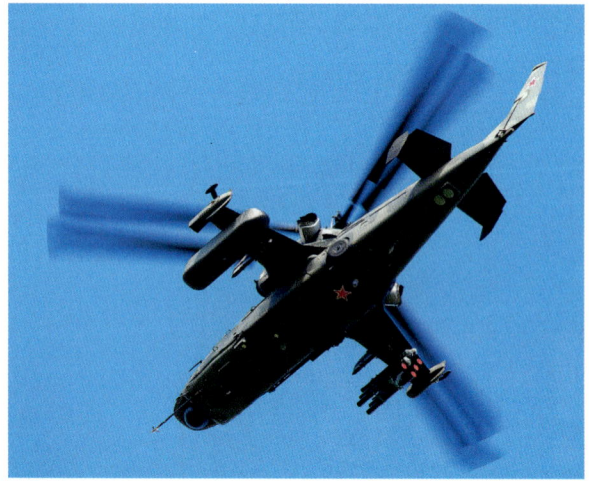

Kamov Ka-52 Alligator	
In service:	2011
Used by:	Russian Aerospace Forces, Egyptian Air Force
Manufacturer:	Kamov JSC and Progress Arsenyev Aviation Company JSCProduced: 1997 to date
Number built:	150+
Specifications	
Propulsion:	2 x Klimov TW3-117VMA / TV3-117VMA
Length:	16m (52ft 6in)
Main Rotor Diameter:	14.50m (47ft 7in)
Height:	4.95m (16ft 3in)
Maximum Take-off Weight:	11,300kg (24,912lb)
Speed:	350km/h (189kts)
Range:	459km (248nm)
Crew:	2
Armament	
Guns:	
1× 30 mm Shipunov 2A42 cannon (hull mounted)	
23 mm UPK-23-250 gun pods	
Hardpoints (to carry a combination of)	
Rockets:	80mm S-8, 122mm S-13 rockets
Missiles:	9K121 Vikhr anti-tank missiles
Vympel R-73 air-to-air missiles	
Kh-25 semi-active laser-guided tactical air-to-ground missiles	
Bombs:	4 × 250kg (550lb) or 2 × 500kg (1,100lb) free-fall bombs

Mil Mi-28

The Russian Apache

When the US began developing the AH-64 Apache in the late 1970s, the Soviet helicopter industry took a close interest, and it was not long before they were offering up their rival designs.

In 1980 the Mil OKB design bureau began work on the helicopter that became the Mi-28. Externally it looked like a derivative of the American Apache with its distinctive stub wing weapon pylons, tandem cockpit and under-nose gun turret.

The Soviet military did not order the helicopter in the 1980s, but Mil OKB was allowed to keep working on the design. In the early 1990s a

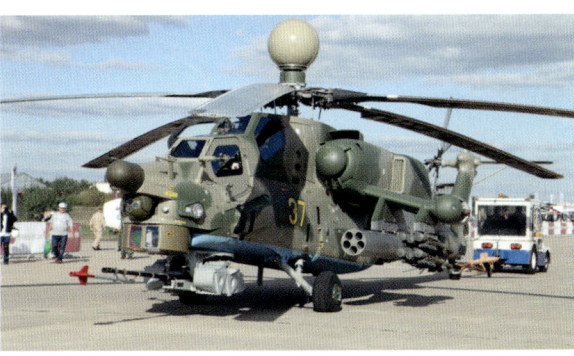

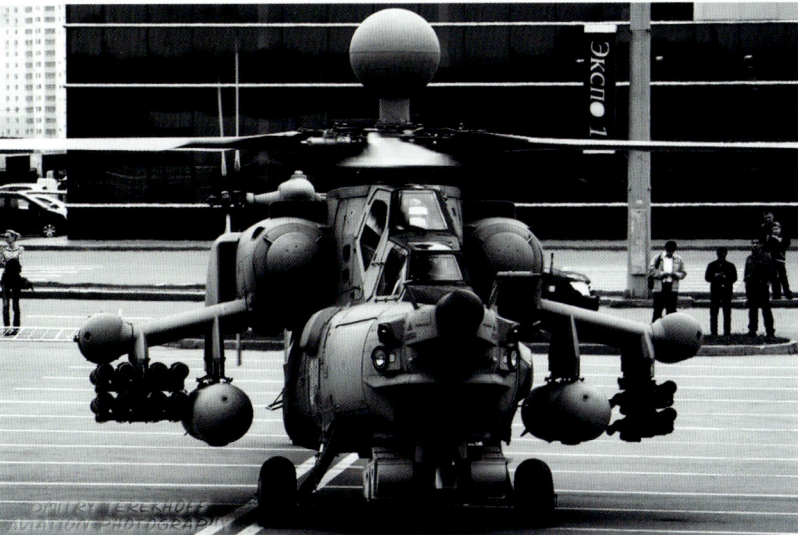

new version, the Mi-28N, or Night, appeared. It was intended to rival the AH-64D Apache Longbow, and it sported a ground surveillance radar mounted above the rotor head and modern night vision sensors. It also featured an advanced suite of weapons including 16 Ataka-V, 9K121 Vikhr and 9M123 Khrizantema anti-tank missiles, and Igla-V and Vympel R-73 air-to-air missiles.

Financial problems meant full-rate manufacturing was not ordered until early in the 21st century and the first production model was delivered in 2006. The helicopter, dubbed the Mi-28NE, has been exported to Algeria and Iraq, and deliveries to the Russian military continue, with more than 100 being in service by 2022.

An updated version, the Mi-28NM, has been under development since 2009 and features more powerful VK-2500P engines, a low-radar signature, extended flight range and advanced weapons control system. The Mi-28NM first flew in 2016 and there are plans to upgrade all the existing Mi-28Ns to the new configuration.

The Mi-28Ns first saw service in Syria in 2016 and they have been used extensively in the war against Ukraine in 2022.

ABOVE: The Mi-28N is the main variant currently in use with the Russian Aerospace Forces. (VITALY V. KUZMIN)

LEFT: The upgraded Mi-28NE is now in production. (DMITRY TEREKHOV)

Mil Mi-28	
In service:	from 2009
Used by:	Russian Aerospace Forces, Iraq, and Algeria
Manufacturer:	Mil OKB design bureau, Rostvertol for final assembly
Produced:	from 1995 onwards
Number built:	126 to date
Specifications	
Powerplant:	2 × Klimov TV3-117 turboshafts
Length:	17.01m (55ft 10in)
Height:	3.82m (12ft 6in)
Max take-off weight:	11,500kg (25,353lb)
Maximum speed:	320km/h (170kts)
Range:	435km (235nm)
Crew:	2 (1 pilot, 1 weapons system operator)
Armament	
Guns:	1 × chin-mounted 30mm Shipunov 2A42 cannon
Hardpoints:	Two pylons to allow a combination configuration of the following weapons:
	16 Ataka-V anti-tank missiles
	9K121 Vikhr anti-tank missiles
	9M123 Khrizantema anti-tank missiles
	8 Igla-V and Vympel R-73 air-to-air missiles
	2 KMGU-2 mine dispensers
	S-8 and S-13 rockets
	Two 23mm UPK-23-250 gun pods

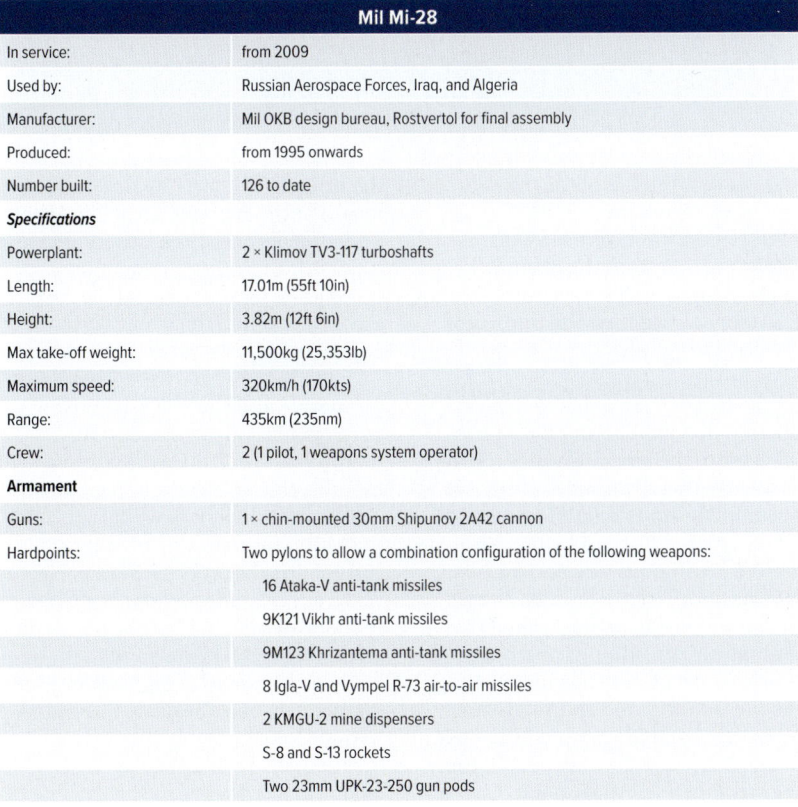

BELOW: Close-in targets are engaged by the Mi-28's 30mm nose cannon. (ALLOCER)

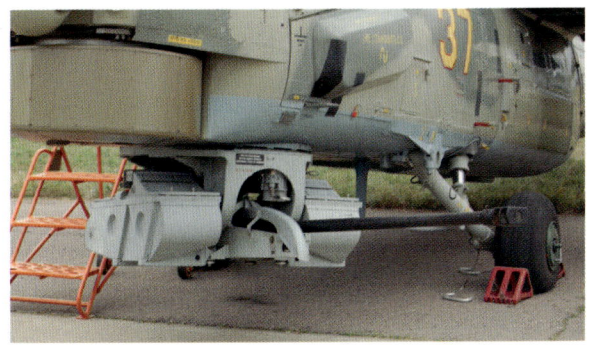

America's Helicopter War

Vietnam 1965 to 1975

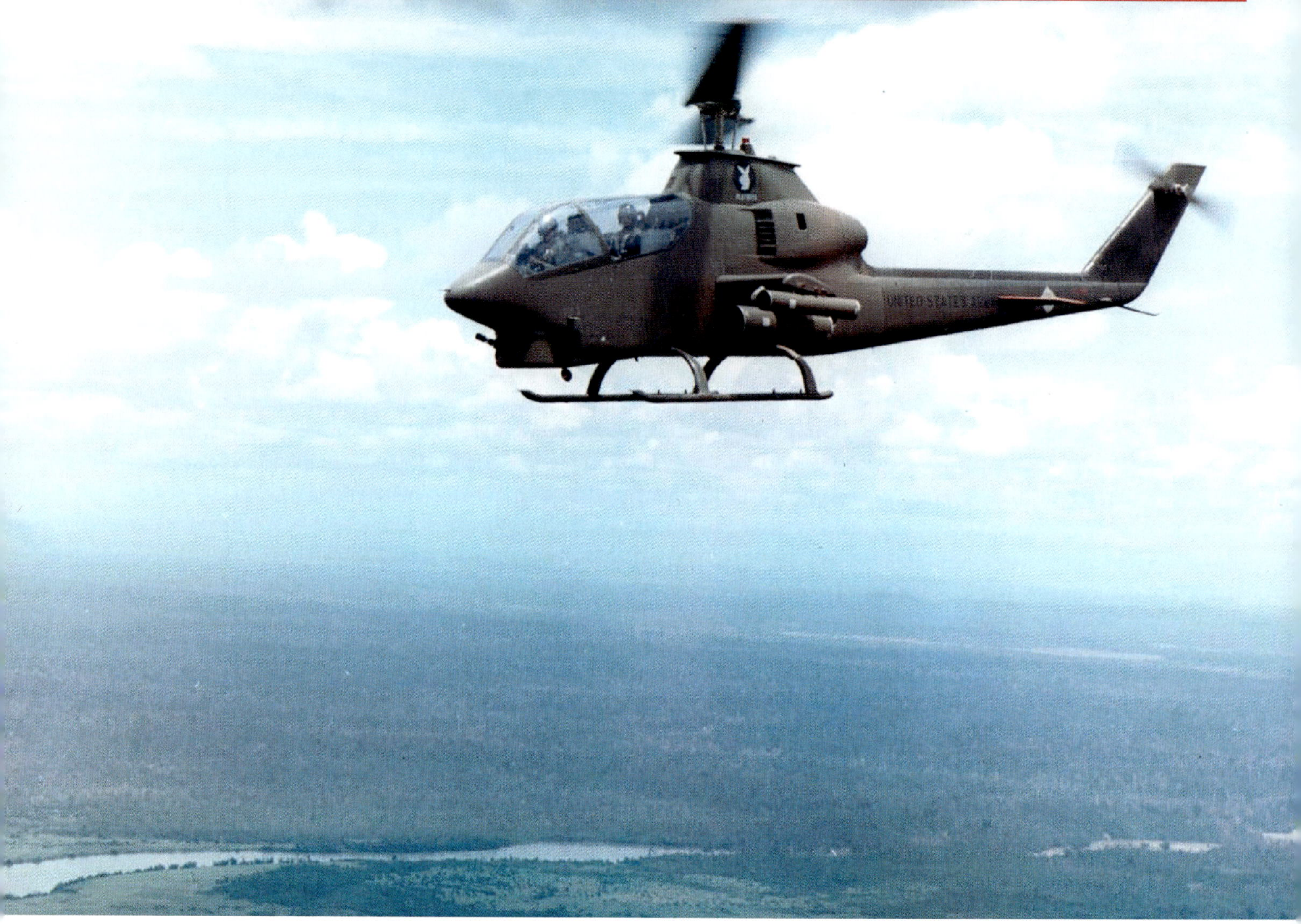

ABOVE: The AH-1G Cobra was the definitive gunship of the Vietnam War and its design set the standard for future attack helicopters. (US ARMY)

US involvement in the Southeast Asian conflict steadily escalated during the first half of 1965 in a bid to roll back advances by Communist forces. By the autumn of that year the US Army's only air mobile division would be in action in the Central Highlands of Vietnam.

A handful of US helicopter units had arrived to support American advisors in the early years of the decade as US President John F Kennedy ramped up support for the government of South Vietnam. Communist Viet Cong guerrillas and North Vietnamese regular troops staged offensives across the south in the early months of 1965, prompting Washington to respond. The then President, Lyndon Johnson, ordered US regular troops to South Vietnam to take the fight to the Communists and prevent the fall of the pro-US Saigon government.

First into action were US Marine Corps units around the northern city of Da Nang. Further to the south, the US Army would bear the burden of the escalating war.

At the end of June 1965, President Johnson approved plans to deploy the first divisional-sized US Army formation, the airmobile division, or as it was officially titled the 11th Air Assault Division (Test). However, US Army chiefs felt the division needed a more prestigious title and on July 1, 1965 it was officially re-titled the 1st Cavalry Division and inherited that famous unit's traditions and battle honours. All of its subordinate air mobile infantry and reconnaissance units subsequently adopted the titles of US Army cavalry units, including the 5th, 7th, 8th, 9th, and 12th Cavalry Regiments. The 7th Cavalry famously fought at the Battle of Little Big Horn under General George Custer. Its 1965 successor regiment took on *Garry Owen* as its march tune, while the 9th Cavalry adopted the iconic Cavalry Stetson hat.

The name changes were a big boost for morale and the newly minted cavalrymen soon started to call themselves the 'Air Cav'. Within a few months, the 1st Battalion, 7th (1st/7th) Cavalry would win new honours under its commanding officer, Lieutenant Colonel Hal Moore. He was a charismatic and dynamic but thoughtful officer who was portrayed on screen by Mel Gibson in the Hollywood movie of his Vietnam War memoir, *We Were Soldiers*. The blond-haired Colonel Moore was jokingly nicknamed 'Yellow Hair' by his troops in a reference to Custer. The

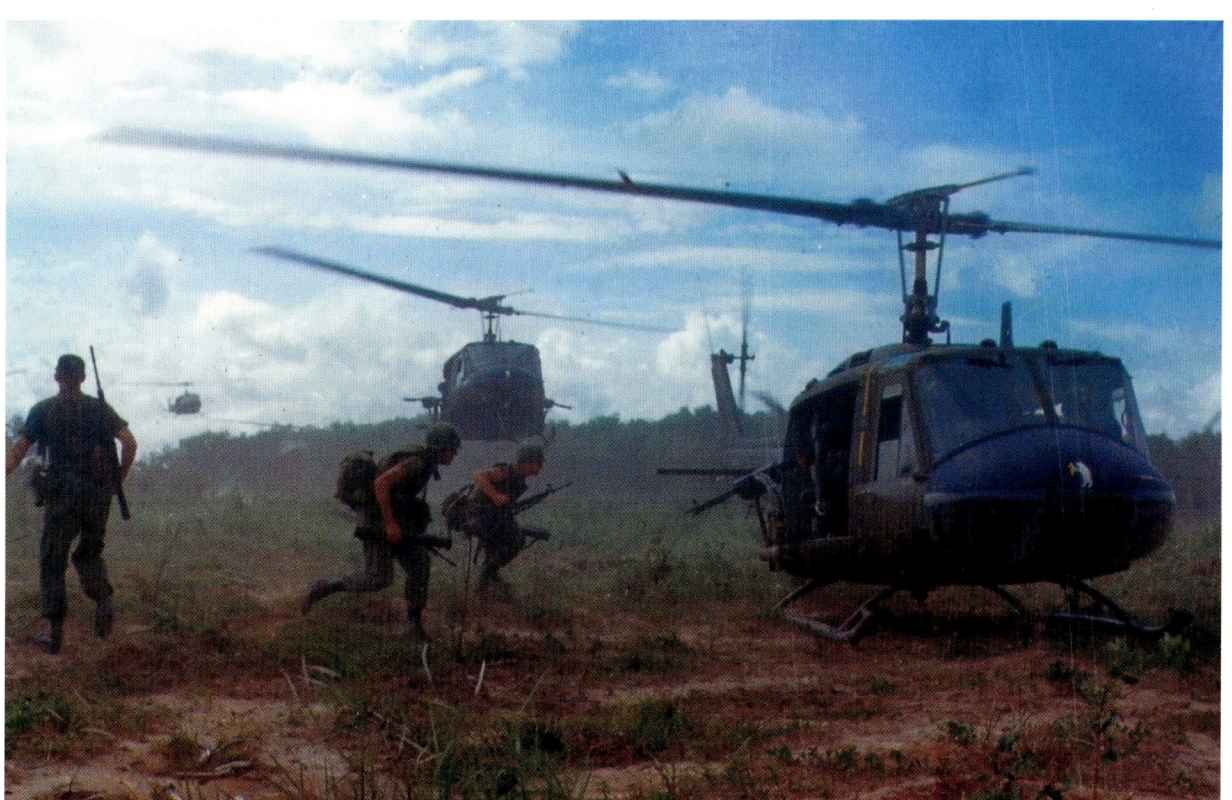

LEFT: The US Army in Vietnam and the iconic UH-1 Huey pioneered airmobile tactics. It was at the heart of all major US operations during the conflict. (US ARMY)

BELOW: The US 1st Cavalry Division's helicopters were transported to Vietnam on board the World War Two-era aircraft carrier, the USS *Boxer*. (US ARMY)

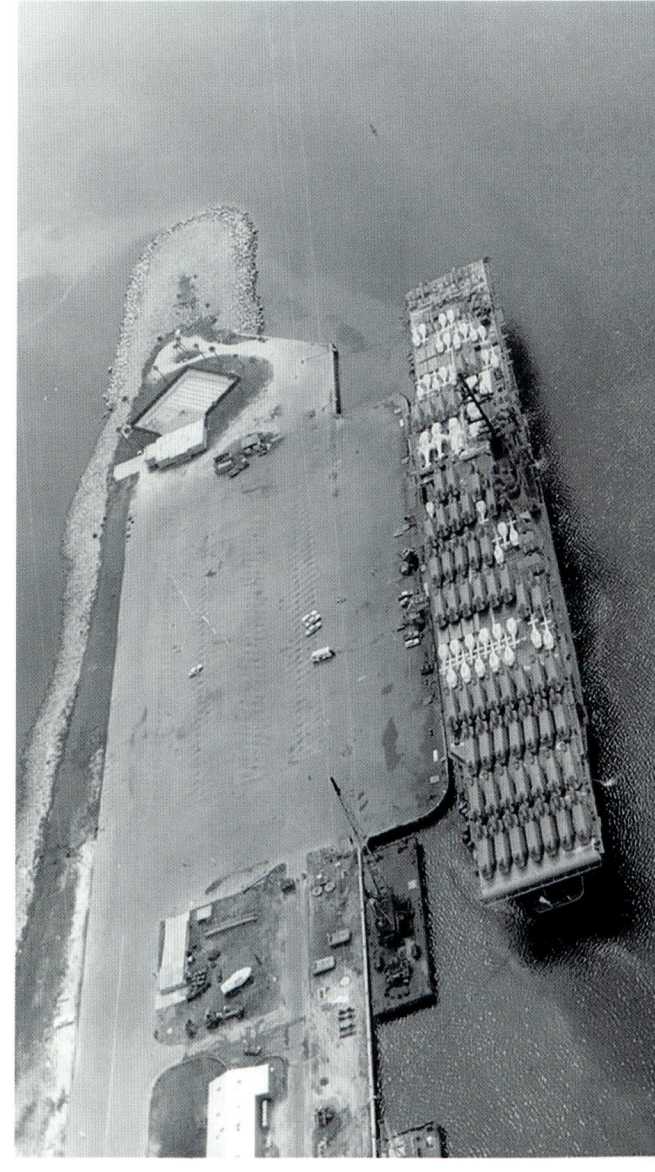

colonel expressed fears that his men could share the fate of their famous predecessors if the US Army's new helicopter-based tactics did not prevail over the North Vietnamese.

The 11th Division had been set up at Fort Benning in Georgia in February 1963 with the mandate to test and trial the use of helicopters to fight on future battlefields. It was no secret that Vietnam was the likely venue for the division's first combat deployment.

Although the new division's organisation looked a lot like a conventional infantry division – it had three brigades, eight infantry battalions, an artillery regiment and support units – everything about it was orientated to air mobility. Helicopters were integrated into every unit and tactical procedure used by the division. The division had its own aviation group, with three battalions of air assault helicopters that in theory could move a whole brigade's worth of troops simultaneously. A contingent of Boeing Vertol CH-47 Chinook heavy lift helicopters were provided to move the fuel, ammunition, and other supplies to the division's forward operating bases.

Airborne firepower, in the shape of armed Bell UH-1 Huey helicopters, was integral to everything the division did. Gunships were incorporated into each of the air assault units to fly escort during air mobile troop insertion missions. The artillery regiment had its own battalion of rocket-armed Hueys to provide fire support when the

division was operating beyond the range of traditional tube artillery support. Armed Hueys and Bell OH-13 Sioux scout helicopters were grouped together in the division's reconnaissance battalion, or air cavalry regiment as it was known. They were the eyes and ears of the division and were tasked with flying over enemy territory to collect intelligence, identify landing zones, or LZs, for air assault operations by the air mobile infantry and strike rapidly at any targets that appeared. The division's reconnaissance unit, the 1st Squadron, 9th (1st/9th) Cavalry made this role its own in Vietnam. It was a hard-hitting, self-contained unit that was first into action to find 'Charlie', as the Viet Cong were nicknamed, or to provide covering fire as the last infantry were extracted by helicopter from a 'hot' landing zone, or LZ, under enemy fire. According to the unit's official history, the 1st/9th Cavalry was responsible for 50% of all enemy soldiers killed by the 1st Cavalry Division during the Vietnam War.

"During the Squadron's time in Vietnam it was 100% mobile with organic transport, which included nearly 100 helicopters," recorded the unit's official history. "[(1st/9th) Cavalry] had three air cavalry troops and each troop had an aero scout platoon, an aero weapons platoon and an aero rifle platoon. The mission of the aero scout platoon was to find the enemy. Until 1968 these platoons used OH-13 observation helicopters but by mid-1968 those ships were replaced » by the faster, more manoeuvrable OH-6A Light Observation Helicopter (LOH, or the Loach). The scouts would skim low over the terrain searching for any sign of enemy movement or activity. The scouts were referred to as the 'White' platoon. The aero weapons, or 'Red' platoon, were initially made up of UH-1B (Huey) gunships until they were replaced by the AH-1G Cobra gunships in 1968. Armed with rockets, miniguns and grenade launchers, the 'Red' gunships joined with the 'White' scout ships to form the 'Pink' team which made up the basic working unit of the squadron in Vietnam. The 'Blue' aero rifle platoon complemented the aerial reconnaissance capabilities of the Pink Team by providing ground reconnaissance. Transported by Huey Slicks, the Blues could be quickly inserted to check sightings by the aerial observer, assess the damage inflicted by the gunships and pursue the enemy. The Squadron's fourth troop, Delta Troop, was a ground cavalry unit with three platoons mounted on wheeled vehicles."

To pull Air Cav operations together, the 1st Cavalry's commanders at all levels down to battalion were provided with their own command Hueys fitted with additional radios so they could choreograph airborne operations as they unfolded.

When the 1st Cavalry sailed for Vietnam in the summer of 1965, it took with it more than 16,000 troops, which was a similar number to the strength of a traditional infantry division, but it only fielded 1,600 vehicles, or half those found in a conventional division. In the place of the legacy trucks and armoured personnel carriers, the 1st Cavalry took 400 helicopters to Vietnam. For the 1960s this was a phenomenal number, and even at the peak of US involvement in Vietnam, in 1968, a standard US infantry division only boasted around 100 helicopters.

The 1st Cavalry was selected to lead the US Army's expanding campaign in Vietnam because the Pentagon thought the division's mobility and firepower would give it an edge over the Viet Cong and their North Vietnamese allies. Up to 1965 the Communist force had relied on light infantry tactics to infiltrate into government-controlled regions and launch surprise attacks to overwhelm isolated detachments of the South Vietnamese ground forces, the Army of the Republic of Vietnam or ARVN. It was hoped that the helicopters of the 1st Cavalry would allow the US Army to turn the tables on the Viet Cong by rapidly inserting US troops inside its territory to either capture key headquarters and supply dumps or force the Communists to mass their troops to counter-attack. Once the Communists had joined battle their troops would become vulnerable to overwhelming US firepower. That, at least, was the theory. It would be put to the test for real in October and November 1965 when the 1st Cavalry was dispatched to Pleiku city in the Central Highlands to

RIGHT: Colonel Hal Moore led the 1st Battalion, 7th Cavalry into the Ia Drang Valley in November 1965. (US ARMY)

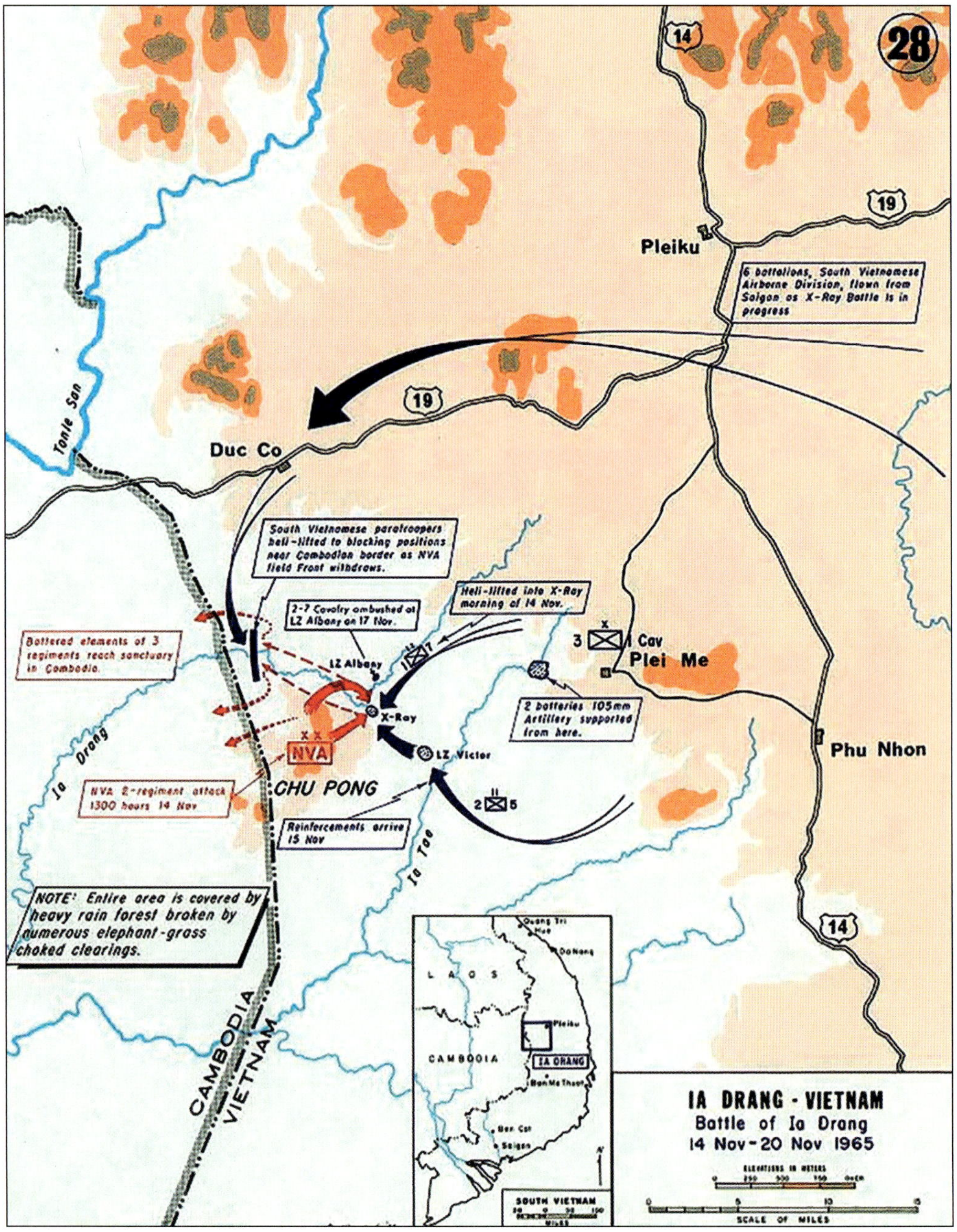

BELOW: The Battle of the Ia Drang Valley. (US ARMY)

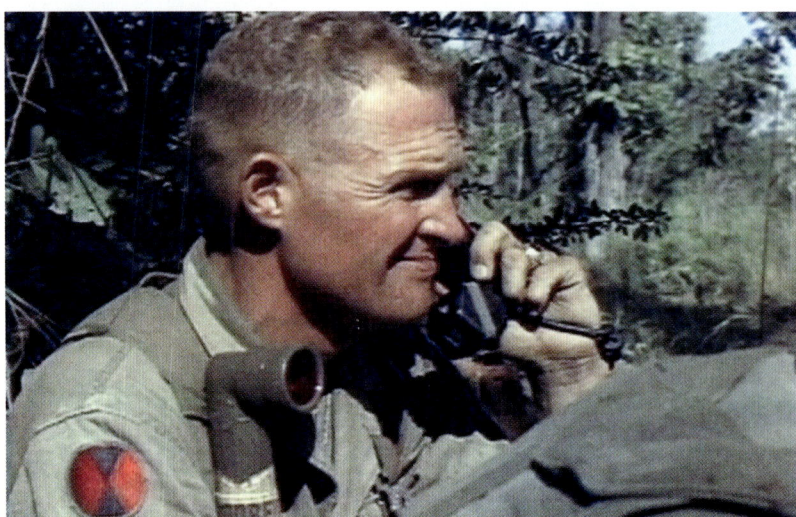

IA DRANG - VIETNAM
Battle of Ia Drang
14 Nov – 20 Nov 1965

counter a suspected build up of North Vietnamese troops.

The first unit of the division on the ground was the 1st/9th Cavalry that was given the mission of finding the enemy. Every day it launched helicopter sweeps over the dense jungle region to try to draw the enemy out into battle, spot potential landing zones and gain an understanding of the terrain. Skirmishes and firefights between the 1st/9th Cavalry and North Vietnamese regular units escalated during October, but the enemy remained elusive.

A major attack by Communist troops on a remote ARVN Special Forces camp north of Pleiku gave the 1st/9th Cavalry its chance to pounce.

Its scout helicopters found a retreating North Vietnamese column in the jungle and within hours of the start of the engagement it had airlifted its rifle platoons into blocking positions to trap the enemy troops. A battle raged over October 30 and into November 1 in which 74 enemy personnel were killed and 37 captured, while five US soldiers were killed and 17 wounded. Once the battle was over the Air Cav troopers discovered a jungle hospital and recovered North Vietnamese army identity cards from the prisoners and enemy dead. This was positive intelligence that the 1st Cavalry was facing a sizable enemy force. The 1st

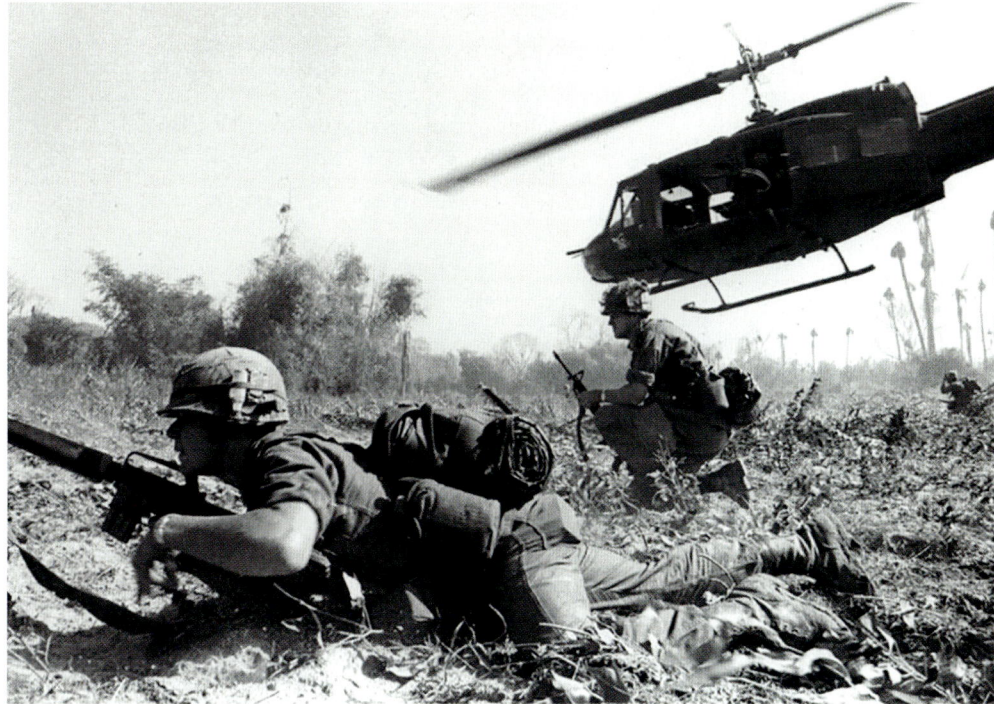

Cavalry planners were now looking at ways to insert more troops into the region in the hope of bringing the enemy to battle. Thanks to 1st/9th Cavalry efforts, a series of landing zones had been identified between Pleiku city and the Cambodian border that could be activated at a few hours' notice once the enemy's main force had been identified.

The 1st/9th Cavalry conducted another ambush operation on November 4 after landing its rifle platoons at night deep inside enemy territory. Some 150 North Vietnamese were reported killed in the intense battle that saw gunships bringing down fire support within 50m of friendly troops.

On November 13, Colonel Moore and his 1st/7th Cavalry were ordered to launch the 1st Cavalry's first-ever battalion-sized air assault operation into the Ia Drang Valley area, where a large concentration of North Vietnamese troops was believed to be based.

After first light on the following morning, four scout Hueys of the 1st/9th Cavalry flew a low-level 'nap-of-the-earth' reconnaissance mission over the target areas to try to find signs of the enemy and confirm the status of the proposed »

ABOVE: US Army UH-D Hueys were the life line from Colonel Moore's isolated troopers during the Battle of the Ia Drang Valley. (US ARMY)

BELOW: Once on the ground the troops of the 1st Battalion, 7th Cavalry had to fight at almost point-blank range because of the thick jungle vegetation. (US ARMY)

1st Cavalry Division Order of Battle Vietnam, October 1965

1st Cavalry Division Headquarters
- 11th General Support Aviation Company (12 x UH-1D)

1st Brigade (Airborne)
- 1st Battalion (Airborne), 8th Cavalry Regiment (airmobile infantry)
- 2nd Battalion (Airborne), 8th Cavalry Regiment (airmobile infantry)
- 1st Battalion (Airborne), 12th Cavalry Regiment (airmobile infantry)

2nd Brigade
- 1st Battalion, 5th Cavalry Regiment (airmobile infantry)
- 2nd Battalion, 5th Cavalry Regiment (airmobile infantry)
- 2nd Battalion, 12th Cavalry Regiment (airmobile infantry)

3rd Brigade
- 1st Battalion, 7th Cavalry Regiment (airmobile infantry)
- 2nd Battalion, 7th Cavalry Regiment (airmobile infantry)

Division Artillery
- 2nd Battalion (Airborne), 19th Artillery Regiment (105mm Howitzers)
- 2nd Battalion, 20th Artillery Regiment (Aerial Rocket) (36 x UH-1B)
- 1st Battalion, 21st Artillery Regiment (105mm Howitzers)
- 1st Battalion, 77th Artillery Regiment (105mm Howitzers)
- Battery E, 82nd Artillery Regiment (Aviation) (12 x OH-13/ UH-1B)

11th Aviation Group
- 1st Squadron, 9th Cavalry Regiment (24 x OH-13, 120 x UH-1B/D) (scout/reconnaissance)
- 227th Aviation Battalion (Assault Helicopter) (60 x UH-1D, 12 x UH-1B gunship)
- 228th Aviation Battalion (Assault Support Helicopter) (57 x CH-47A)
- 229th Aviation Battalion (Assault Helicopter) (60 x UH-1D, 12 x UH-1B gunship)
- 17th Aviation Company (CV-2/C-7 Caribou transport aircraft)
- 478th Aviation Company (4 x CH-54)

Divisional Support Command
- 15th Medical Battalion
- 15th Supply & Services Battalion
- Aerial Equipment Supply Company (Airborne)
- 15th Administrative Company
- 27th Maintenance Battalion
- 8th Engineer Battalion
- 13th Signal Battalion
- 15th Transportation Battalion
- 545th Military Police Company
- 191st Military Intelligence Detachment
- 371st Army Security Agency Company

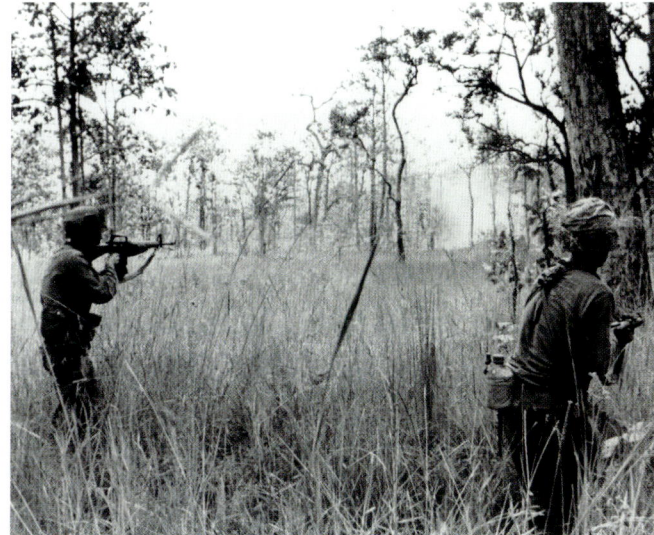

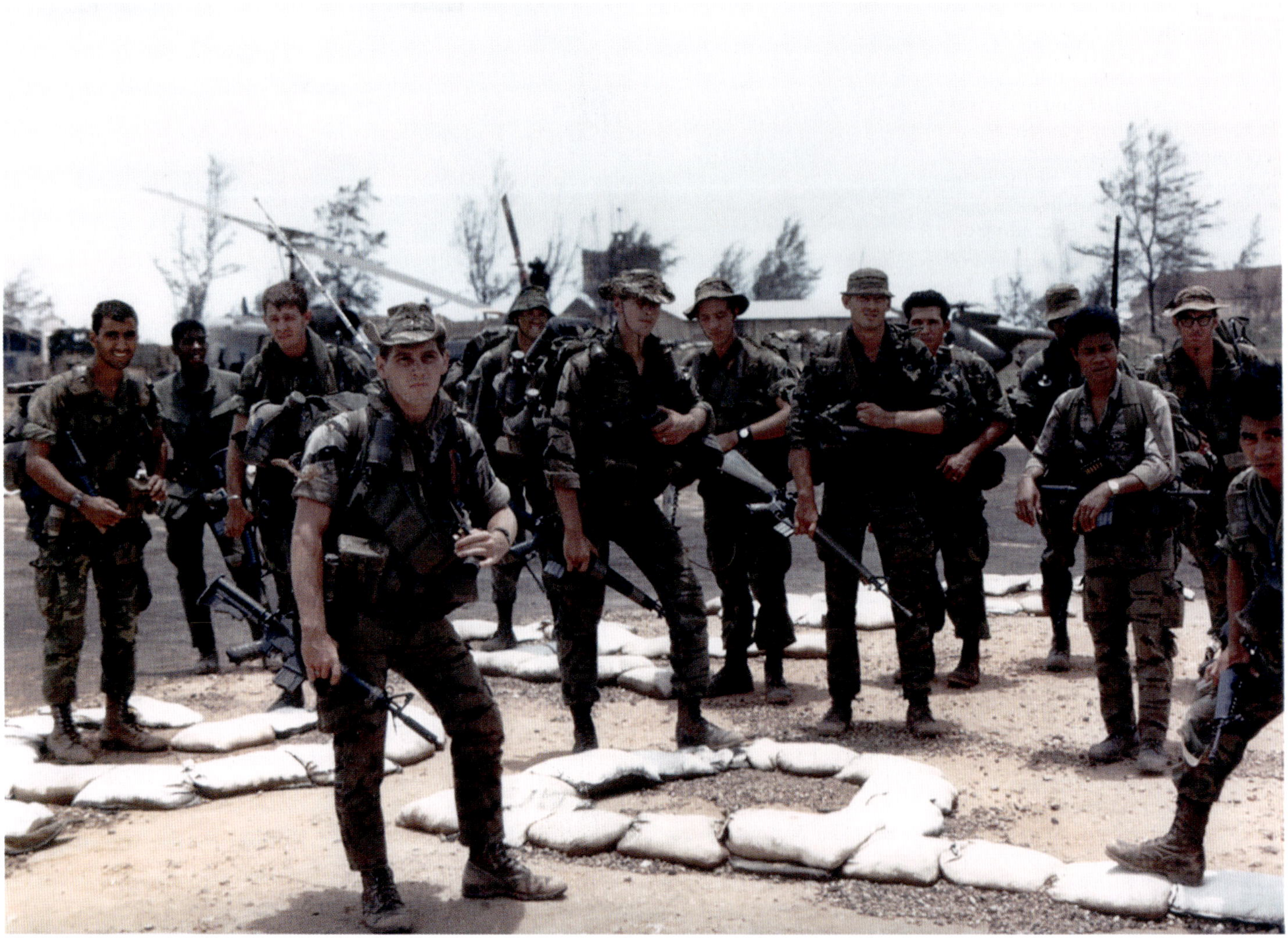

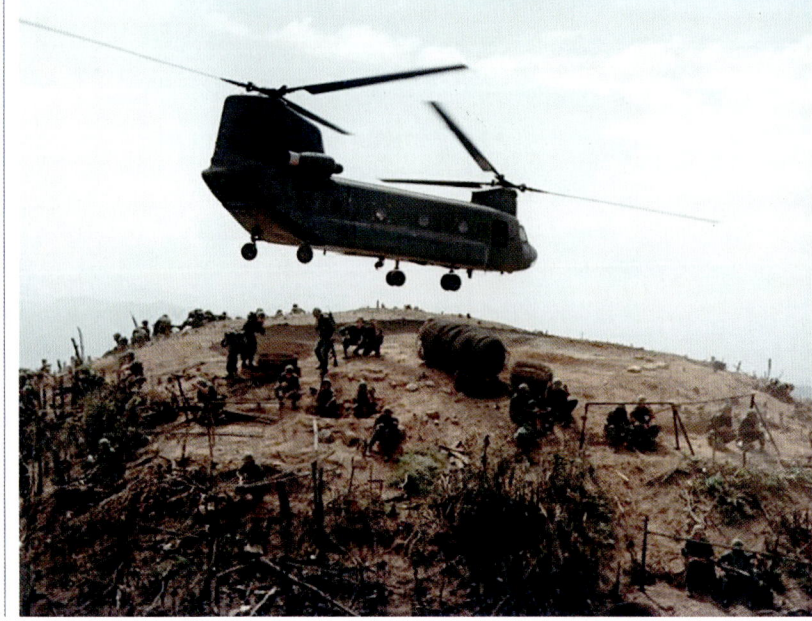

ABOVE: Long-range reconnaissance patrols of the 1st Cavalry Division were flown by helicopter deep into Viet Cong-held territory to try to find enemy troop positions.
(US ARMY)

RIGHT: The mighty CH-47 Chinook moved all of the 1st Cavalry Division's supplies and ammunition to forward operating bases to keep its troops and UH-1s in the fight.
(ICEMANWCS)

landing zones. After a 40-minute flight, the scouts returned to Colonel Moore's forward operating base at Plei Me. They did not take any fire or spot any enemy troops. More importantly, they reported that one of the landing zones, code name LZ X-Ray, looked the most suitable because it could accommodate up

to 10 Hueys at time, maximising the number of soldiers Colonel Moore could move in each wave of helicopter lifts.

Within minutes of receiving the reports from the scout team, Colonel Moore had issued his orders and the gunship and troop transport Hueys were spinning up, preparing to take

off to fly the 1st/7th Cavalry to LZ X-Ray.

"At 10.17am [105mm] artillery preparatory fires [around LZ X-Ray] began," recorded a US Army history of the battle. "Thirteen minutes later the leading elements of Company B lifted off the Plei Me airstrip with a thunderous roar in a storm of red dust. With volleys of artillery fire slamming into the objective area, the 16 Hueys – four platoons of four each – filed southwestward across the midmorning sky at 2,000ft. Two kilometres out, they dropped to treetop level. The aerial rocket artillery gunships [of 2nd Battalion, 20th Artillery (Airmobile)] meanwhile worked X-Ray over for 30 seconds expending half of their loads, then circled nearby, available on call. The escort gunships [of the 229th Aviation Battalion (Airmobile)] came next, rockets and machine guns blazing, immediately ahead of the lift ships. As the lead helicopters braked for the assault landing, their door gunners and some of the infantrymen fired into the trees and tall grass. Lunging from the ships the men of Company B, Colonel Moore among them, charged into the trees, snap-firing at likely enemy positions. By 10.48am the helicopters were already returning to Plei Me for the rest of Company B and advance contingents of Company A."

The air assault phase of the operation proved anti-climatic. There were no Communist troops dug-in around the fringe of the landing zone, ready to open fire as the first helicopters disgorged their troops. The calm would not last long. Elements of three North Vietnamese regiments were nearby and they were immediately ordered to strike at the Americans who had just landed in their midst.

The next two days saw the 1st/7th Cavalry fight for its life as the Communist troops attempted to overwhelm its position. LZ X-Ray was a flat clearing with scrub trees, anthills and thick elephant grass stretching out to the edge of the jungle. Colonel Moore set up his tactical headquarters in the centre of the clearing next to a small resupply landing zone that could take two Hueys at a time. His troops fanned out to form a perimeter and they started to probe into the jungle.

By afternoon, the first contacts had been reported around the perimeter and soon waves of North Vietnamese were attacking the US troops. One platoon was cut off and the rest of the Cavalrymen went firm in their positions and tried to repel the human wave charges of Communist troops.

The 1st/7th Cavalry's command team called up air and artillery fire.

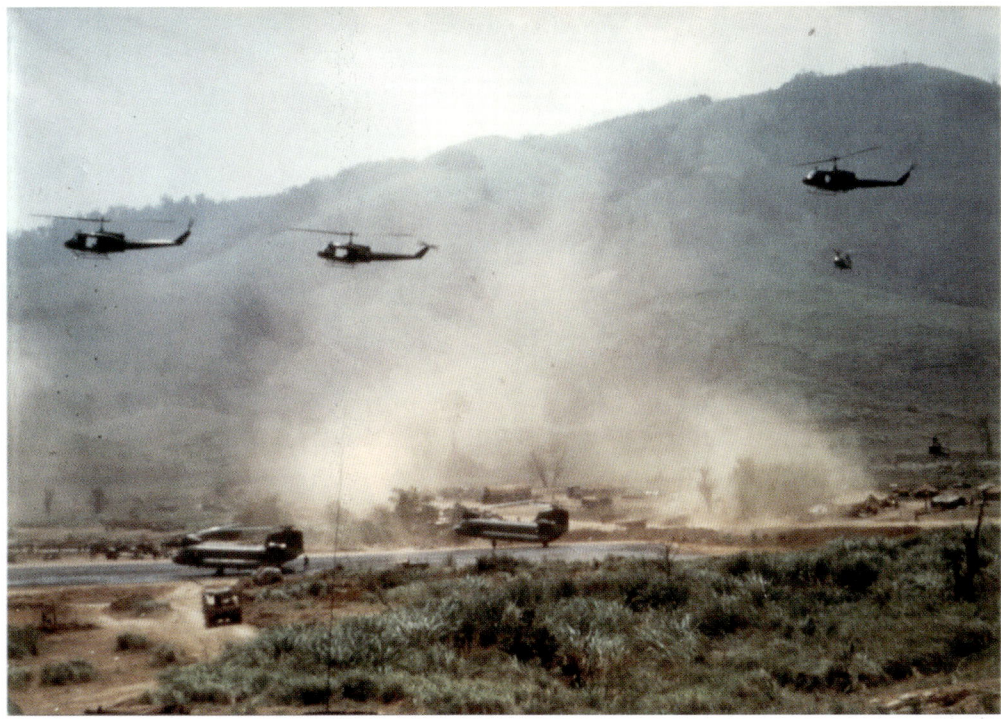

Soon USAF fast jets were rolling in to bomb enemy troop concentrations and artillery fire was raining down. Completing the fire support were Huey gunships that blasted enemy positions with rockets and machine guns. This continued through the afternoon as wave after wave of attackers surged towards the tight US perimeter. It took time for the gunship crews and USAF strike pilots to pinpoint the enemy positions underneath the jungle canopy, but once they were fully orientated the air and rocket strikes became more accurate. Ground controller and helicopter scouts began to spot Communist troops moving down tracks to join the battle and those enemy reinforcements were soon being attacked from the air.

On LZ X-Ray, a shuttle of Hueys was bringing in ammunition for the hardpressed Cavalrymen and »

ABOVE: After the first battles in the Ia Drang Valley, the 1st Cavalry operated across Vietnam until 1971, often deploying rapidly by helicopter when a crisis developed. (ICEMANWCS)

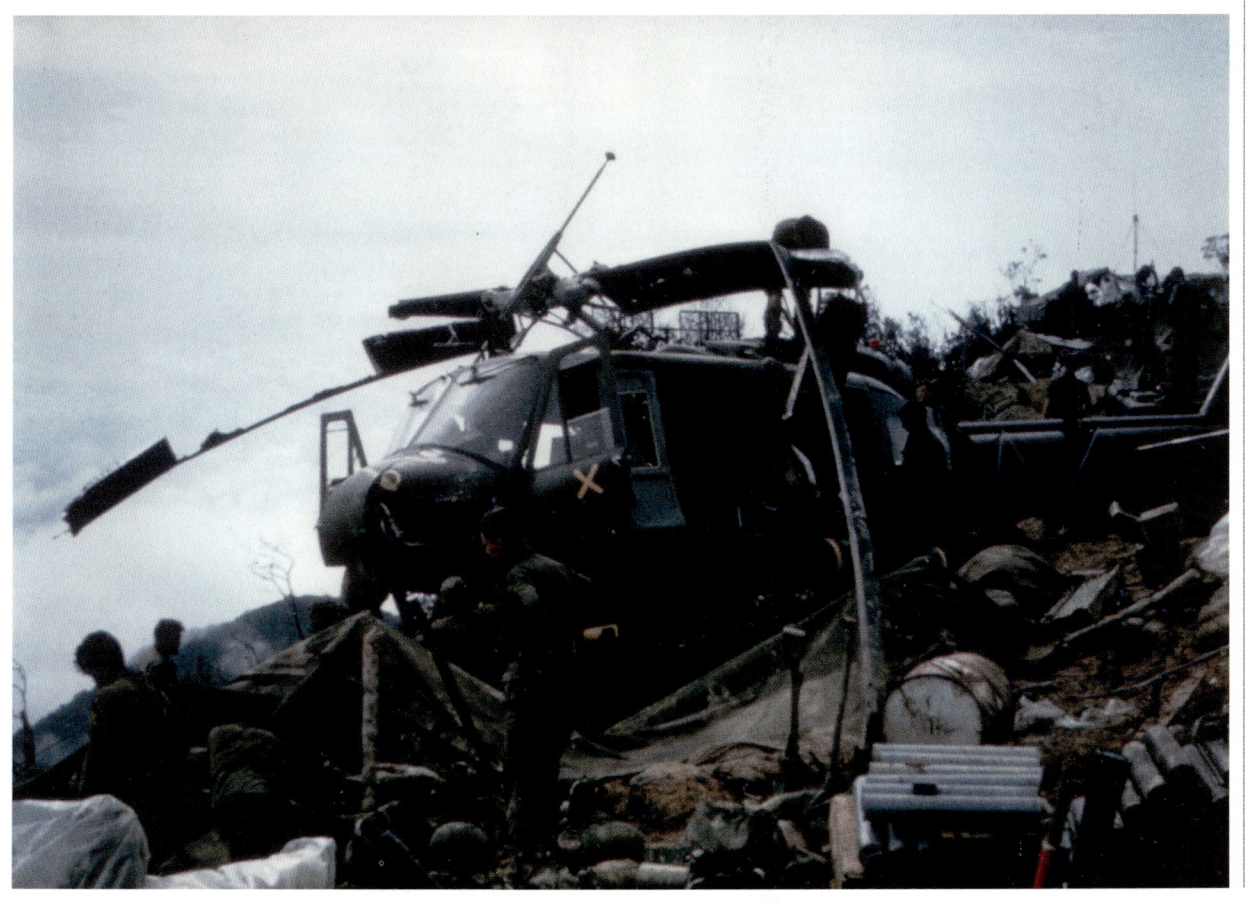

LEFT: The US Army lost nearly 7,000 UH-1 Hueys in Vietnam and more than 3,000 of their crews were killed in action. (ICEMANWCS)

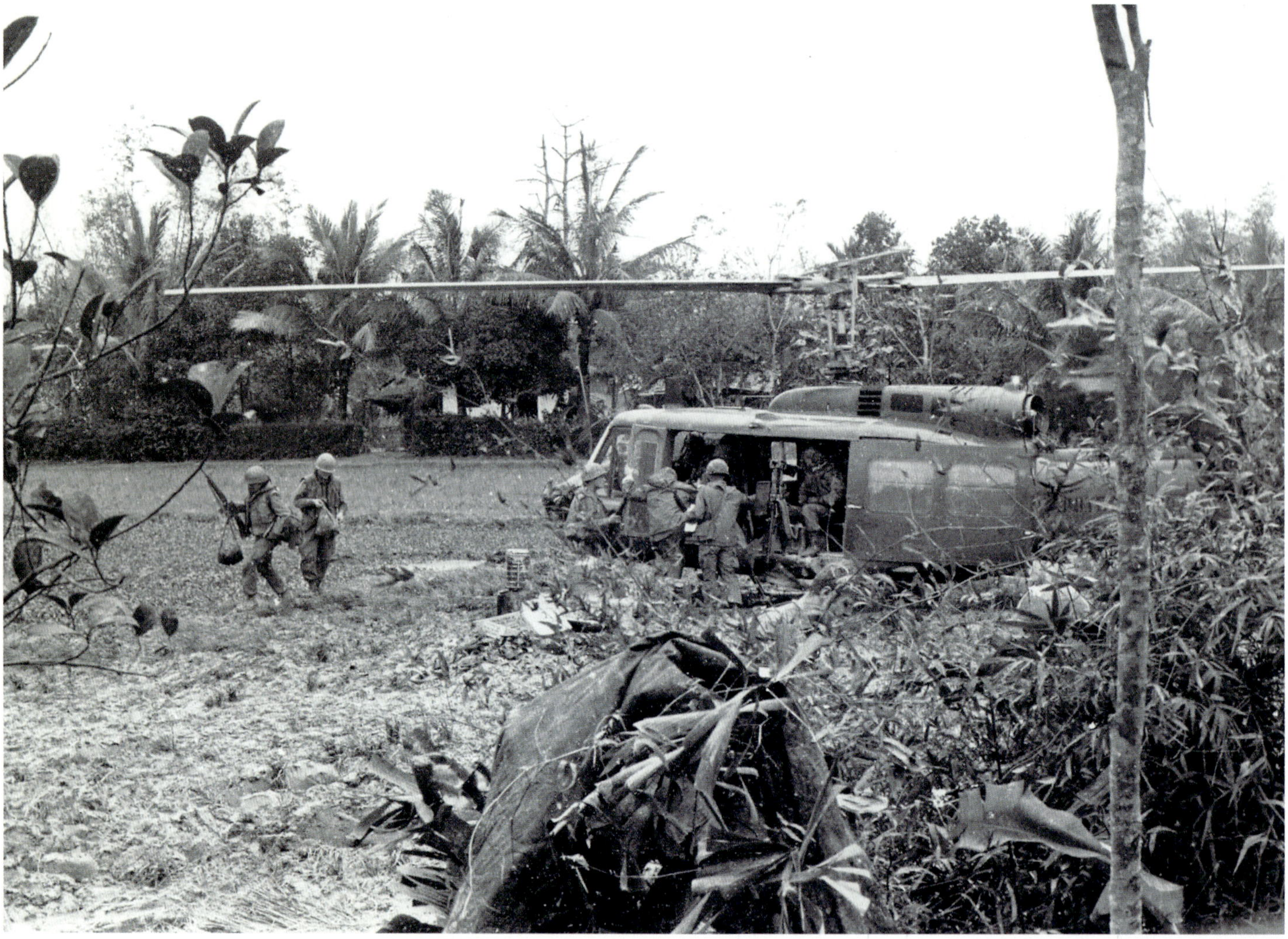

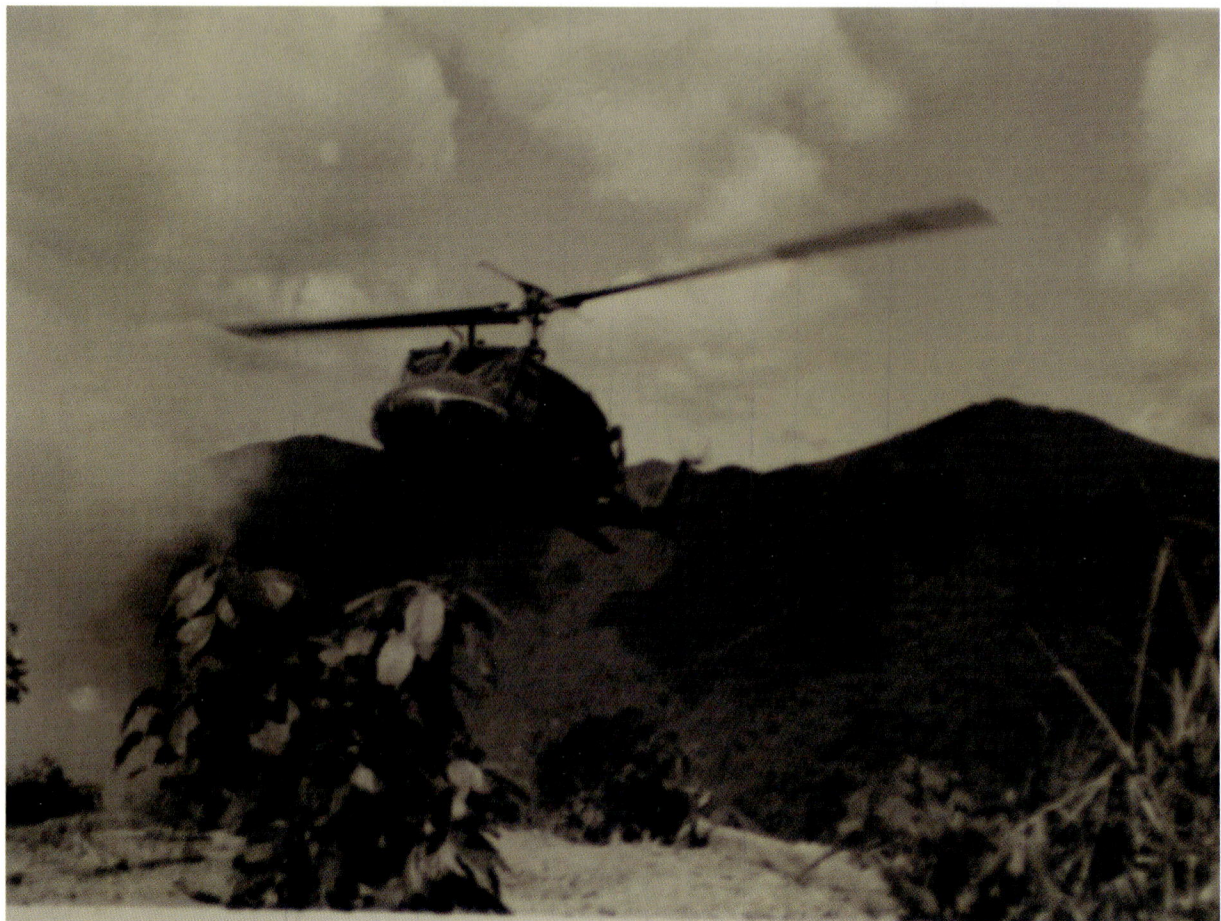

ABOVE: The 1st Cavalry Division's helicopters spearheaded a major operation in 1968 to recapture Hue during the Tet Offensive. (US ARMY)

RIGHT: The 101st Airborne Division was the second divisional-sized airmobile formation in Vietnam. (US ARMY)

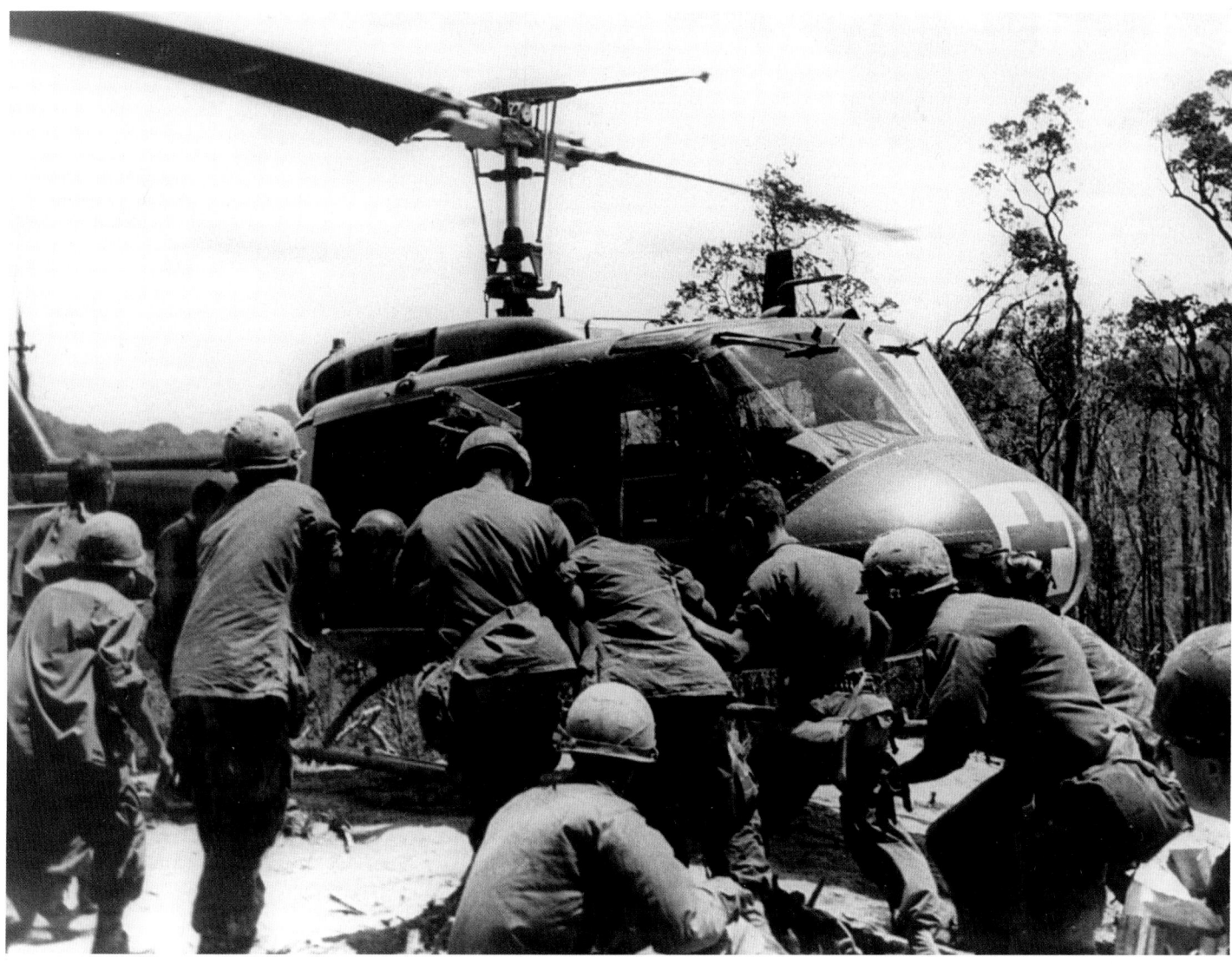

lifting out the wounded. Enemy fire swept the landing zone, damaging several Hueys, but they kept coming. Only two were damaged and unable to lift off again. After the battle was over, they were taken out by Chinook for repair.

Communist machine gunners hit a USAF Douglas A-1E Skyraider making a low-level pass over the battlefield. However, when the enemy troops tried to seize the crashed A-1E, a Huey gunship swept in and destroyed the aircraft.

Night prevented the air support from continuing and during the darkness Colonel Moore and his men had to rely on artillery fire for protection. At dawn the battle resumed again, with more human wave attacks coming in a bid to overrun the US lines. Again, Colonel Moore and his command team choreographed strike jets and Huey gunships to keep the enemy at bay. The Aerial Rocket Artillery Hueys did the heavy lifting during this phase of the battle, putting down barrages of rockets on concentrations of enemy troops moving into attack positions.

Just before 08.00am the battle reached its climax. In a bid to make it impossible for the US to use its airpower and artillery, the Communists surged forward to within grenade-throwing range of the Cavalry lines. US commanders popped smoke on their positions so the gunship pilots could identify the friendly lines, and this allowed them to put down rockets within a few dozen metres of the Cavalrymen. This barrage broke the back of the Communist attack. Later in the morning the Communists pulled back, leaving hundreds of their dead behind. Colonel Moore estimated that more than 600 North Vietnamese soldiers had died in the battle.

Colonel Moore and his men did not share the fate of the Cavalry's predecessors at the Little Big Horn. Gunships, fast jet air and artillery support kept the Communist troops at bay and the Huey Slick pilots maintained a non-stop flow of ammunition heading into LZ X-Ray, as well as bringing out wounded Cavalrymen.

Senior US commanders were full of praise for Colonel Moore and his Cavalrymen. The top US commander in Vietnam, General William Westmoreland, stated: "The ability of the Americans to meet and defeat the best troops the enemy could put on the field of battle was once more demonstrated beyond any doubt, as was the validity of the US Army's airmobile concept."

Moore was less certain, later commenting that: "The peasant soldiers [of North Vietnam] had withstood the terrible high-tech fire storm delivered against them by a superpower and had at least fought the Americans to a draw. By their yardstick, a draw against such a powerful opponent was the equivalent of a victory."

General Westmoreland and the Pentagon immediately requested that more helicopters and air cavalry units be sent to Vietnam. Over the next seven years the number and size of helicopter-equipped US Army units surged. At the peak of the war there were two air assault divisions, the 1st Cavalry Division and 101st Airborne Division (Air Assault), in Vietnam. Each had more than 400 helicopters to allow them to manoeuvre across the battlefield by air. And each US Army division had its own »

ABOVE: As US troops were withdrawn from 1969, the 101st Airborne Division took on an increasing burden of combat operations in Vietnam. (US ARMY)

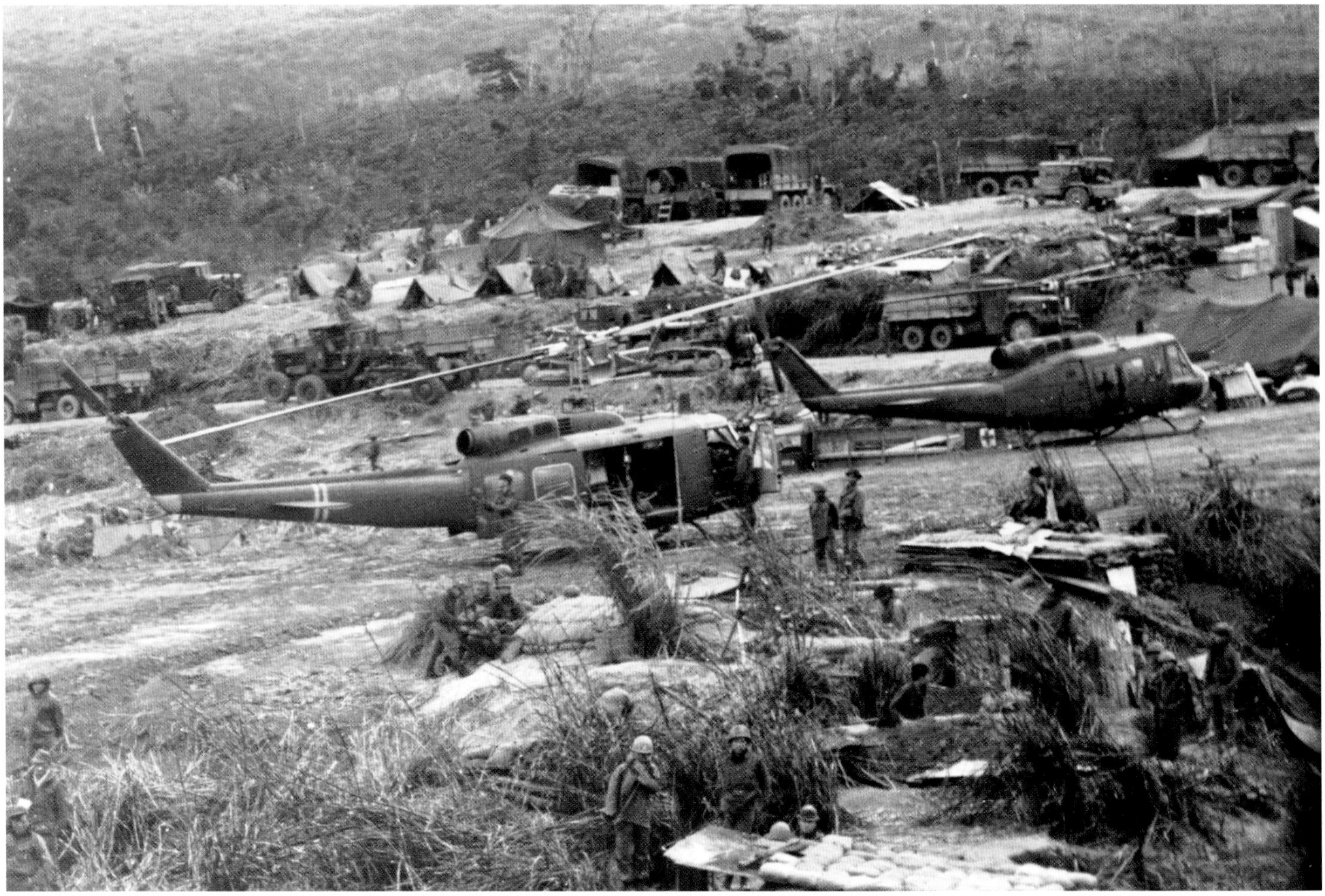

ABOVE: The 101st Airborne Division massed the largest concentration of helicopters ever seen in the Vietnam War to support Operation Lam Son 719, a drive by the South Vietnamese ARVN into Laos in February 1971. (USMC)

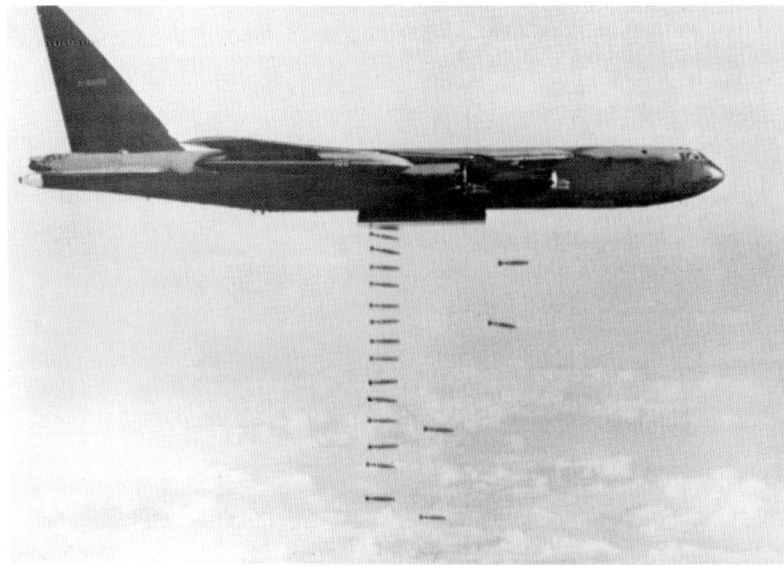

RIGHT: Lavish US firepower, including USAF B-52 'Arc Light' carpet bombing strikes, laid on to support Operation Lam Son 719. (USAF)

air assault battalion to allow it to conduct local airmobility operations around its own area of responsibility. There were scores of independent, or corps level units, including reconnaissance, rocket artillery, troops transport and heavy lift, and these could be assigned to units for specific operations. New or enhanced helicopters were brought into service to boost the capability of the Air Cav.

At the same time, the North Vietnamese learned how to defeat the American's helicopters. They brought bigger and more powerful anti-aircraft guns south and acquired SA-7 Strela shoulder-launched man-portable surface-to-air missiles from the Soviet Union. In 1971, the US and the ARVN launched their largest ever air assault operation into Laos in a bid to cut the famous Communist supply line, known as Ho Chi Minh Trail. This would turn into the toughest test of the Air Cav in the whole of the Vietnam War.

Operation Lam Son 719 was supposed to showcase the US policy of Vietnamization, as the handover of the war to the ARVN was dubbed by the Pentagon. Two ARVN combat divisions, backed by an ARVN armoured brigade, were concentrated in the north of Vietnam, close to Laos, for the offensive across the border. US ground combat troops were not allowed to cross into Laos, so the US military was restricted to providing fast jet air, artillery, helicopters, and logistical support.

To support the ARVN offensive, the US 101st Airborne Division's aviation group and several other US Army and US Marine Corps aviation units were moved to the old USMC base at Khe Sanh and several other forward operating bases during January 1971. This would prove to be the biggest concentration of attack helicopters in the entire Vietnam War.

For the operation, the 101st Airborne's two assault helicopter battalions were reinforced with three other Huey-equipped battalions and the division's reconnaissance unit, the 2nd Squadron, 17th (2nd/17th) Cavalry Regiment, was augmented by four additional troops, or companies, of AH-1G Cobras. A USMC Cobra unit also supported a USMC transport helicopter squadron. In total, some 750 US helicopters were committed to the battle and almost every single machine received some damage »

ABOVE: AH-1G Cobras of the 2nd/17th Cavalry flew deep into Laos to prepare the battlefield for the arrival of the main ARVN infantry units from South Vietnam. (US ARMY)

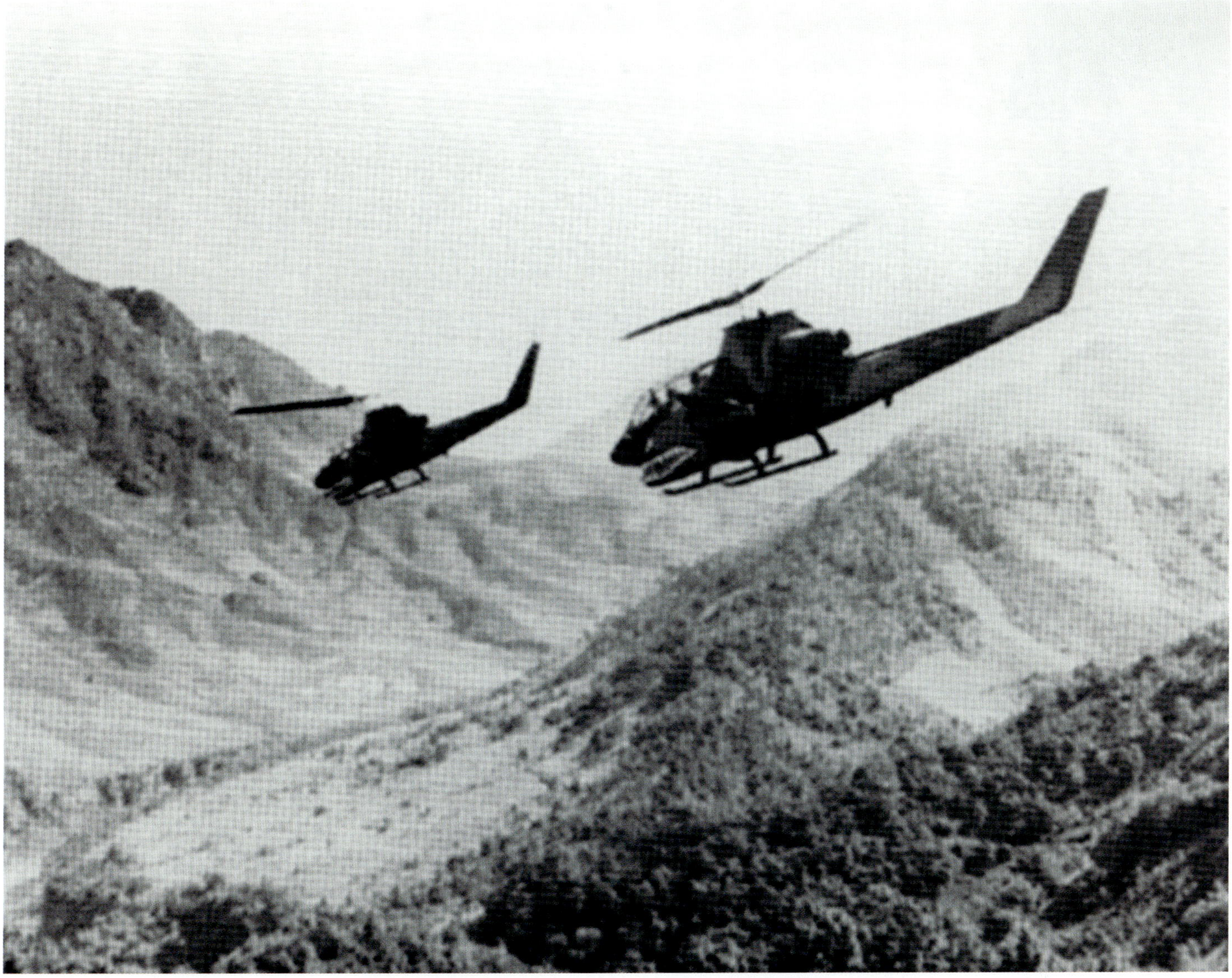

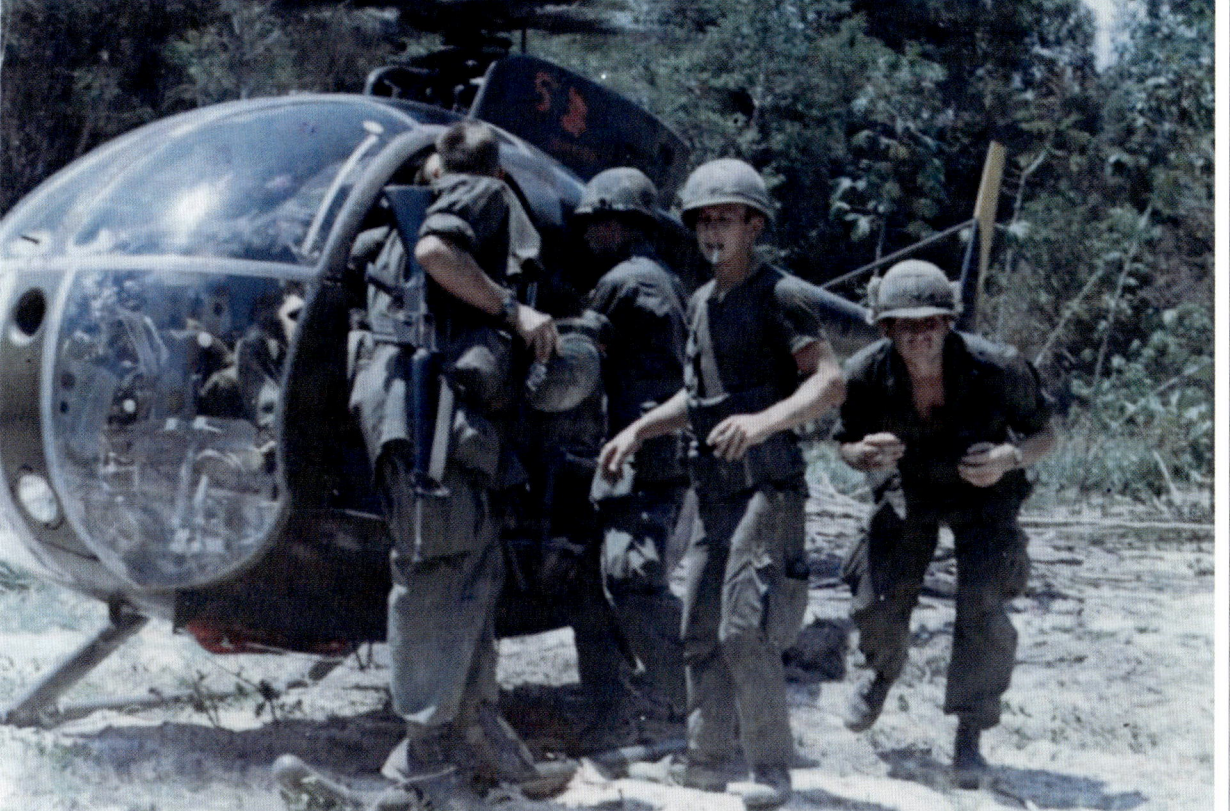

LEFT: By 1971 the OH-6 Loach was the main scout helicopter in US Air Cav units, working in tandem with AH-1G gunships. (US ARMY)

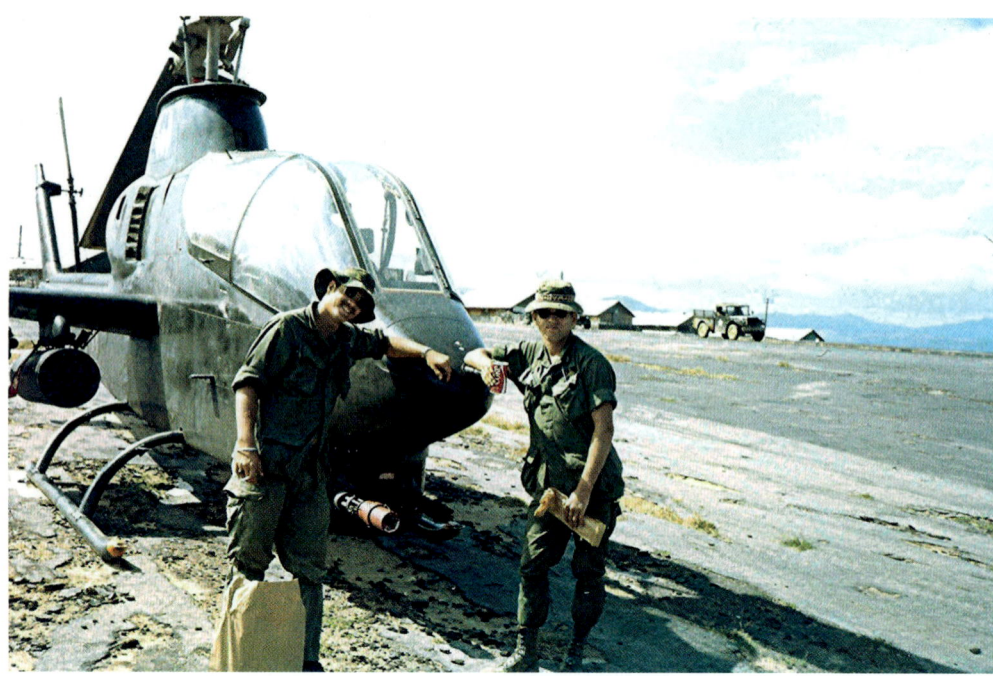

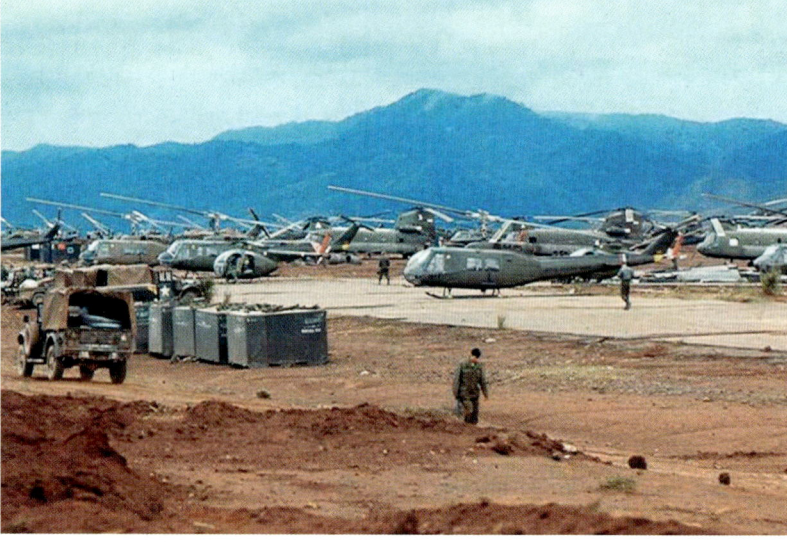

during the operation. The USAF and US Navy promised to fly 200 strike sorties a day over the battlefield, while some 34 US Army heavy artillery pieces were also positioned to fire into Laos.

Unfortunately, the North Vietnamese had received plenty of advance intelligence of the offensive and had positioned some 22,000 regular troops, backed up by between 170 and 200 23mm to 100mm calibre anti-aircraft guns, to try to protect the Ho Chi Minh Trail. The ARVN and its US allies were about to poke a hornet's nest.

The 2nd/17th Cavalry was heavily involved in the offensive. First, it screened the assembly of the attack force in northern Vietnam and then scouted into Laos to look for landing zones for ARVN troops. US and ARVN commanders had set their sights on capturing the town of Tchepone, some 50km inside Laos, which was believed to be surrounded by jungle supply bases and North Vietnamese troop positions. Phase one of Operation Lam Som 719 kicked off on February 8, 1971, with five battalion-sized ARVN air assault operations to capture landing zones to the north and south of Route 9, the main east-west road to Tchepone. These were soon reinforced by artillery airlifted by Chinooks and, in effect, became advanced fire bases. As this was underway an ARVN tank column pushed along Route 9.

US Hueys, escorted by Cobras, successfully landed the first wave of ARVN troops on their objectives but the American helicopters were soon coming under sustained anti-aircraft fire. North Vietnamese troops quickly organised counter-attacks and

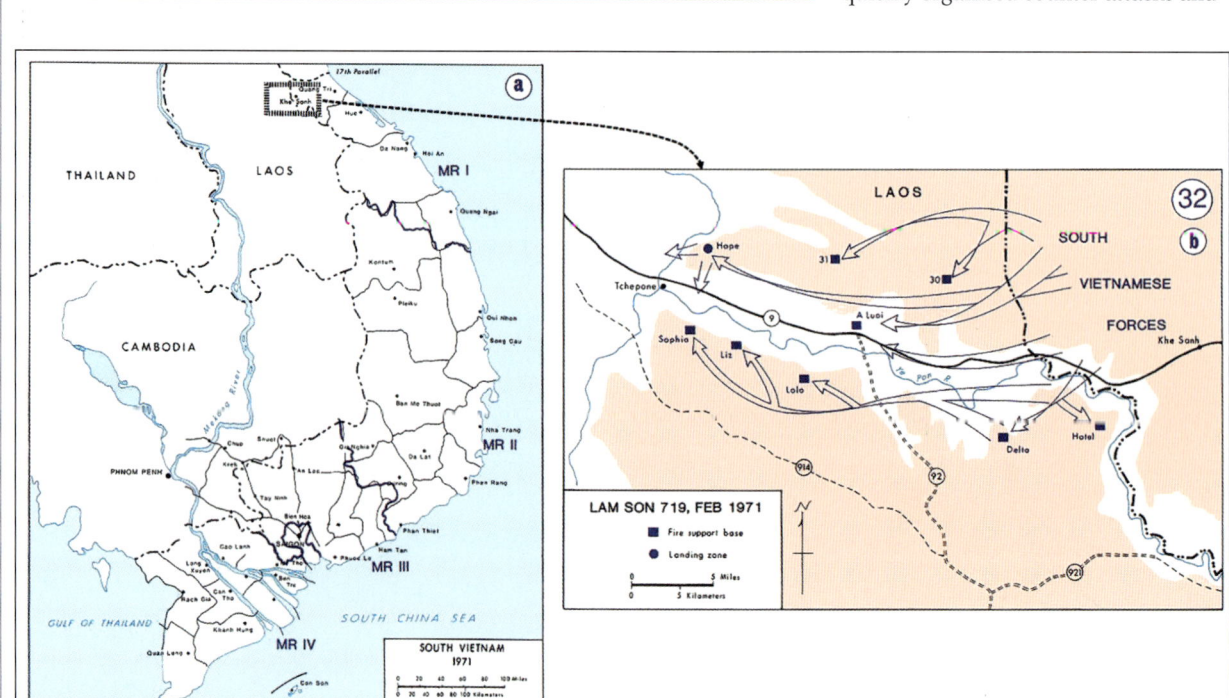

LAM SON 719, FEB 1971
■ Fire support base
● Landing zone
0   5 Miles
0   5 Kilometers

SOUTH VIETNAM 1971

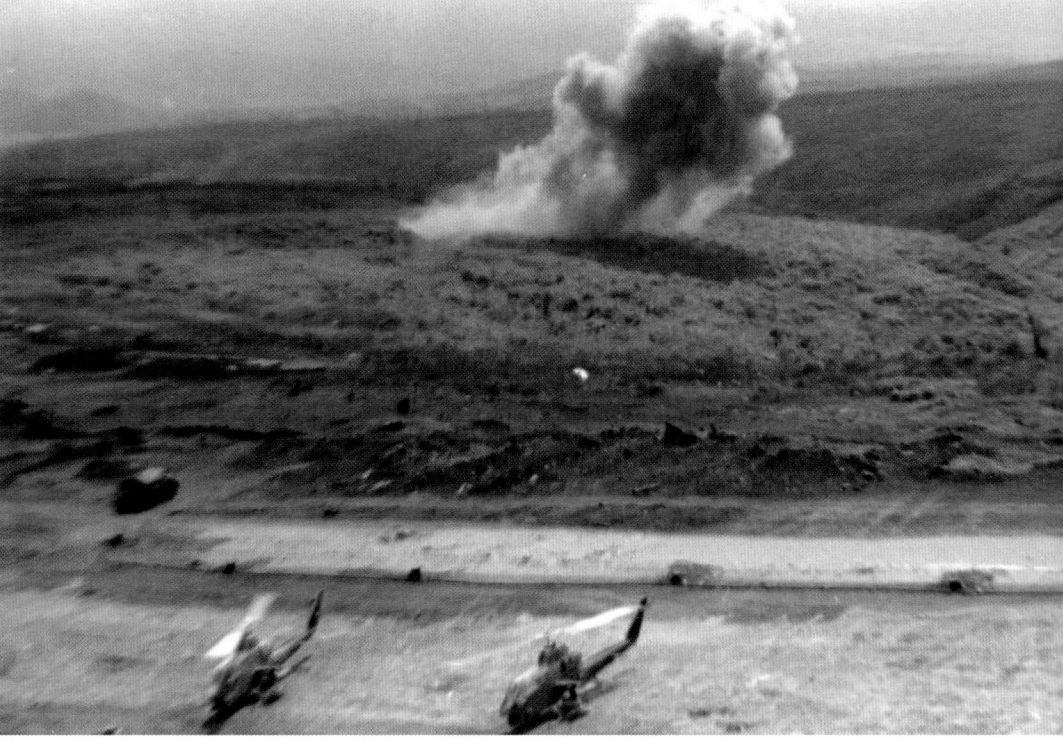

US Army and USMC Major Aviation Units Operation Lam Son 719/Dewey Canyon, January-March 1971

Headquarters US XXIV Corps

101st Combat Aviation Group

101st Aviation Battalion (Assault Helicopter) (60 x UH-1DH, 12 x AH-1G)

158th Aviation Battalion (Assault Helicopter) (60x UH-1D/H)
- D Company, 227th Aerial Weapons Battalion (12 x AH-1G)

159th Aviation Support Helicopter Battalion (36 x CH-47, 4 x CH-54)

4th Battalion, 77th Field Artillery (Aerial Rocket Artillery) (36 x AH-1G)
- B Battery, 2nd Battalion, 20th Aerial Rocket Artillery Regiment (12 x AH-1G)

14th Aviation Battalion
- 71st Assault Helicopter Company (20 x UH-1D/H, 6 x UH-2C gunship)
- 116th Assault Helicopter Company (20 x UH-1D/H, 6 x UH-2C gunship)
- 174th Assault Helicopter Company (20 x UH-1D/H, 6 x UH-2C gunship)
- 132nd Aviation Support Helicopter Company (12 x CH-47)

223rd Aviation Battalion
- 48th Assault Helicopter Company (UH-1D/H, 4 x AH-1G)
- 173rd Assault Helicopter Company (UH-1D/H, 4 x AH-1G)
- 282nd Assault Helicopter Company (20 x UH-1D/H, 12 x UH-2B/C gunship)
- 238th Aerial Weapons Company (12 x AH-1G)

2nd Squadron, 17th Air Cavalry
- A Troop, 2nd Squadron, 17th Cavalry Regiment (9 x AH-1G, 10 x OH-6)
- B Troop, 2nd Squadron, 17th Cavalry Regiment (9 x AH-1G, 10 x OH-6)
- C Troop, 2nd Squadron, 17th Cavalry Regiment (9 x AH-1G, 10 x OH-6)

Attached units for Op Lam Son 719
- 235th Aerial Weapons Company (24 x AH-1G)
- B Troop, 7th Squadron, 1st Cavalry Regiment (9 x AH-1G, 10 x OH-6)
- C Troop, 7th Squadron, 17th Cavalry Regiment (9 x AH-1G, 10 x OH-6)
- D Troop, 3rd Squadron, 5th Cavalry Regiment (9 x AH-1G, 10 x OH-6)
- D Company, 158th Aviation Battalion (Assault Helicopter) (12 x AH-1G)

67th Medical Group
- 237th Medial Detachment (UH-1D/H)
- 571st Medical Detachment (UH-1D/H)

1st Marine Air Wing, USMC
- Marine Heavy Helicopter Squadron 463 (20 x CH-53D)
- Marine Light Helicopter Squadron 367 (14 x AH-1G)

operation involved 120 US Hueys delivering two ARVN battalions to a landing zone 65km inside Laos. A US Army pilot said this objective was the "most hostile air defence environment encountered in the entire war". Good tactics and gunship support from escort Cobras and fast air meant only one Huey was lost in the initial insertion operation. Sustaining the ARVN troops in these isolated bases proved more problematic, as the

Communists started to mass anti-aircraft guns on the flight routes around the fire bases.

The extraction of the ARVN troops was now ordered and the US helicopter force was mustered to lift out the South Vietnamese. The last battalion was extracted on March 25, as Communist troops were overrunning its position. US Hueys made repeated runs, covered by Cobras, to bring out the last troops. »

ABOVE: Communist artillery struck back at forward operating bases that housed US Army and USMC helicopters, interrupting re-supply flights during Operation Lam Son 719. (USMC)

BELOW: Thousands of South Vietnamese ARVN troops were flown into Laos on US Army Hueys. (USMC)

effectively penned the ARVN troops inside their positions. In an ominous development, the Communists brought up PT-76 light tanks and managed to overrun one of the AVRN fire bases. US helicopters flew mission after mission to support the ARVN troops, but they were facing unrelenting fire from well-positioned anti-aircraft guns. In one day alone, 10 US helicopters were shot down. One US helicopter pilot commented after the battle, "In Vietnam you have to hunt the enemy. But in Laos man, they hunt you."

To break the stalemate, US command decided to pull out some of the hard-pressed troops and re-insert them in new landing zones on high ground overlooking Tchepone. USAF Boeing B-52 Stratofortresses were brought in between March 3 and 6 to prep the landing zones ahead of the insertion. The most westerly

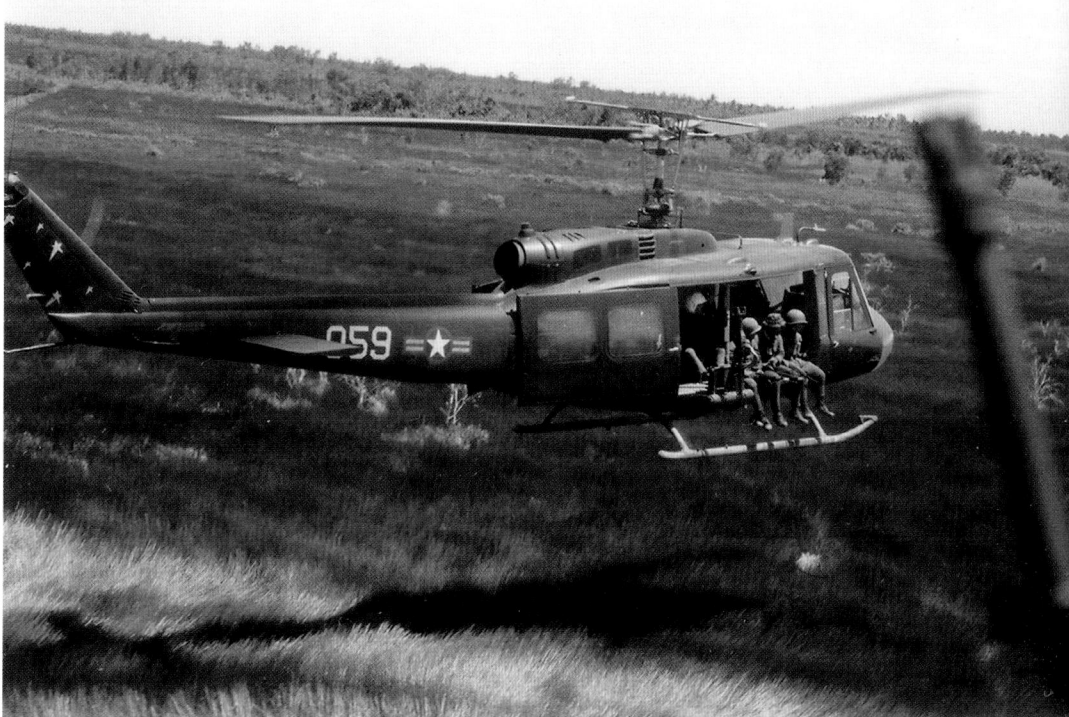

RIGHT: USMC CH-53D Sea Stallions joined the aerial re-supply effort to keep ARVN units in Laos fighting. (USMC)

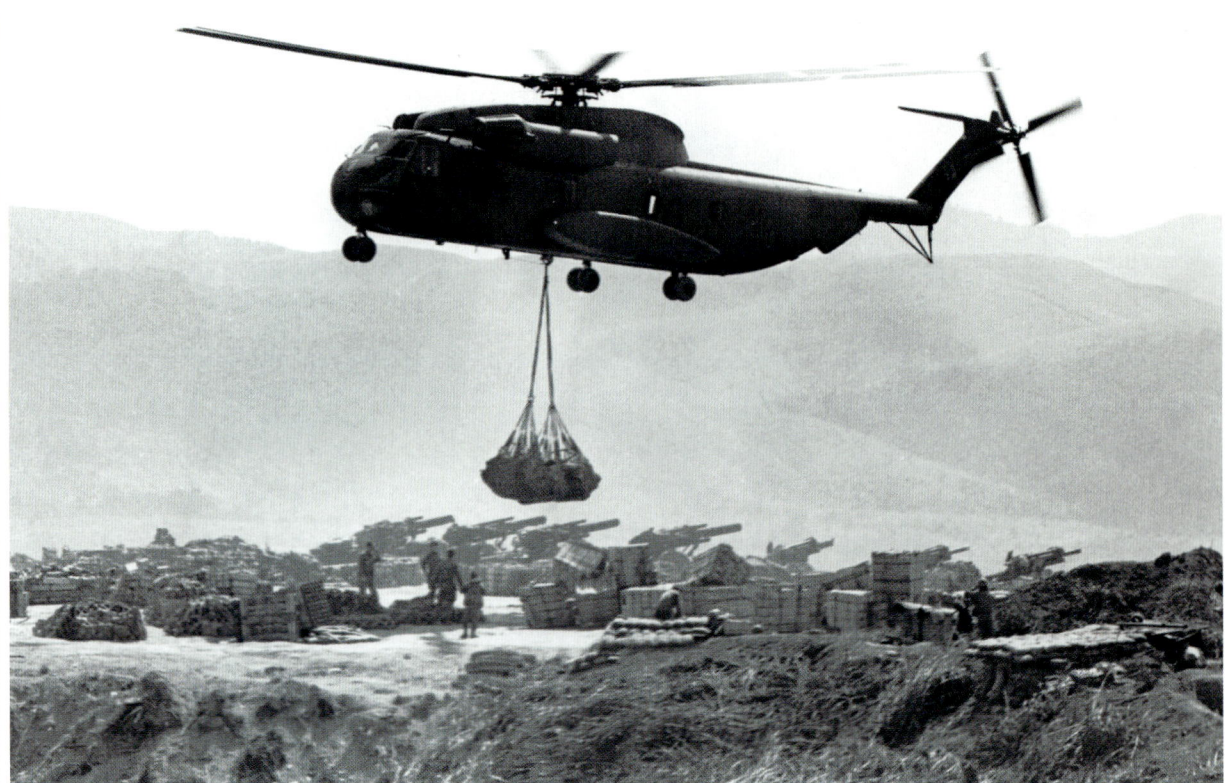

BELOW LEFT: After its success in Vietnam, the US Army moved to fit the TOW missile to its AH-1 Cobras. (USAF)

BELOW RIGHT: TOW-equipped UH-1 played an important role in defeating the 1972 Communist Spring offensive. (US ARMY)

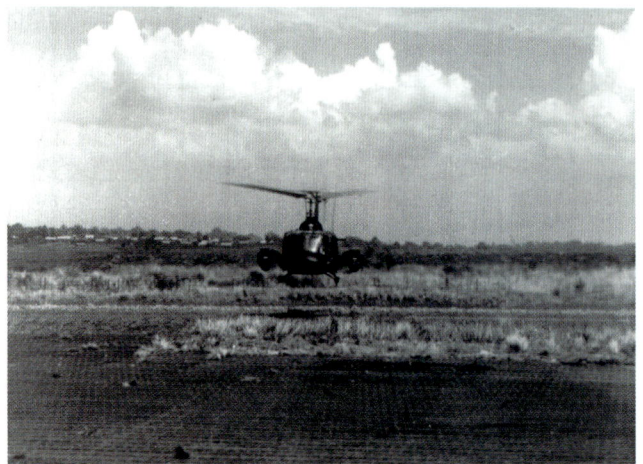

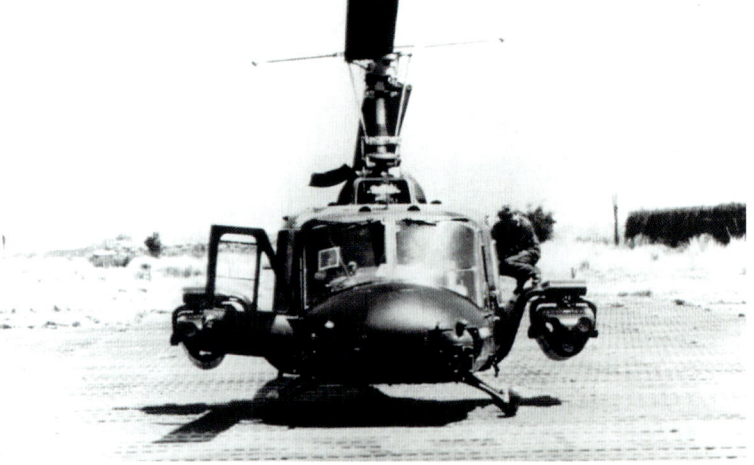

RIGHT: The first-ever tanks to be knocked out by helicopter-launched wire-guided anti-tank missiles were destroyed by the TOW-equipped UH-1s in 1972. (US ARMY)

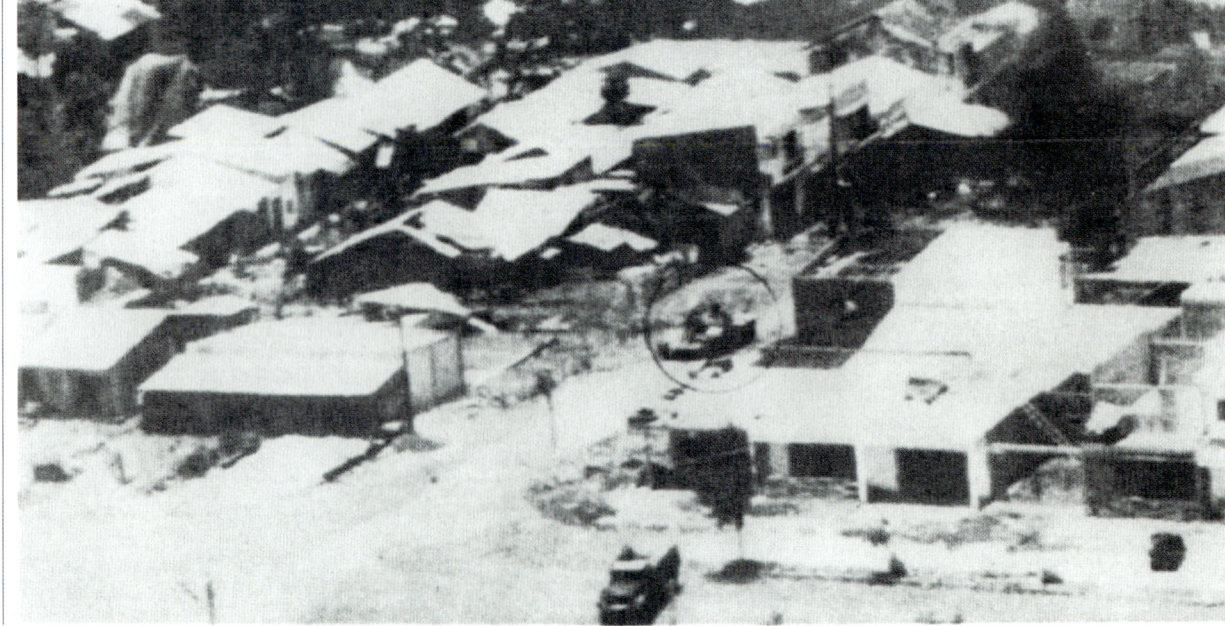

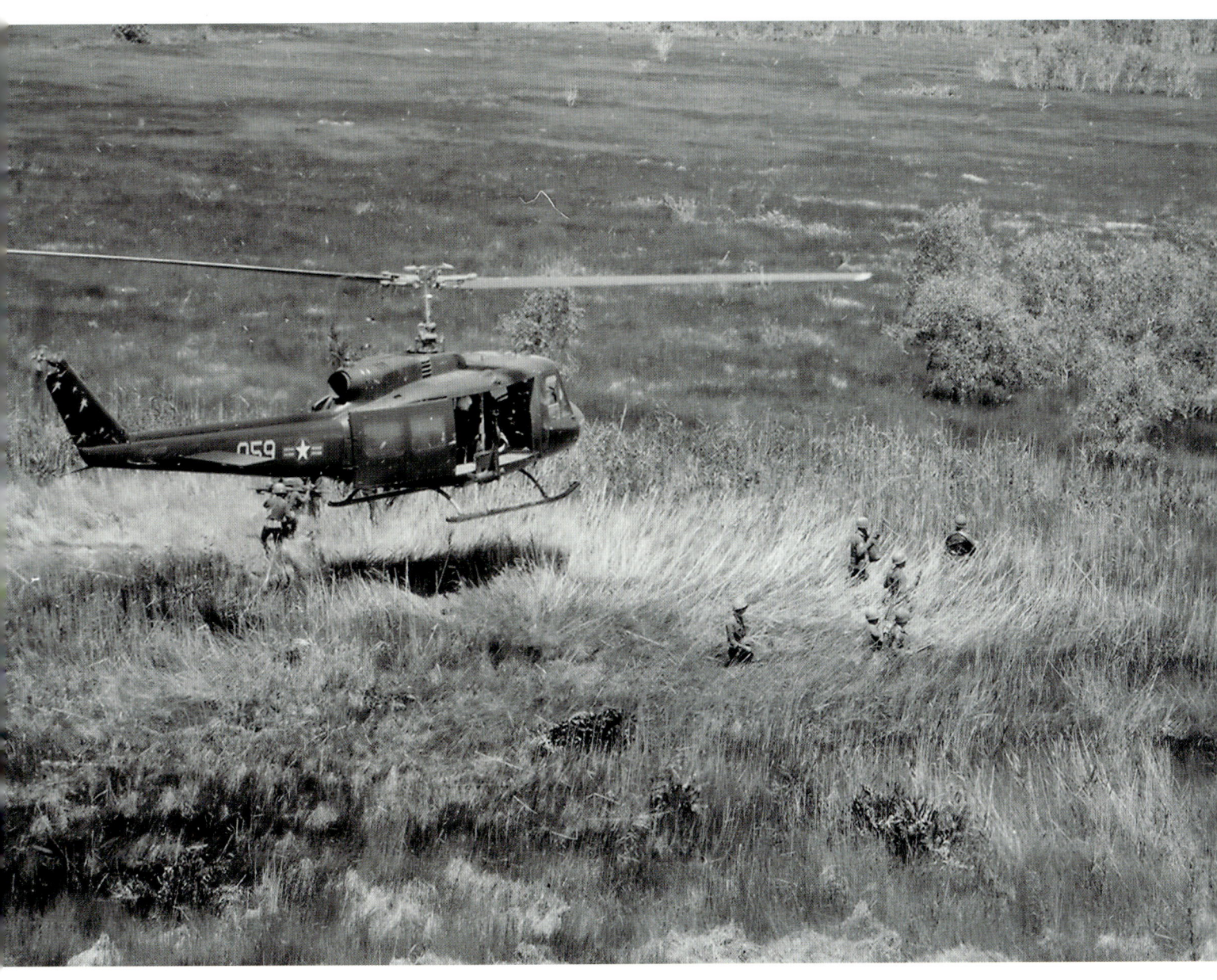

Lam Son 719 was hailed a major success, having destroyed or captured 20,000 tons of ammunitions, 12,000 tons of rice, 106 tanks, 1,500 crew-served weapons, 76 artillery pieces and 405 trucks. ARVN losses were heavy with more than 1,700 of its troops being killed and 6,600 wounded. The US lost 215, with 1,148 wounded, and 38 missing in action.

Helicopters were hit particularly hard, with more than 80 being lost in action, including 50 Hueys and 20 AH-1Gs shot down in Laos. Some 72 helicopter aircrew members were killed, 59 wounded and 11 reported missing. Another 26 helicopters were lost in South Vietnam. Almost every US helicopter took battle damage, with 618 being hit. The US helicopter casualties prompted criticism, but US commanders stressed that when compared to the number of sorties flown and the heavy defences encountered, they were not unbearable. In total, US Army helicopters flew 164,422 sorties during the 67 days of Operation Lam Som 719,

including 34,173 gunship and 17,887 air cavalry sorties.

Operation Lam Som 719 was clearly a stand-up conventional battle, rather than a counter-insurgency fight that the US military was used to in South Vietnam. US air mobile operations had come a long way from the battle in the Ia Drang Valley in 1965 in terms of scale, complexity, and ambition. The appearance of North Vietnamese tanks was a new development, and the US Army was very concerned that its attack helicopters did not have the anti-armour weapons to take them on.

The light PT-76s that appeared during Operation Lam Som 719 were eventually neutralised by a combination of artillery, airstrikes and well-aimed rockets from gunships, but US Army commanders realised it was only a matter of time before heavier Communist armour appeared. A crash programme was launched to mount the wire-guided BGM-71 TOW missile on a UH-1B as an interim measure until the much-vaunted AH-56 Cheyenne entered service. The first of

these helicopters arrived in Vietnam in early 1972, just in time to be used in action to halt the Communist Spring Offensive. 1st Combat Aerial TOW Team, which was code named Hawk's Claw, was called into action for the first time on May 2 to engage four US-made M-41s that had been pressed into service by Communist troops. It successfully knocked them out near An Loc. Twelve days later the Hawk's Claw helicopters got the chance to go into action against Soviet-supplied tanks attacking Kontum. Communist infantry, backed by PT-76 light tanks and T-54 main battle tanks, tried to overrun the city but the attack faltered after the missile-armed helicopters picked off the advancing tanks.

The Huey-TOW combination proved very effective over the next month in several other engagements. Tank killing by helicopter had been shown to work. The US Army decided to modify its AH-1 Cobras to fire the TOW missile. The late and over budget AH-56 Cheyenne was cancelled.

Moscow's First Helicopter War

The Soviet Invasion of Afghanistan 1979-1989

For a decade Soviet troops fought a brutal war against Afghan insurgents in a doomed bid to prop up the pro-Moscow government in Kabul. This war saw the Soviets for the first time make extensive use of helicopters in combat and it also saw the combat debut of the Mil Mi-24 attack helicopter.

The first phase unfolded in December 1979 with Russian airborne troops and Spetsnaz, or special force, units staging a coup d'main (strategic raid or strike) in the Afghan capital and other provincial cities to seize the centres of government and military power and install local leaders loyal to Moscow. The head of the Afghan government died as Soviet Spetsnaz stormed the presidential palace.

Over the next two years resistance to the new regime and the Soviet presence grew in the countryside, with local insurgents, known as the Mujahideen, attacking isolated garrisons, and ambushing Soviet supply convoys.

By 1982, the Soviet high command was determined put down the uprising and set in train a series of multi-division operations to surround and then sweep into Mujahideen strong holds. The biggest and most ambitious of these were launched into the Panjshir Valley, which the insurgents used as a base to attack the main supply route from Kabul back to the Soviet border.

More than 100 Soviet helicopters, including Mil Mi-8 troop transports, Mi-6 heavy lift helicopters and Mi-24 gunships, were massed for the operation that kicked off with insertion of airborne battalions into the valley, behind the Mujahideen defence lines. Soviet tanks and motorised infantry units pushed up the main roads into the valley, trapping the Mujahideen. Fire support from the Mi-24s and the newly arrived Sukhoi Su-25 Rook ground attack jets prevented the insurgents neutralising the airborne forces' bridgeheads. Rather than risk destruction, the Mujahideen slipped away into the mountains to fight another day. Throughout the rest of the year, small detachments of Soviet troops were inserted by helicopter across the mountains to conduct search and destroy sweeps for isolated insurgent bands.

The success of the Soviet helicopters in these Panjshir battles prompted the expansion of their use elsewhere in

RIGHT: The Mi-24 received its baptism of fire in Afghanistan in 1980. (US DOD)

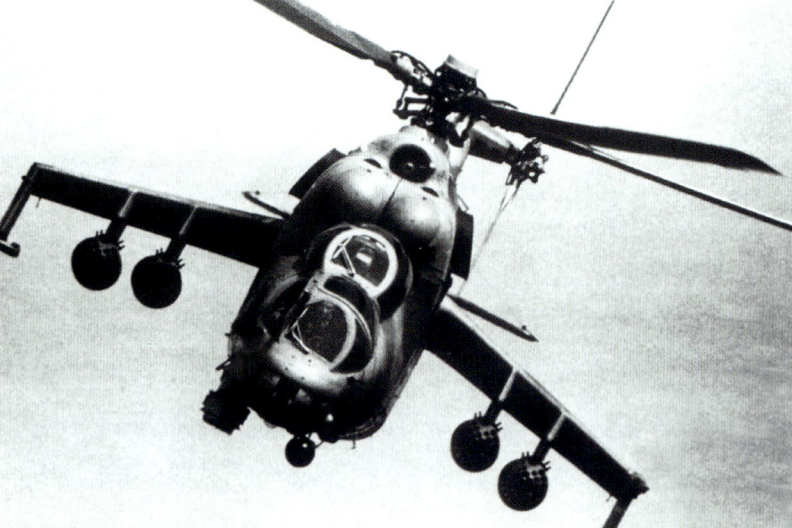

RIGHT: Soviet Spetsnaz units spearheaded air assault operations into insurgent held territory. (MIKHAIL EVSTAFIEV)

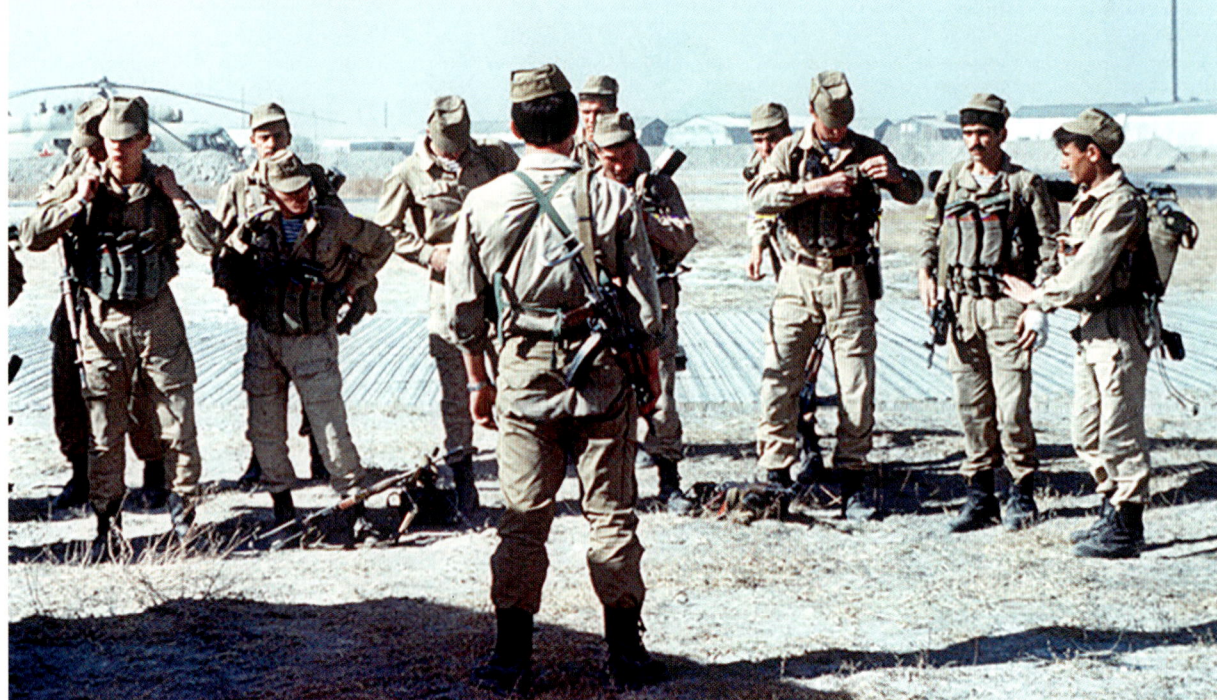

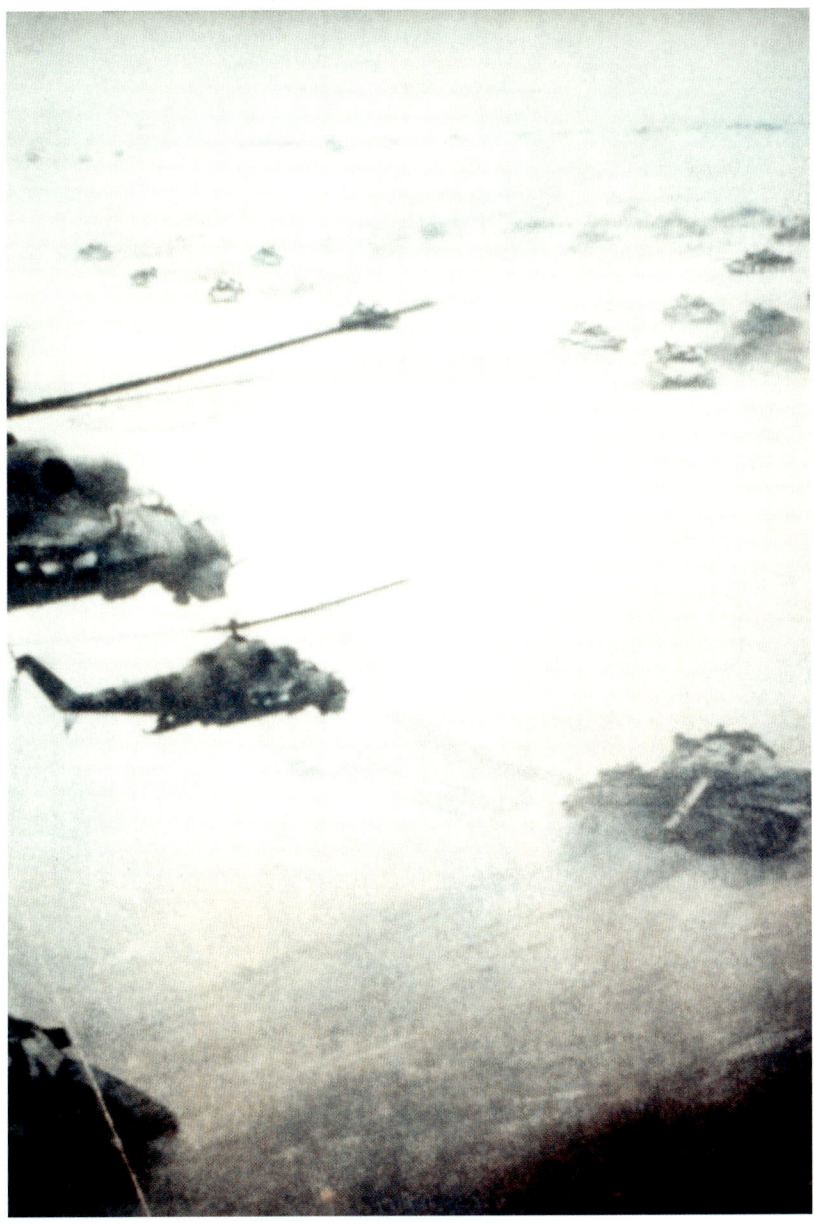

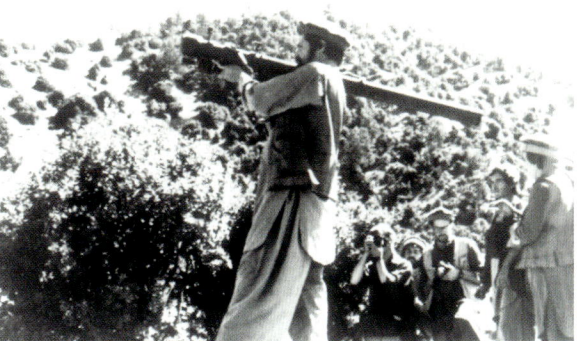

ABOVE: US-supplied man-portable surface-to-air missiles arrived in Afghanistan from 1986 to challenge Soviet air supremacy. (US DOD)

LEFT: Mi-24s were much in demand flying top cover for Soviet military convoys around Afghanistan. (US DOD)

evacuate casualties. Not surprisingly, the Mujahideen's backers in Washington DC, London and Islamabad were keen to neutralise the ability of the Soviet helicopters to operate at will. From 1986 onwards, British-made Blowpipe and US-made Stinger shoulder-launched surface-to-air missiles, known as manpads, were supplied to the Mujahideen, via Pakistan.

In the 1980s these weapons were credited with shooting down hundreds of Soviet helicopters and aircraft. Subsequent analysis has indicated just under 100 missiles actually found their mark, with around half of those losses being helicopters. As soon as the manpads appeared the Soviets started fitting decoy flares to their helicopters and using more aggressive tactics to dodge the missiles. The Mujahideen ended up firing several hundred missiles at Soviet helicopters, but they were such poor shots the vast majority of them missed.

When the last Soviet combat troops left Afghanistan in February 1989 the world was on the brink of a major shock. By the end of the year the Berlin Wall had fallen and within two years the Soviet Union had collapsed. The successor Russian army, however, would never go to war again without the support of large numbers of helicopter gunships.

BELOW: In the 21st century the US-formed Afghan Air Force operated dozens of Mi-35s and they were flown by several pilots who had originally served in the Soviet-era Afghan air arm.
(US DOD/COMBAT CAMERA)

Afghanistan. Soviet garrisons were set up outside each major city and each was provided with its own helicopter regiment, comprising a mixed force of Mi-6s, Mi-8/17s and Mi-24s that were able support search and destroy operations in the countryside. At its peak, between 1985 and 1988, the Soviet helicopter force boasted 140 Mi-24, 105 Mi-8/17s and 40 Mi-6s.

Helicopter-borne assault operations were routinely launched across Afghanistan as the Soviets tried to keep a lid on the growing insurgency. Helicopter gunships also provided top cover for truck convoys delivering supplies to remote garrisons. By the mid-1980s, the Soviets had become experts at positioning fuel supplies in their small forward operating bases so helicopter crews could drop down to refuel and ensure they had the endurance to stay on station, far from their home bases.

Soviet helicopter gunship pilots gained a reputation for daredevil flying in the extreme climate.

They were renowned for their low-level passes to put rockets and cannon fire down on Mujahideen positions. The presence of Mi-24s was usually enough to suppress insurgent fire to allow Mi-8/17s to get in to a landing zone to delivery vital supplies or

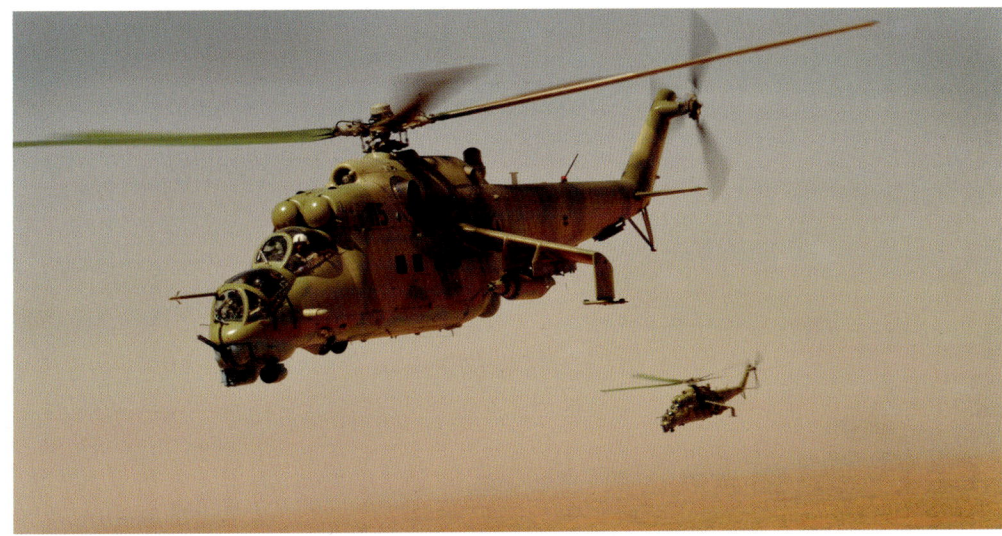

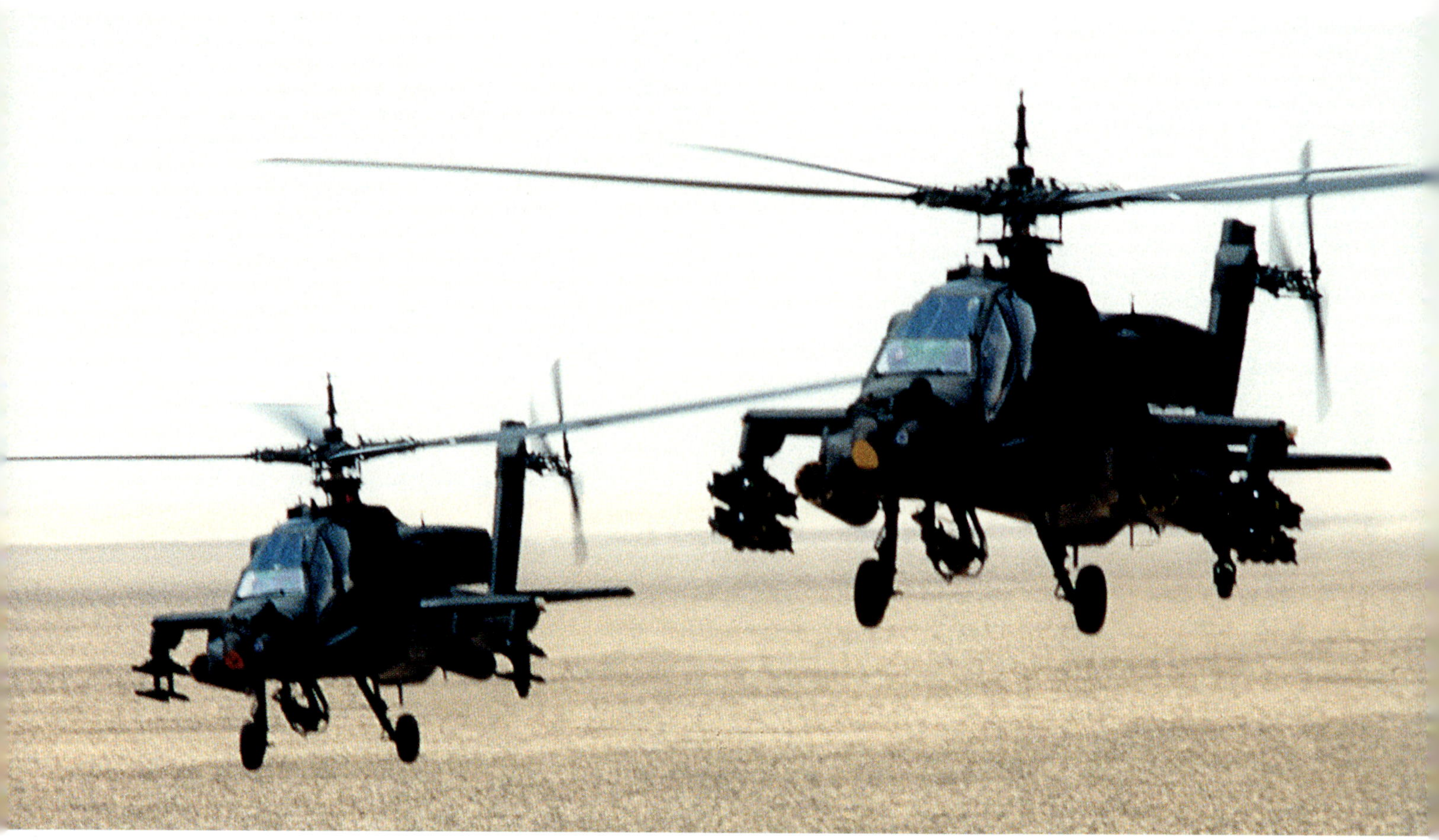

Apache Dawn

US Army Aviation during the 1991 Gulf War

ABOVE: A US Army AH-64A Apache on the prowl over the Iraqi desert. (US DOD/COMBAT CAMERA)

"There were just row after row of AH-64A Apaches – they stretched all along the ramp at Dharhan Air Base. I didn't know we had that many helicopters!" So said a US Army officer in August 1990.

On August 8, 1990, a constant stream of US Air Force Lockheed C-5 Galaxy transport aircraft started arriving at the Saudi Arabian air base to deliver hundreds of US Army helicopters. By the start of the US-led offensive to recapture Kuwait in January 1991 more than 1,600 US Army helicopters were operating in support of coalition units throughout the Middle East.

Ever since the Vietnam War, the US Army had invested heavily in rotary wing hardware and developed a concept of operations – AirLand Battle – to integrate helicopters closely with ground units. AirLand Battle called for units, from battalions

RIGHT: General Norman Schwarzkopf devised the US offensive that devastated the Iraqi army occupying Kuwait. (US DOD/COMBAT CAMERA)

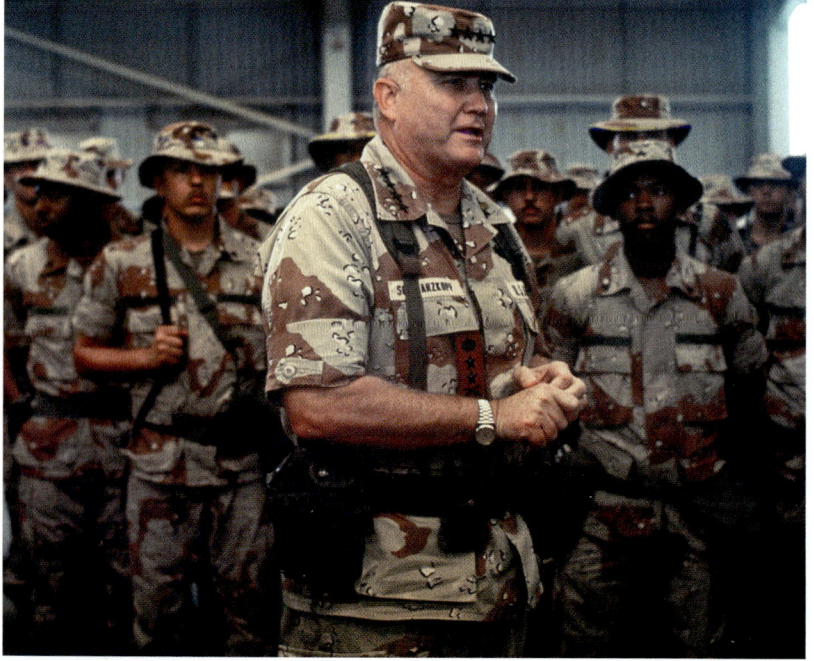

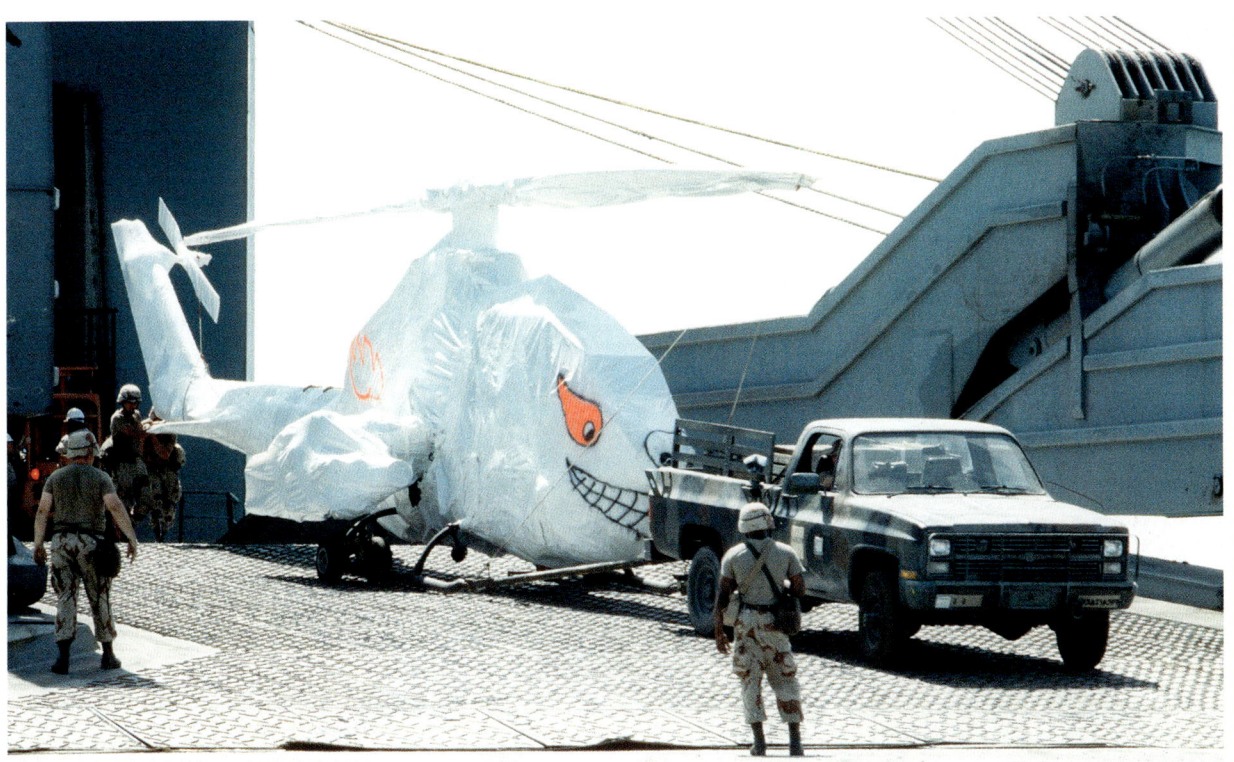

up to army corps, to penetrate deep into the enemy's rear to surround and eventually destroy their main force. The concept envisaged helicopters being used to lift troops behind enemy lines, move supplies forward to advancing ground units and destroy enemy armour with surprise missile attacks. Terrain, night, or severe weather would not provide the enemy with shelter or safe haven because of the widespread use of night vision equipment, advanced radar sensors and electronic surveillance.

By 1990 each US Army division-sized formation had been provided with a combat aviation brigade equipped with attack, troop and cargo transport helicopters to enable it to put AirLand Battle into practice. Divisions also had a cavalry squadron for reconnaissance, which combined scouts equipped with both armoured vehicles and helicopters. Each corps headquarters was provided with its own independent aviation brigades, which included two battalions of Apache, to give corps commanders the ability to strike deep behind the frontline at the enemy's second echelon forces. The US Army also had a unique airmobile unit, the 101st Airborne Division (Air Assault), which was trained and equipped to conduct strategic helicopter operations far behind enemy lines.

Between August and October 1990, seven aviation brigades and numerous small support helicopter units were deployed to Saudi Arabia under the command of the US Army's XVIII Airborne Corps. First to arrive on the USAF C-5s were the helicopters of the 160th Special Operations Aviation Regiment, but they were only a down payment. In the early days of the Gulf crisis, after the Iraqi invasion of Kuwait, US Army commanders were worried that Saddam Hussein would order his tank division to head south to seize Saudi Arabia's oil fields. Top priority was therefore given to getting anti-armour forces to Saudi Arabia. So, the aviation package of the US Army's 82nd Airborne Division's ready brigade was made double its usual size for its new mission to Saudi Arabia. It landed at Dhahran on August 8 with 15 AH-64A, 15 Sikorsky UH-60 Blackhawk utility helicopters and eight Bell OH-58C/D scout helicopters. Within three weeks the remainder of the 82nd Airborne's aviation brigade was on the ground in Saudi Arabia's vulnerable eastern province with more than 100 helicopters. They were soon flying patrols up to the Kuwaiti border to watch for any incursions by Iraqi troops.

Beginning on August 16, advanced elements of the 101st Airborne arrived in Saudi Arabia, reinforced by ➤➤

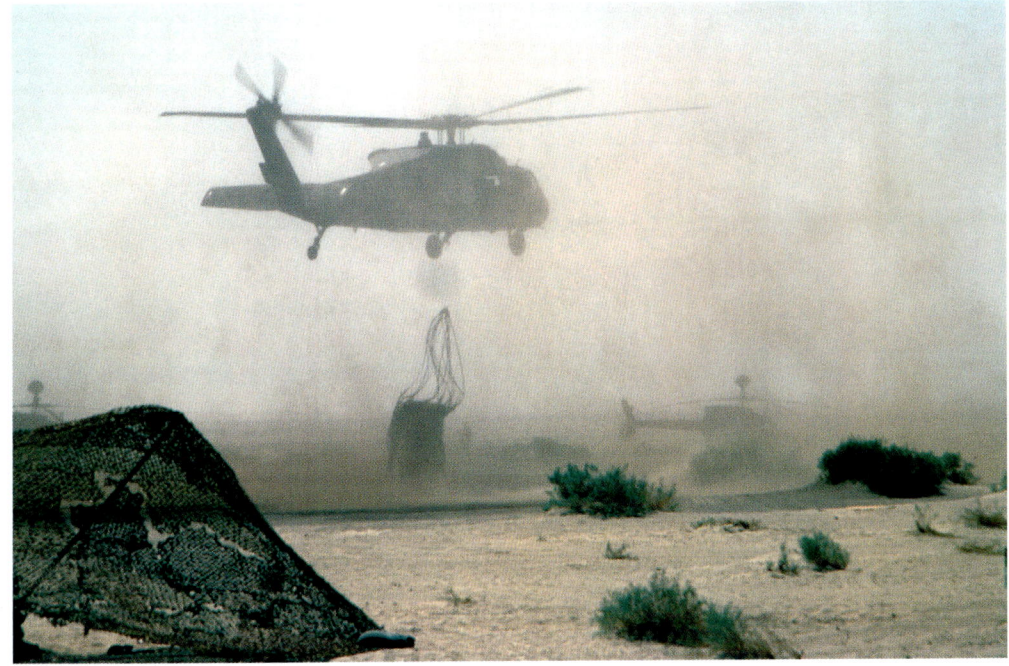

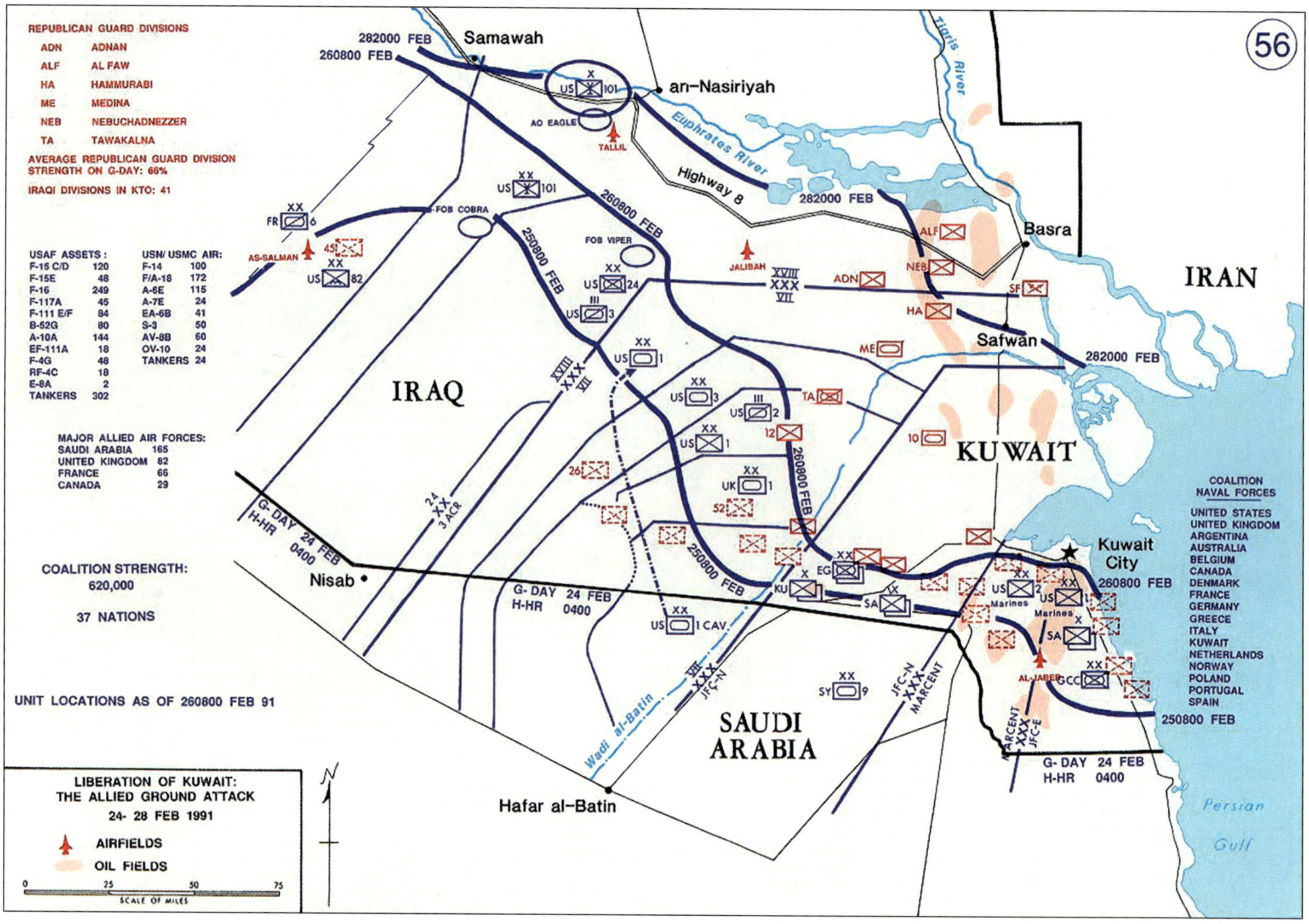

Map

56

REPUBLICAN GUARD DIVISIONS
ADN ADNAN
ALF AL FAW
HA HAMMURABI
ME MEDINA
NEB NEBUCHADNEZZER
TA TAWAKALNA
AVERAGE REPUBLICAN GUARD DIVISION
STRENGTH ON G-DAY: 66%
IRAQI DIVISIONS IN KTO: 41

USAF ASSETS:		USN/ USMC AIR:	
F-15 C/D	120	F-14	100
F-15E	48	F/A-18	172
F-16	249	A-6E	115
F-117A	45	A-7E	24
F-111 E/F	84	EA-6B	41
B-52G	80	S-3	50
A-10A	144	AV-8B	60
EF-111A	18	OV-10	24
F-4G	48	TANKERS	24
RF-4C	18		
E-8A	2		
TANKERS	302		

MAJOR ALLIED AIR FORCES:
SAUDI ARABIA 165
UNITED KINGDOM 82
FRANCE 66
CANADA 29

COALITION STRENGTH:
620,000

37 NATIONS

UNIT LOCATIONS AS OF 260800 FEB 91

COALITION
NAVAL FORCES

UNITED STATES
UNITED KINGDOM
ARGENTINA
AUSTRALIA
BELGIUM
CANADA
DENMARK
FRANCE
GERMANY
GREECE
ITALY
KUWAIT
NETHERLANDS
NORWAY
POLAND
PORTUGAL
SPAIN

IRAN
IRAQ
KUWAIT
SAUDI ARABIA
Persian Gulf

Samawah
an-Nasiriyah
Basra
Safwan
Nisab
Kuwait City
Hafar al-Batin

Euphrates River
Tigris River
Highway 8
Wadi al-Batin

LIBERATION OF KUWAIT:
THE ALLIED GROUND ATTACK
24- 28 FEB 1991

▲ AIRFIELDS
OIL FIELDS

0   25   50   75
SCALE OF MILES

ABOVE: General Schwarzkopf's plan to defeat the Iraqi army. (US DOD/COMBAT CAMERA)

additional Apaches from the 2nd Battalion, 299th Aviation Regiment from its home garrison in Germany. The division's 317 helicopters, including 36 Apaches and 21 Bell AH-1F Cobras, arrived by sea on US Navy fast transport ships and they were soon moved up the coast to the 'Screaming Eagles' bases near the port of Dammam.

The US build-up of helicopter forces was not yet complete. In the weeks that followed, the aviation brigades of the 24th Infantry Division (Mechanised) and 1st Cavalry Division, each with 18 Apaches and 40 other helicopters, began arriving in Saudi Arabia. On top of that, the 12th Aviation Brigade with 36 more Apaches was sent to the Middle East from its bases in Germany.

During this phase of Operation Desert Shield, the US and coalition commanders focused on defending Saudi Arabia from an expected Iraqi incursion. The idea was that the Apache battalions would fly up to the Kuwaiti border and engage advancing Iraqi tank columns with their laser-guided AGM-114 Hellfire missiles. As this holding action was

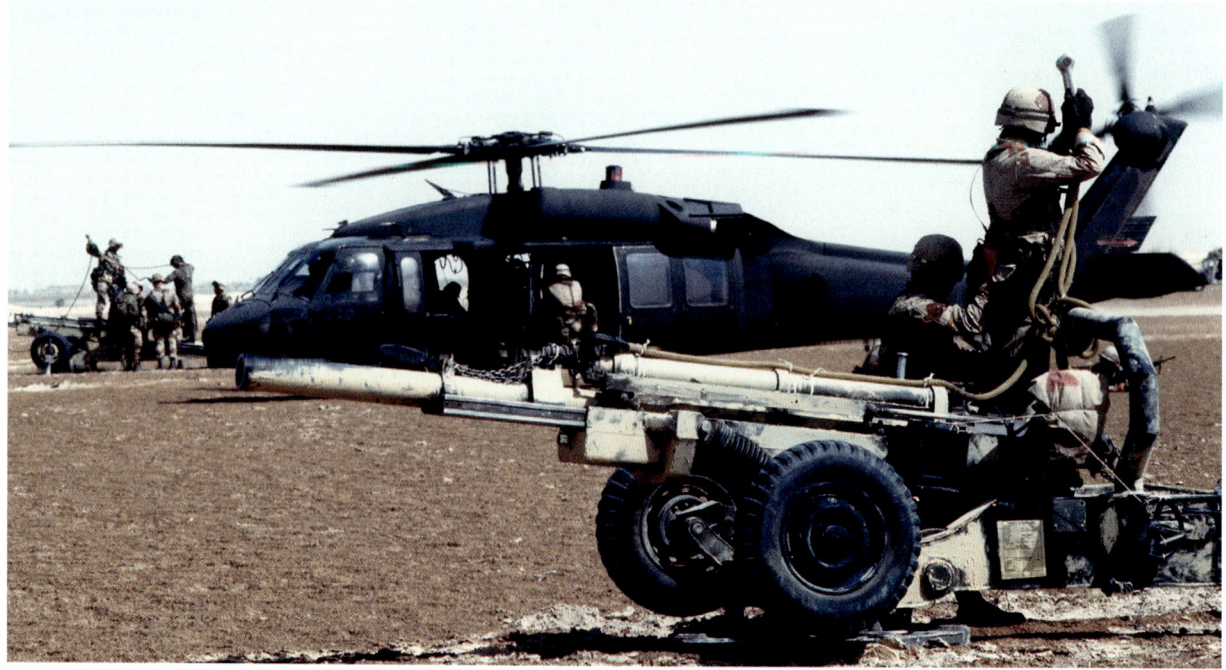

RIGHT: 101st Airborne Division troopers practice to under-sling their 105mm howitzers from UH-60 Blackhawks during the build-up to the ground invasion. (US DOD/COMBAT CAMERA)

underway, the 101st Airborne was to manoeuvre out into the desert in an aerial outflanking strike.

While this concept looked good on paper, the US Army helicopter crew had to quickly work out how to fly in the extreme desert environment. The featureless terrain made it difficult for the pilots to use their night vision goggles and many lost situational awareness, leading to several of them flying into the ground. Fine dust also created huge dust clouds when helicopters tried to land or take off, which again disorientated pilots. This was a similar phenomenon to that experienced when flying in snowy conditions, known as a 'white out'. In the desert they were called 'brown outs'. Eventually, the pilots mastered the conditions and when winter approached flying conditions improved.

Prior to its deployment to Saudi Arabia, the Apache had developed a notorious reputation for unreliability. This, however, was due to a shortage of spare parts in frontline units. When AH-64 units were ordered to Saudi Arabia, the locker of spare parts was opened and plane-loads of replacements flowed to the Middle East. Soon, AH-64 units in Saudi Arabia were reporting availability levels in excess of those attained in peacetime. In some cases, rates of over 90% were reported. The movement of critical spare parts from the dockside to frontline Apache units was also helped by Boeing CH-47D Chinook heavy lift helicopters being assigned to keep supplies flowing.

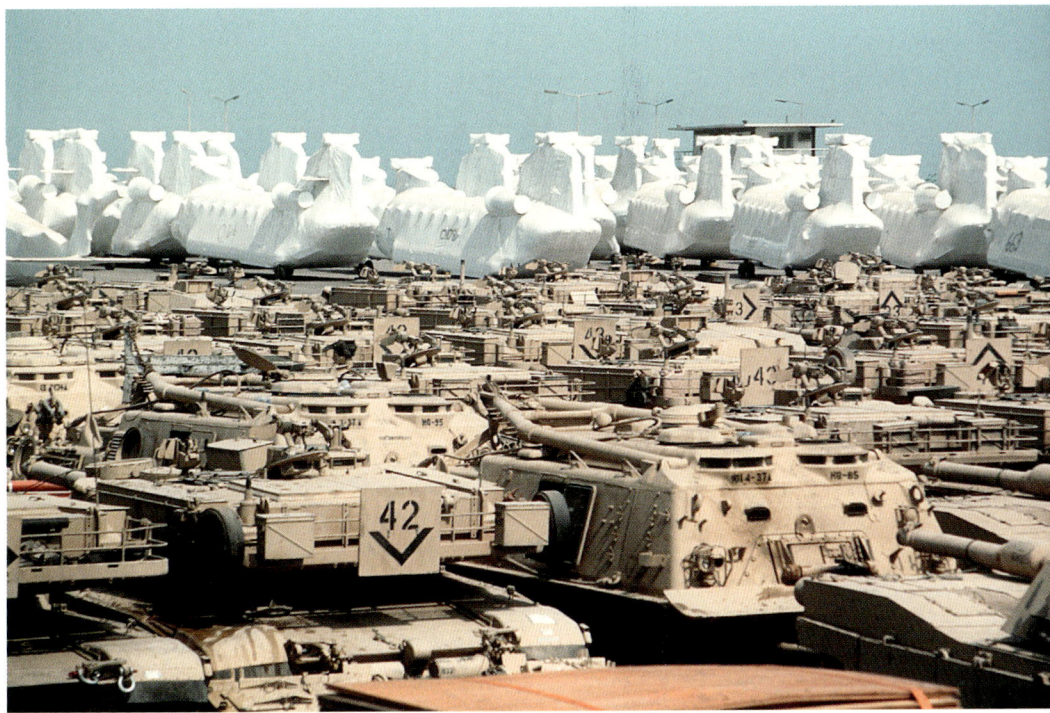

To give US forces in the Middle East an offensive capability, US President George H W Bush ordered the deployment of the US Army VII Corps to Saudi Arabia from Germany. This armour-heavy formation took a formidable force of more than 300 helicopters with it. Its two armoured division's aviation brigades each mustered two battalions of Apaches, while the 1st Infantry Division (Mechanised) only had one battalion of Apaches. To provide VII Corps with a deep strike capability, the 11st Combat Aviation Brigade was dispatched to Saudi Arabia.

VII Corps started to arrive in Saudi ports during the final weeks of December 1990 and over the next month its divisions moved out into tactical assembly areas near Hafar al Batin, just south of the point where the Saudi-Kuwaiti-Iraqi borders meet. The airfields at Al Qaysumah and King Khalid Military City became key hubs for US helicopters. Further out to the west, the XVIII Airborne Corps concentrated its helicopters at the airfield at Rafha and desert air strips. »

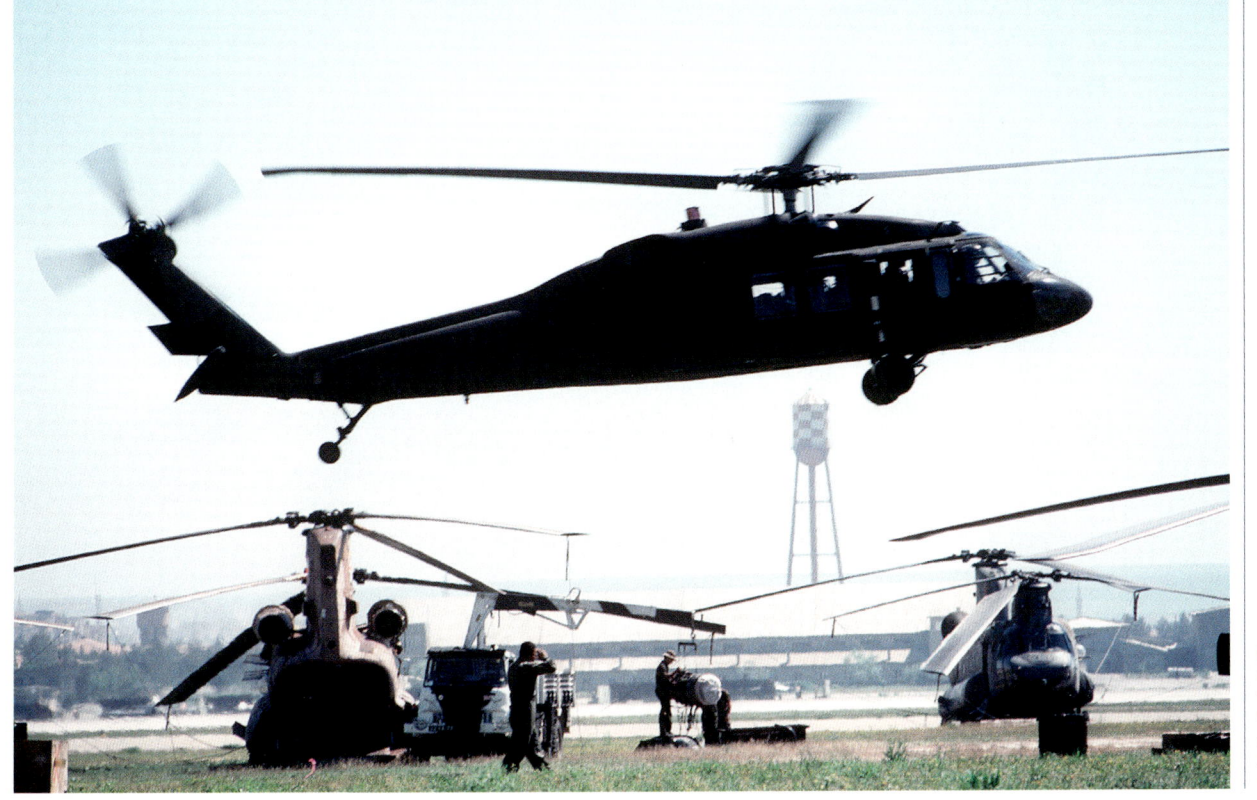

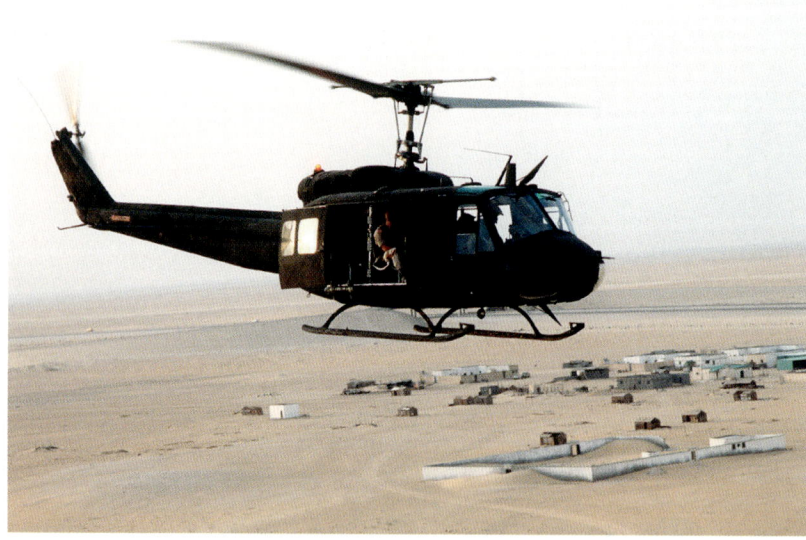

Major Helicopter Units US XVII Airborne Corps in Operation Desert Strom, February 1991		
3rd Armored Cavalry Regiment		
• 4th (Aviation) Squadron (25 x AH-1F, 25 x OH-58D, 18 x UH-1H)		
12th Aviation Brigade		
• 3rd Battalion, 227th Aviation Regiment (18 x AH-64A)		
• 5th Squadron, 6th Cavalry Regiment (18 x AH-64A)		
101st Aviation Division (Air Assault) Aviation Brigade		
• 1st Battalion, 101st Aviation Regiment (18 x AH-64A)		
• 3rd Battalion, 101st Aviation Regiment (18 x AH-1F)		
• 2nd Battalion, 229th Aviation Regiment (Task Force Viper)		
• 2nd Squadron, 17th Cavalry (AH-1F, OH-58C)		
82nd Airborne Division Aviation Brigade		
• 1st Battalion, 82nd Aviation (18 x AH-64A)		
24th Infantry Division (Mechanised) Aviation Brigade		
• 1st Battalion, 24th Aviation Regiment (18 x AH-64A)		
French 6th Dauget Light Armoured Division		
• 3e Régiment d›Hélicoptères de Combat		
• 5e Régiment d›Hélicoptères de Combat		
• 1er Régiment d›Hélicoptères de Combat		
Operated a mix of 60 x SA342M Gazelle, 14 x SA341F Gazelle, 14 x SA341/F Gazelle and 38 SA330B Puma		

ABOVE: The iconic UH-1 Huey still served in US Army aviation units in utility and support roles in 1990 and went to war again during Operation Desert Storm. (US DOD/COMBAT CAMERA)

US helicopter units had to set up several forward operating bases, or FOBs, at some very primitive locations, and extensive engineering support was needed to make them hospitable and operational. Makeshift revetments were created by bulldozing sand berms around helicopter disposal areas, weapon dumps and fuel pillows. These desert bases were occupied until the start of the ground offensive when the US aviation brigades went into mobile mode and followed in the wake of the armoured spearheads. Fuel tankers, ammunition trucks and command vans then moved behind the ground troops, setting up forward air refuelling points (FARPs) and then leap frogging them forward as the advance continued.

By the eve of the land phase of Operation Desert Storm on February 24, the US Army had deployed a massive force of helicopters in the Middle East, including 278 AH-64As, 131 AH-1F/Ss, 299 UH-60, 64 UH-60V, 24 EH-60, 295 OH-58C, 92 UH-58D, 314 UH-1 and 127 CH-47s.

It fell to US Army AH-6As of the 1st Battalion, 101st Aviation Regiment to fire the opening shots of the 1991 Gulf War at 2.38am on January 17. Eight US Army Apaches, accompanied by two USAF Special Operations Sikorsky MH-5J Pave Lows of Task Force Normandy, headed out into the Iraqi desert before the war had officially begun. They crossed the Iraqi border at low level and then headed 80 miles

inside Saddam Hussein's country to attack two radar sites that covered a key section of air space. Once destroyed, coalition aircraft was able to penetrate deep into Baghdad and take the Iraqi air defences around the city by surprise.

The Pave Lows led the way using their satellite navigation systems to lead the AH-64As to their targets and, right on H-Hour, four Apaches blasted each radar site with their Hellfire missiles. In a sign of the times, video imagery of the highly accurate strikes was recorded by the AH-64As' night vision systems and later played to the media at a Pentagon press conference.

The US Central Command chief, General Norman Schwarzkopf,

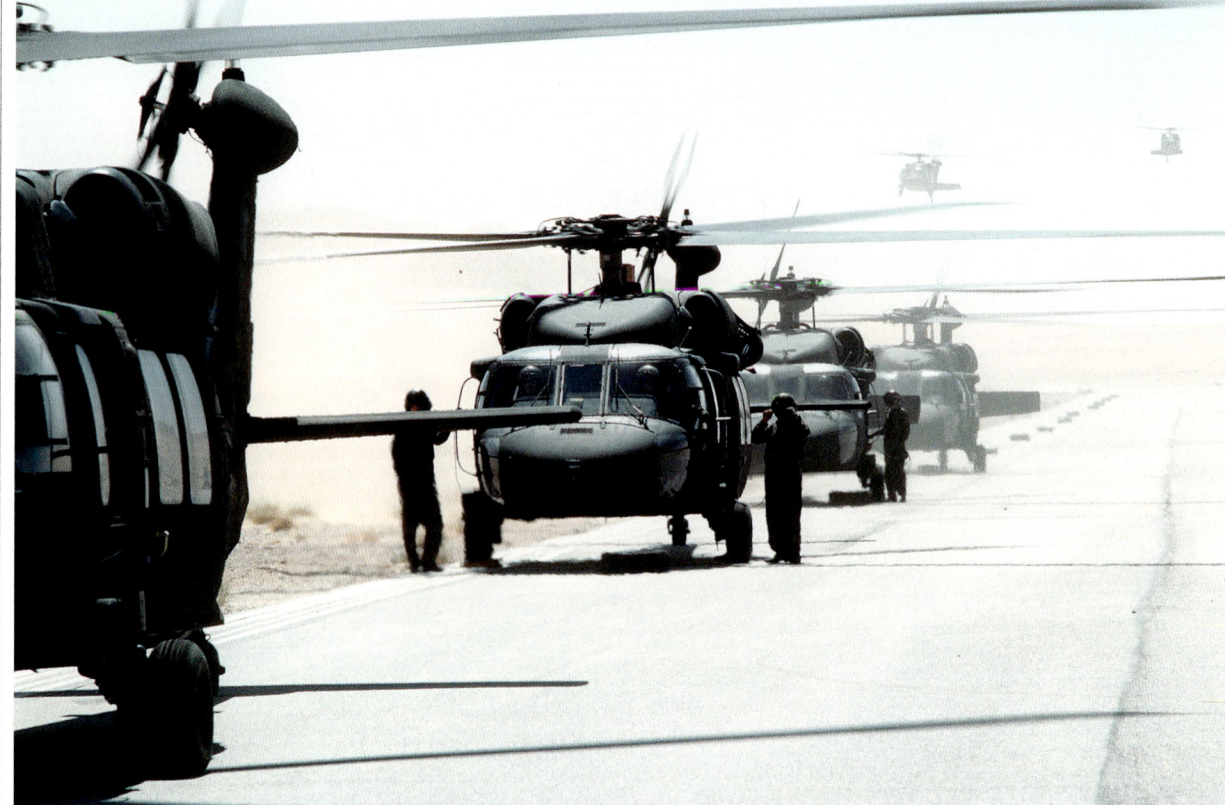

RIGHT: XVIII Airborne Corps helicopter units began moving to remote desert air strips in January 1991 in preparation for their air assault operation into Iraq. (US DOD/COMBAT CAMERA)

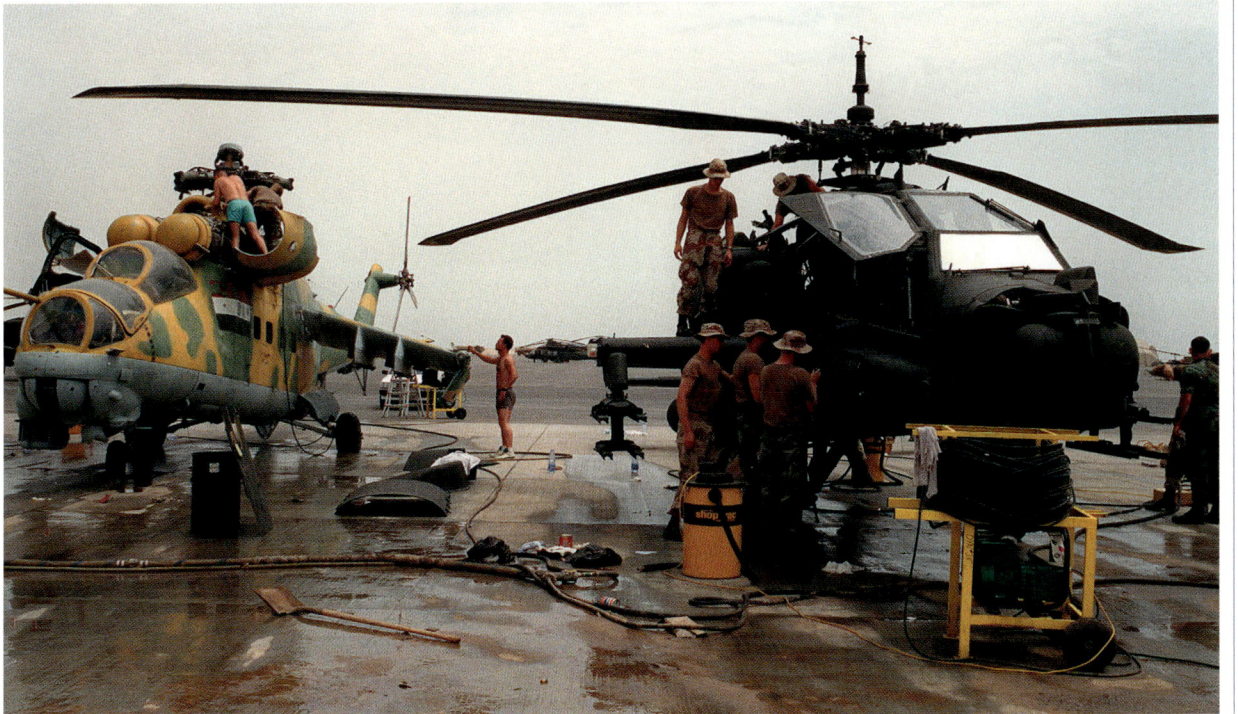

devised an audacious plan to defeat the Iraqi army occupying Kuwait, as well as the armoured reserves of Saddam Hussein's Republican Guard sitting back astride the Kuwait-Iraq border. To paraphrase the head of the US Joint Chiefs of Staff General Colin Powell, the idea was to "cut off and kill" the Iraqi army.

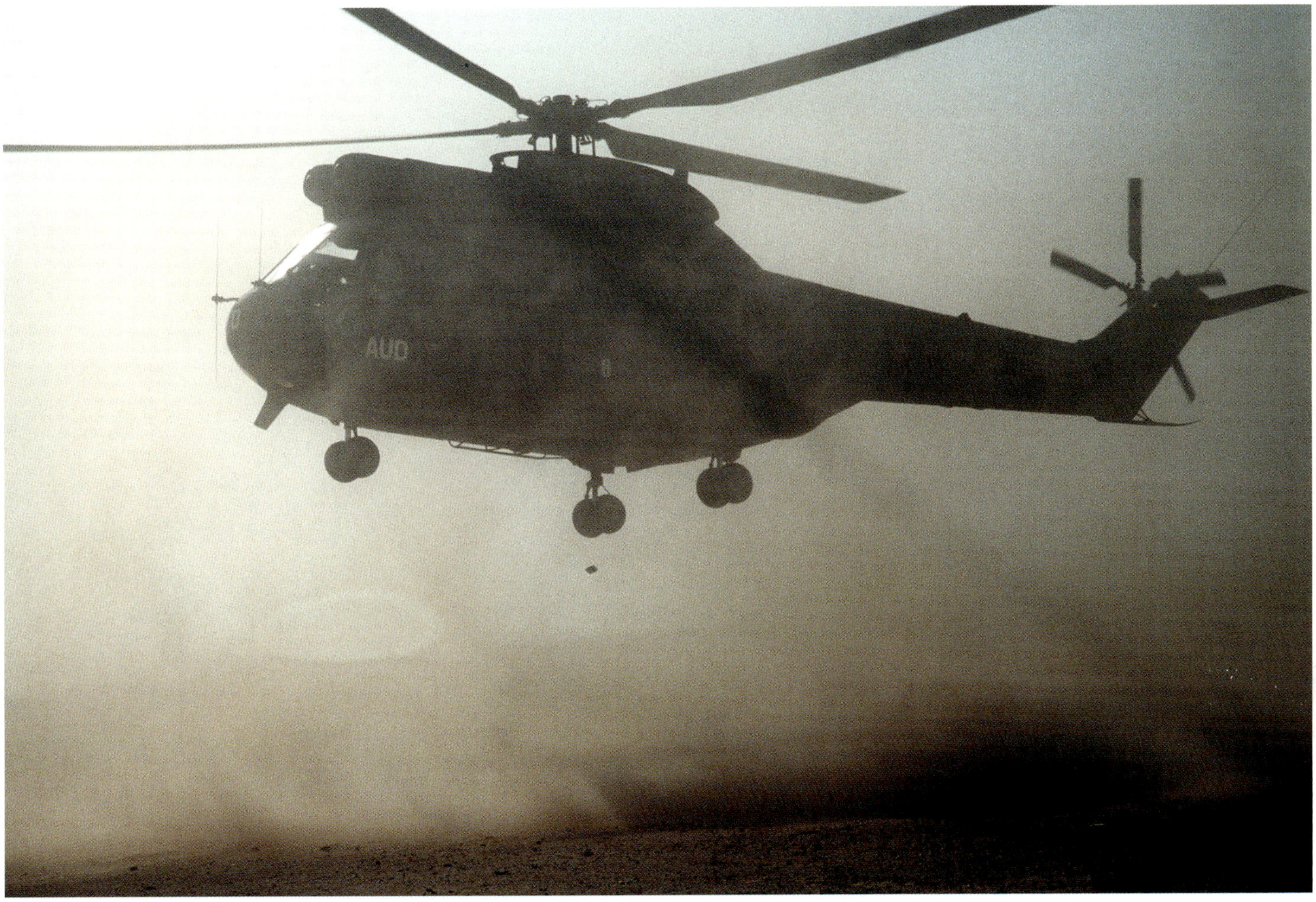

To close the ring around the Iraqis, XVIII Airborne Corps, comprising US and French airmobile forces, were to advance deep into the Iraqi army's rear area, using helicopters as their main means of transport. On February 14, reconnaissance missions started to fly deep into the Iraqi desert to try to pinpoint the main enemy

positions. A French Light Army Aviation (ALAT) Aérospatiale Puma helicopter fitted with an experimental Orchidée battlefield surveillance radar flew 24 missions to keep XVIII Airborne Corps objectives under surveillance. Several Iraqi tank and vehicle columns were detected by the French helicopters. US Army »

ABOVE: French ALAT Puma helicopters were assigned to support the US XVIII Airborne Corps' air assault operation.
(US DOD/COMBAT CAMERA)

LEFT: AH-64A units expected to be confronted by Iraqi Mi-24s once they entered Iraqi air space, but Saddam Hussein's attack helicopters remained on the ground and the only Mi-24s encountered were those captured on the ground.
(US DOD/COMBAT CAMERA)

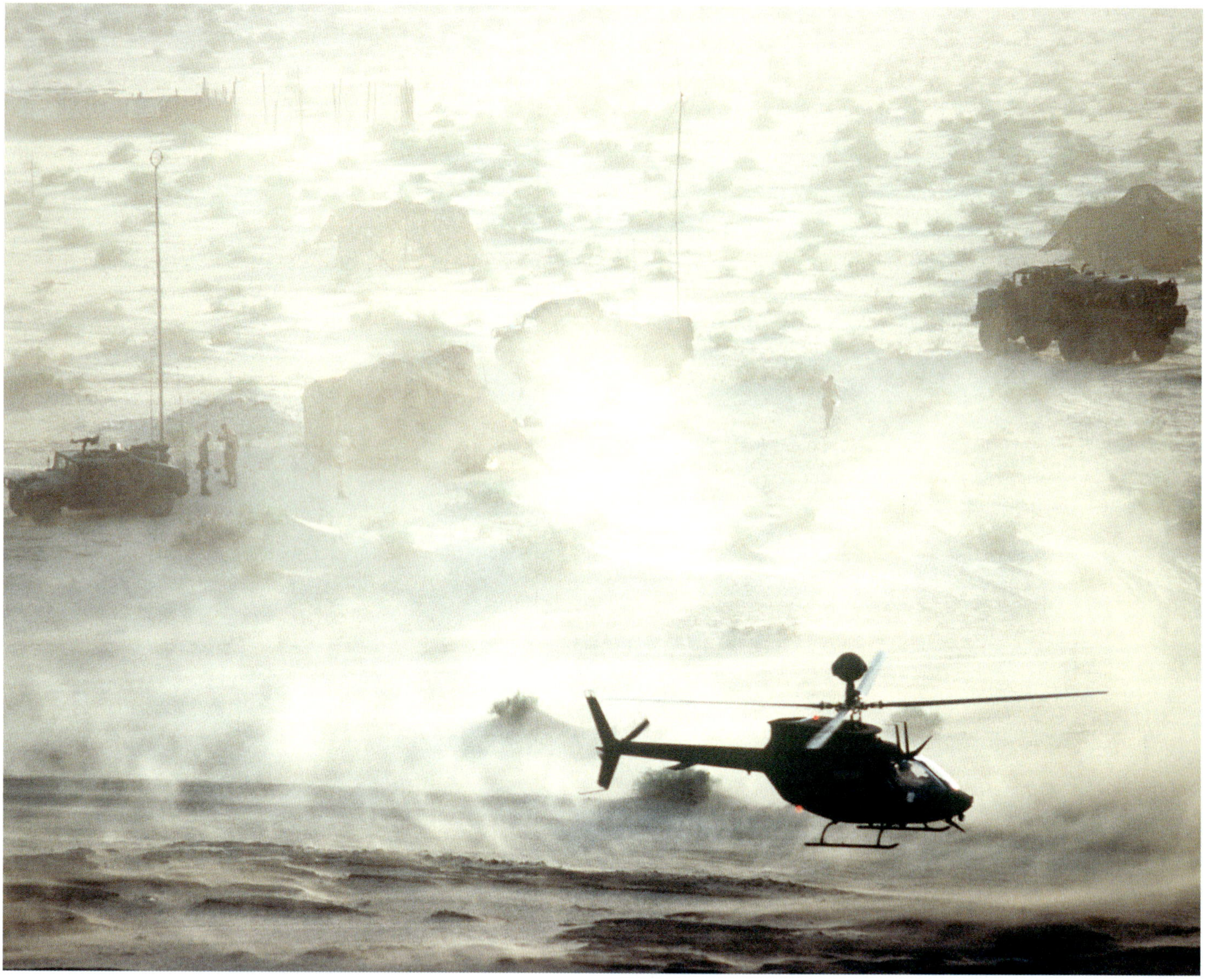

ABOVE: US helicopter units spent the build up to the ground invasion in forward operating bases out in the Saudi desert.
(US DOD/COMBAT CAMERA)

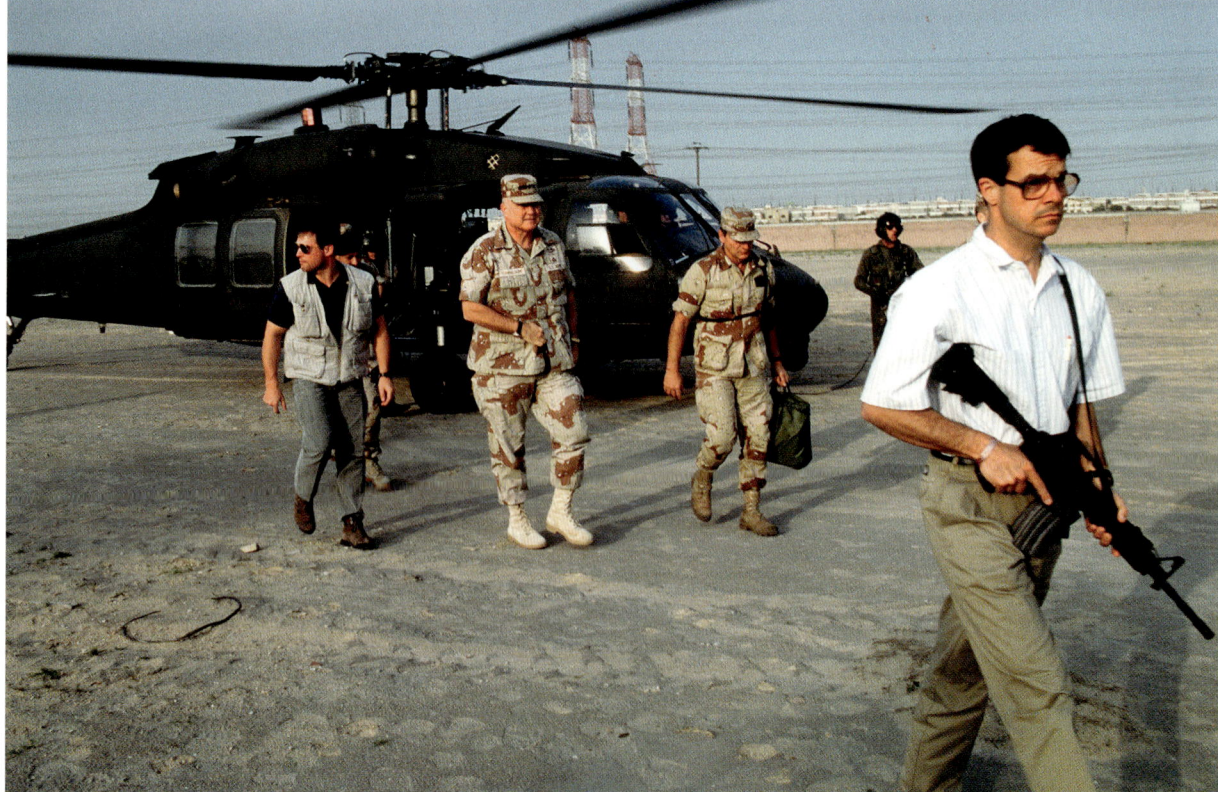

ABOVE: US helicopter units spent the build up to the ground invasion in forward operating bases out in the Saudi desert.
(US DOD/COMBAT CAMERA)

RIGHT: General Schwarzkopf flew up to the frontline in the days before the ground attack to make sure his commanders and their troops were ready for the coming battle.
(US DOD/COMBAT CAMERA)

Apache and USAF Fairchild A-10A Warthog tank busters were called in to attack them.

USAF Boeing B-52 Stratofortress heavy bombers were now carpet-bombing Iraqi positions on a daily basis and Iraqi morale was already starting to waver in the face of this unrelenting pounding. XVIII Airborne Corps helicopters were criss-crossing the desert with great regularity and in one famous incident, on February 20, a whole Iraqi battalion tried to surrender to the 101st Airborne. The US plan called for the XVIII Airborne Corps to leap frog forward into the Euphrates valley, via several FOBs. To prevent surprises, small reconnaissance teams were landed by helicopters close to the proposed FOBs to ensure there were no Iraqi troops nearby and give warning of Iraqi threats in the area.

The build-up of XVIII Airborne Corps and its helicopters was protected by the tanks and infantry of the 24th Division deployed along the Iraqi border. Its OH-58s and Apaches flew patrols to monitor Iraqi positions. These helicopters were in action against Iraqi border posts on January 30 and February 18, including designating targets for destruction with laser-guided Copperhead artillery rounds.

G-Day or Ground Day was set for February 24 by General Schwarzkopf. At 7.25am the 101st Airborne's 1st Brigade lifted off on the first main attack of XVIII Airborne Corps' advance, to seize Objective Cobra. A formation of 67 UH-6s, 30 Chinooks and UH-1Hs headed 80km into Iraq and landed unopposed on a piece of empty desert. A-10As and AH-1Fs escorted the transport helicopters as they flew northwards at low level. Before the air assault troops landed, the escorting strike jets and gunships started to bombard a small Iraqi infantry position 2km from Objective Cobra. An artillery battery was landed by Chinook and it was soon in action against the Iraqi infantry. Within minutes of the start of this bombardment the Iraqis surrendered to the circling AH-1Fs.

Feverish work then began to transform Objective Cobra into a fully fledged FOB to enable the next phase of the operation to get underway. A shuttle of CH-47s, flying back and forth from Rafha airfield, brought in more troops, artillery, fuel, and ammunition. Soon the 101st and 12th Aviation Brigades had moved their Apache units into Objective Cobra. They were rapidly re-armed and refuelled and sent out to hunt for Iraqi tanks and artillery along the Euphrates valley. Pairs of OH-58Ds patrolled the desert in every direction looking for targets and then calling up Apaches to hit them. Each Apache battalion established its own FARPs and began to rotate its companies through them so fully armed and »

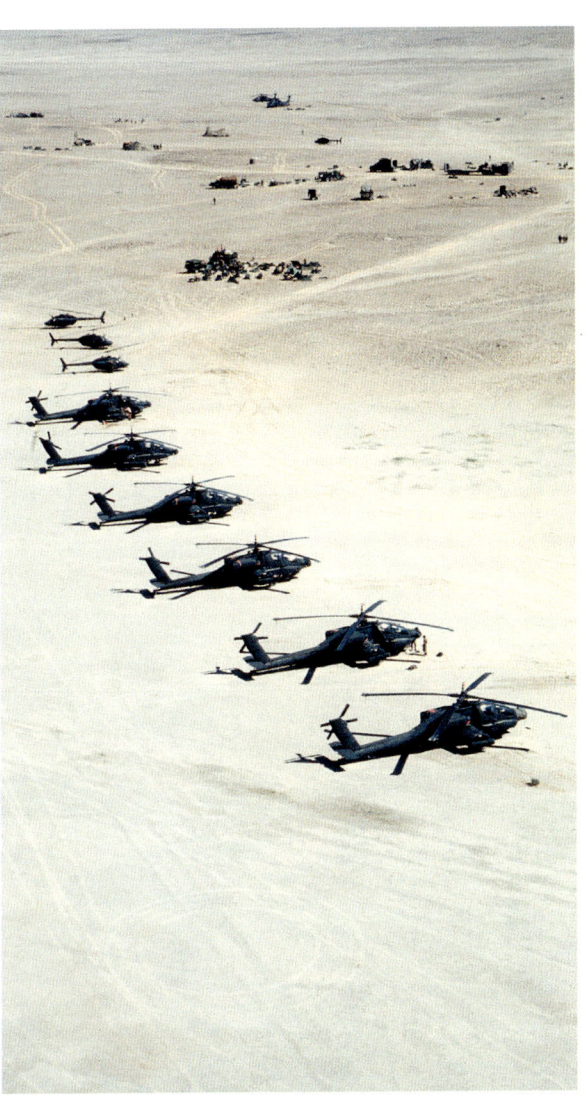

ABOVE: XVIII Airborne Corps advanced its AH-64A units through a series of Forward Arming and Refuelling Points to keep them in the fight.
(US DOD/COMBAT CAMERA)

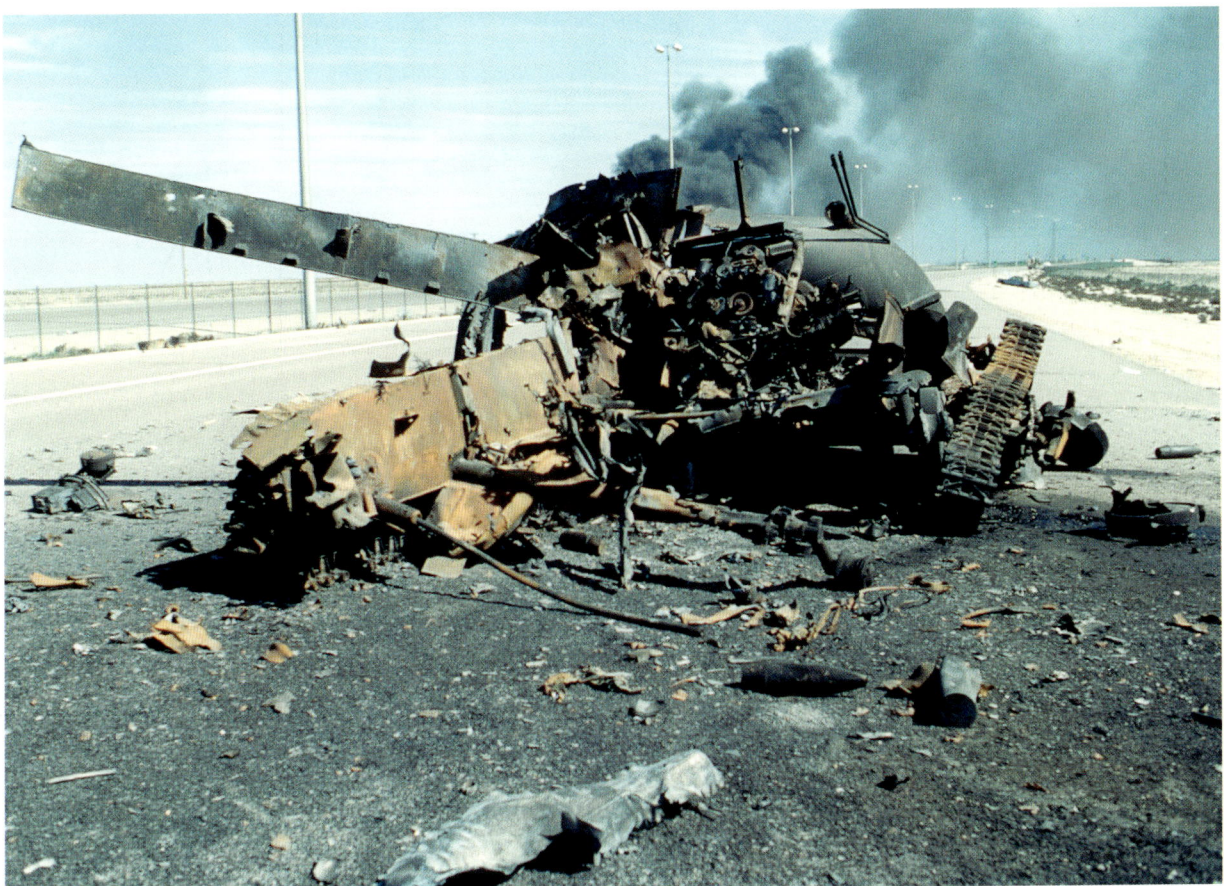

LEFT: Iraqi tanks were soon being destroyed in large numbers after the AH-64As starting patrolling deep behind enemy lines.
(US DOD/COMBAT CAMERA)

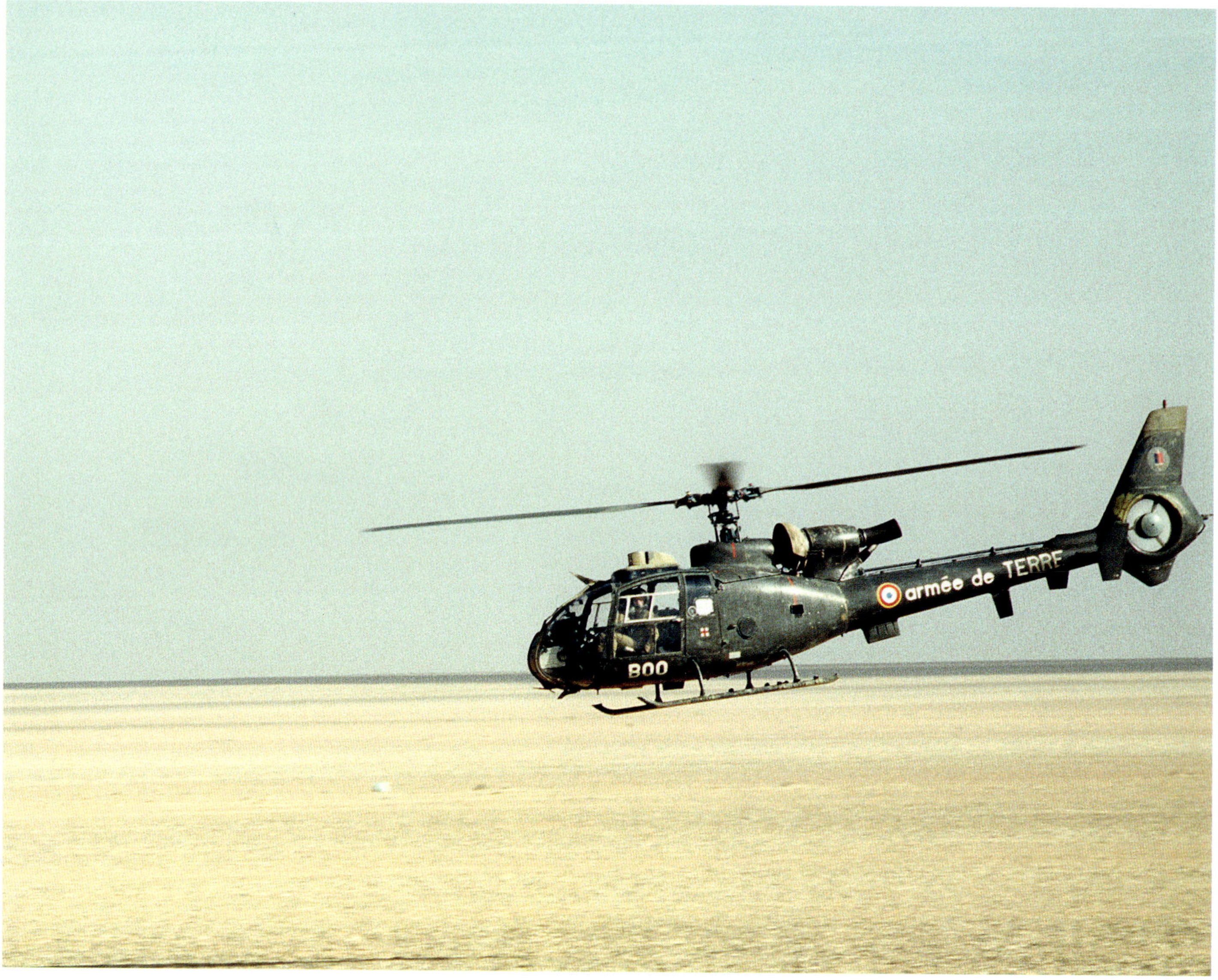

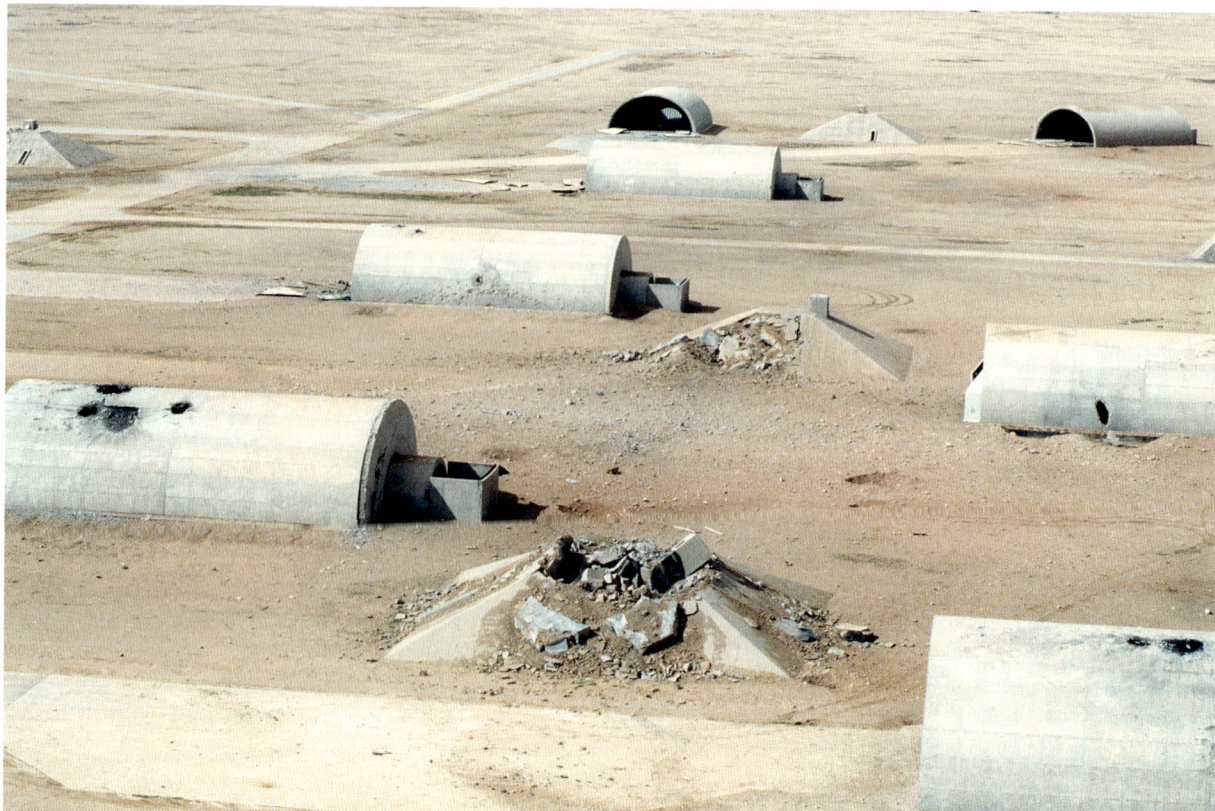

ABOVE: French ALAT Gazelle helicopters led the advance on As Salman Air Base. (US DOD/COMBAT CAMERA)

RIGHT: When French and US troops arrived at As Salman, they found the base devastated and the defenders quickly surrendered. (US DOD/COMBAT CAMERA)

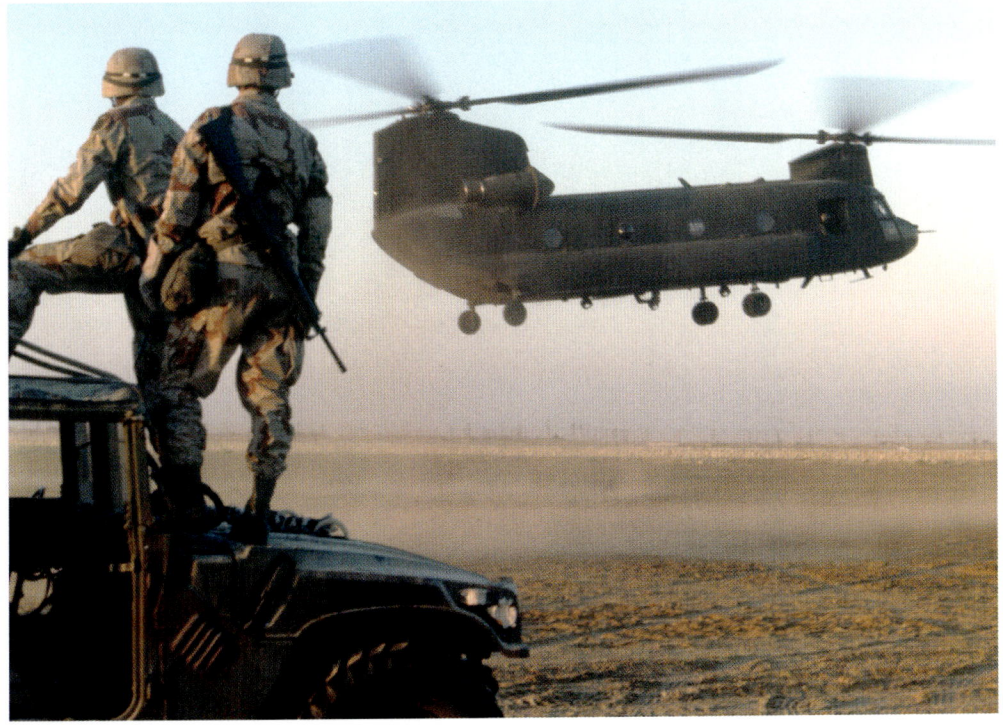

fuelled AH-64As were always in the air, ready to strike.

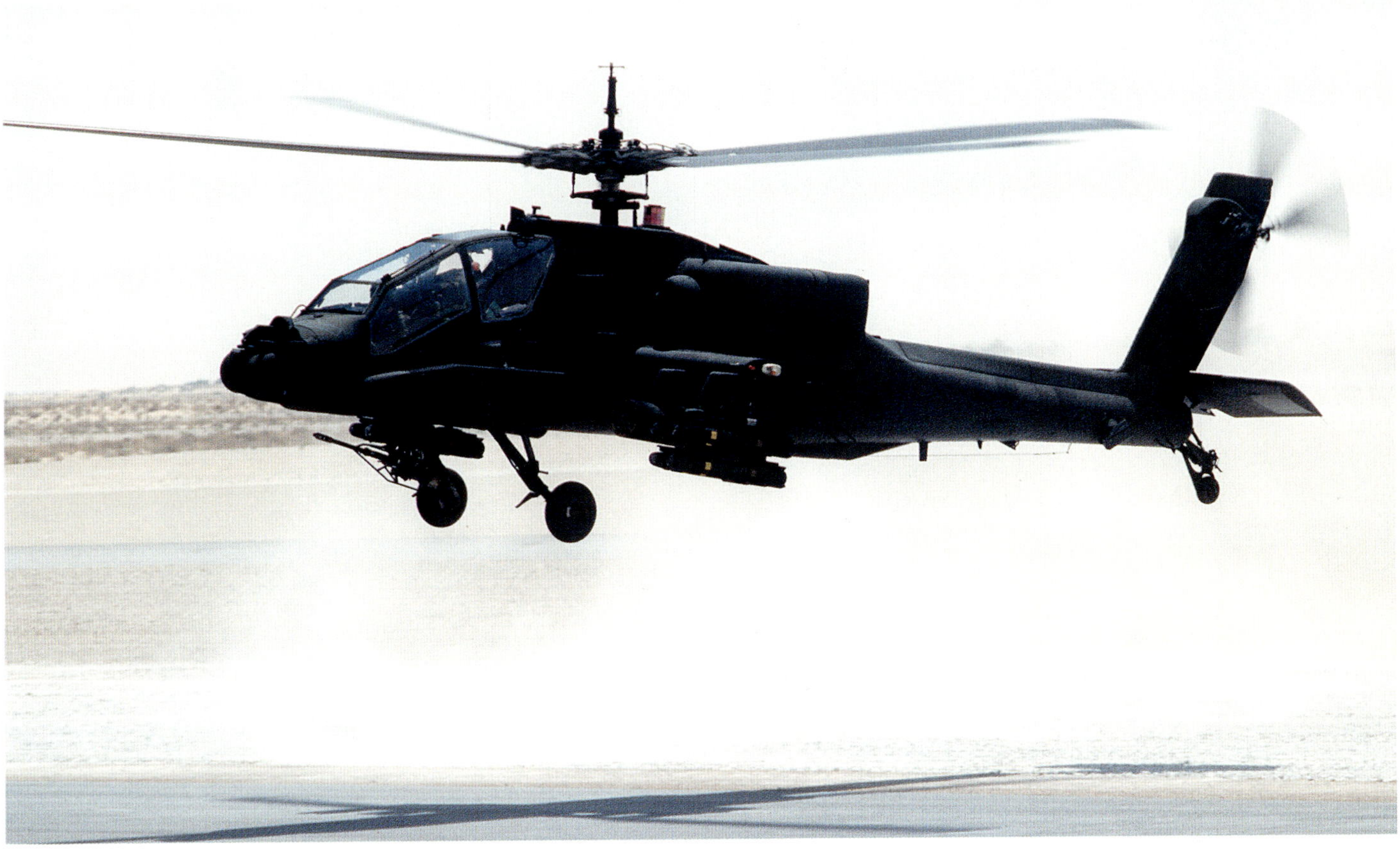

By the afternoon of February 25, the 101st Airborne's 3rd Brigade was ready to launch on the next phase of the advance to the Euphrates. At 3.00pm 66 UH-60s took off carrying 1,000 airborne troopers to seize five new FOBs near the town of Al Khidr on Highway 8, which linked the southern city of Basra with Baghdad. By first light on February 26, the 3rd Brigade was firmly established, and US Army combat engineers were at work demolishing road bridges to cut this key Iraqi supply route.

A huge dust storm engulfed southern Iraq on February 26 and soon 30 knot winds had effectively grounded all of XVIII Airborne Corps' helicopters and its fixed-wing air support. Fortunately, the Iraqi high command had little idea what the Americans were doing and there were no counter-attacks to strike at the lightly armed units of the 101st Airborne.

The weather cleared on February 27 and the 101st Airborne was able to launch three battalions of infantry on dozens of UH-60s to seize Objective Viper, 159km to the east of Objective Cobra. Apaches from the 101st and 12th Aviation Brigade escorted the air assault but there was no opposition. The only US casualties of the day were the crew of a 101st Airborne medical evacuation UH-60 that was diverted in an attempt to rescue a USAF Lockheed F-16 Fighting Falcon

pilot who has been shot down just behind enemy lines. The helicopter was shot down and five crew killed, while three others were taken prisoner. Despite this setback, XVIII Airborne Corps and its two brigades of Apaches were now positioned deep behind enemy lines, ready to join the crucial battle that was looming over the next 24 hours as VII Corps engaged the Republican Guard.

Coming up behind the 101st Airborne were the tanks of the 24th Division, and by the early hours of February 27 they had driven across the desert to the Euphrates valley.

While the bulk of XVIII Airborne Corps headed eastwards to join the battle with the Republican Guard, its western flank was protected by the French Daguet, or Dagger, Division, and the US 82nd Airborne Division. To clear the way the 82nd Airborne's two Apache battalions, backed by USAF jets, staged a strike on Iraqi tanks and artillery defending »

ABOVE: Once XVIII Airborne Corps was established in Objective Cobra, AH-64A units were launched to strike at Iraqi troops in the Euphrates valley. (US DOD/COMBAT CAMERA)

BELOW: CH-47 Chinooks shuttled forward to deliver fuel, ammunitions, and spare parts to Objective Cobra to keep XVIII Airborne Corps' AH-64A units fighting. (US DOD/COMBAT CAMERA)

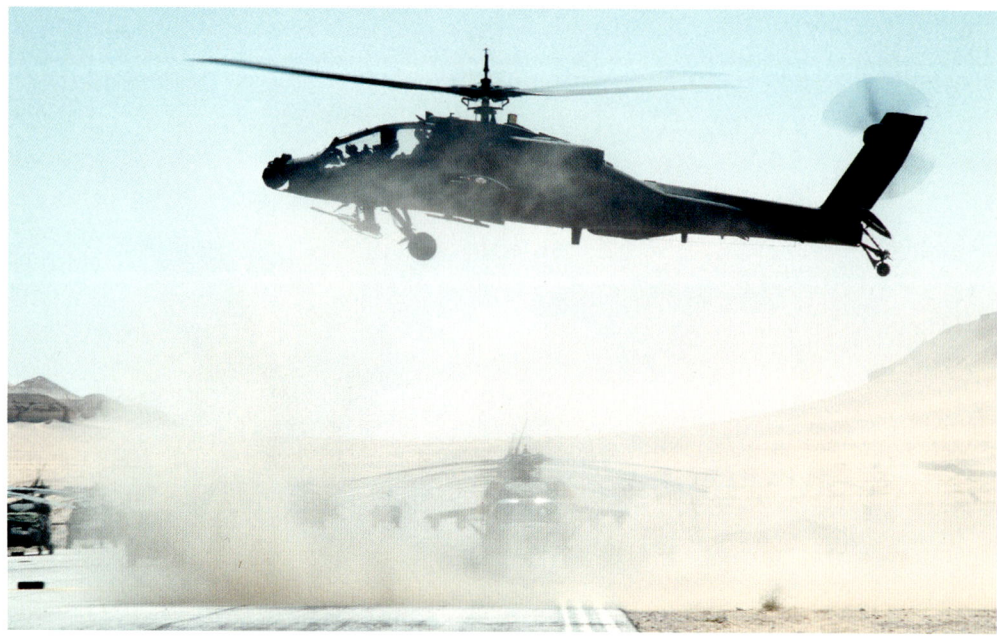

ABOVE: Apaches of the 12th Aviation Brigade joined the 101st Airborne's AH-64As for the deep strike raids into the Euphrates valley. (US DOD/COMBAT CAMERA)

As Salman Air Base on the night of February 18. More strike missions followed during the next day as the Apaches bombarded the Iraqi division spread out between the air base and the Saudi border.

When the Daguet Division's armoured columns crossed the border, ALAT Aérospatiale Gazelles flew ahead of them at low level. Formations of 30 French helicopters swarmed over the desert engaging any Iraqi positions they encountered with HOT wire-guided missiles. During the advance, the French helicopters knocked out 127 tanks, vehicles, and bunkers. By the time

the French Foreign Legion drove through the gates of As Salman Air Base, the Iraqi 45th Division had ceased to exist as a fighting force. The French troops and the 82nd Division spent the rest of the war rounding up prisoners.

The VII Corps was General Schwarzkopf's heavy punch and it had been given one objective – destroy the Republican Guard's tank divisions positioned in the Iraq-Kuwait border region.

Even before the ground invasion proper started, VII Corps attack helicopters were in action as part of the concerted coalition effort to

hammer frontline Iraqi units. The aim was to render these troops 50% combat effective by G-Day. As well as blasting frontline positions, the Apaches were sent on patrols deep behind Iraqi lines to overfly the routes their parent divisions were expected to take to reach the Republican Guard. Crews videoed their missions to play back to senior commanders and intelligence analysts after they returned to their bases. During one of these missions, on February 16, an Apache of the 1st Battalion, 1st Aviation Regiment became disorientated and engaged US Army vehicles. This was the only friendly

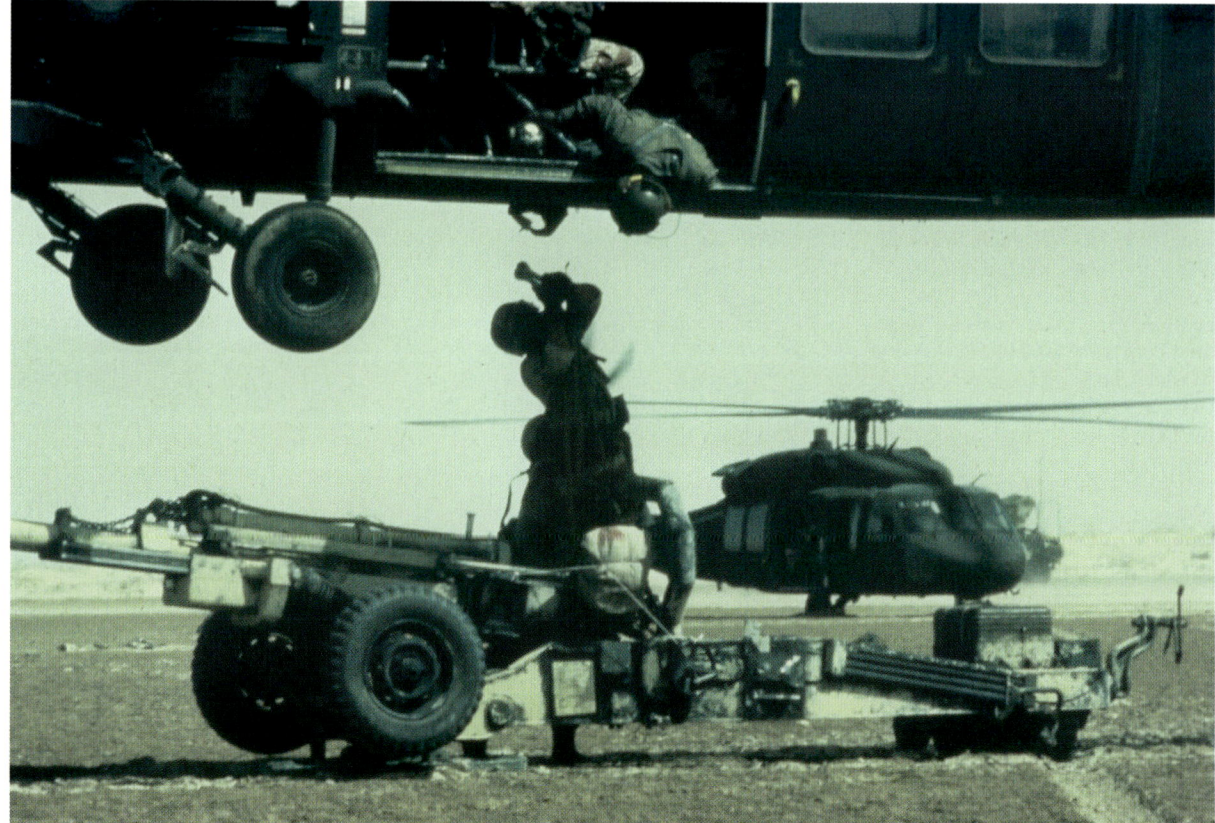

RIGHT: 105mm howitzers were flown forward to enhance the protection of Objective Cobra. (US DOD/COMBAT CAMERA)

fire incident involving AH-64As during Operation Desert Storm.

The VII Corps advance got underway on February 24, with the 1st Infantry Division (Mechanised) overrunning the Iraqi border defence line. This was cleared in a few hours and then the 2nd Armored Cavalry Regiment charged into Iraq in a dash to find the Republican Guard. Its scout patrols of AH-1Fs and OH-58Ds flew low level across the desert 30km ahead of the regiment's tanks. The 11th Aviation Brigade was held on strip alert ready to launch a mass Apache attack if the 2nd Cavalry found a target.

In the early hours of February 25, the 2nd Cavalry's scout helicopters discovered an Iraqi armoured division and called in air strikes to devastate its tanks. That division was soon rolled over and VII Corps continued its advance.

The first contact with the Republican Guard was made on the morning of February 26 by the 2nd Cavalry's helicopters but they were unable to call down sustained air strikes due to the huge sand storm engulfing southern Iraq. The 1st Armored Division's scout OH-58Ds and AH-1Fs had managed to find units of the Republican Guard when one of the Cobras was caught in the sand storm. It crashed right in front of Iraqi positions but the crew was successfully rescued by ground scouts.

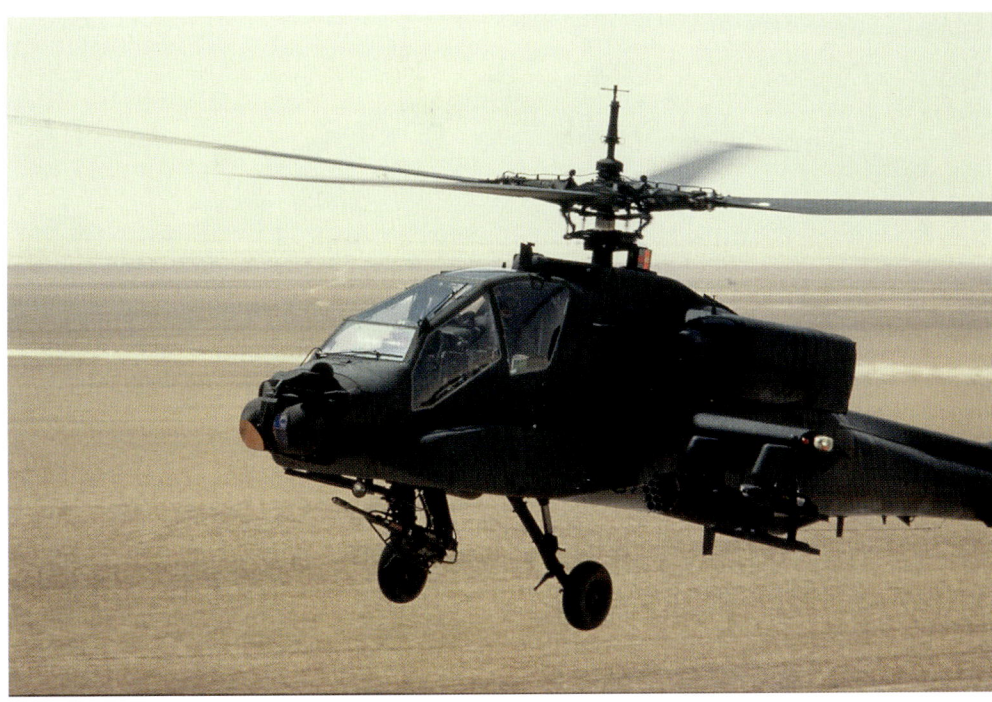

US helicopter operations in and around the Republican Guards were put on hold until the storm lifted.

VII Corps planners were now manoeuvring the 1st and 3rd Armored Divisions to bring their tanks up to assault the Republican Guard. The two US divisions swung into a line facing eastward, with the 1st Division on the left and 3rd Division on the right. By late afternoon the storm was lifting, and 1st Division's

Apaches were launched to strike at a reserve Republican Guard brigade. Meanwhile, Abrams tanks went toe-to-toe with the T-72 tanks of the Medina and Tarrakalma Divisions. The 11th Aviation Brigade's Apaches were then sent into action around 9.00pm against targets 40km behind the front.

The next day would be pivotal. In the early hours of February 27, the 11th Brigade went into action again, hitting »

ABOVE: Apache units from the 11th Aviation Brigade provided aerial firepower to support the armoured divisions of VII Corps. (US DOD/COMBAT CAMERA)

BELOW: VII Corps tank columns stretched as far as the eye could see once they crossed into Iraq on February 24. (US DOD/COMBAT CAMERA)

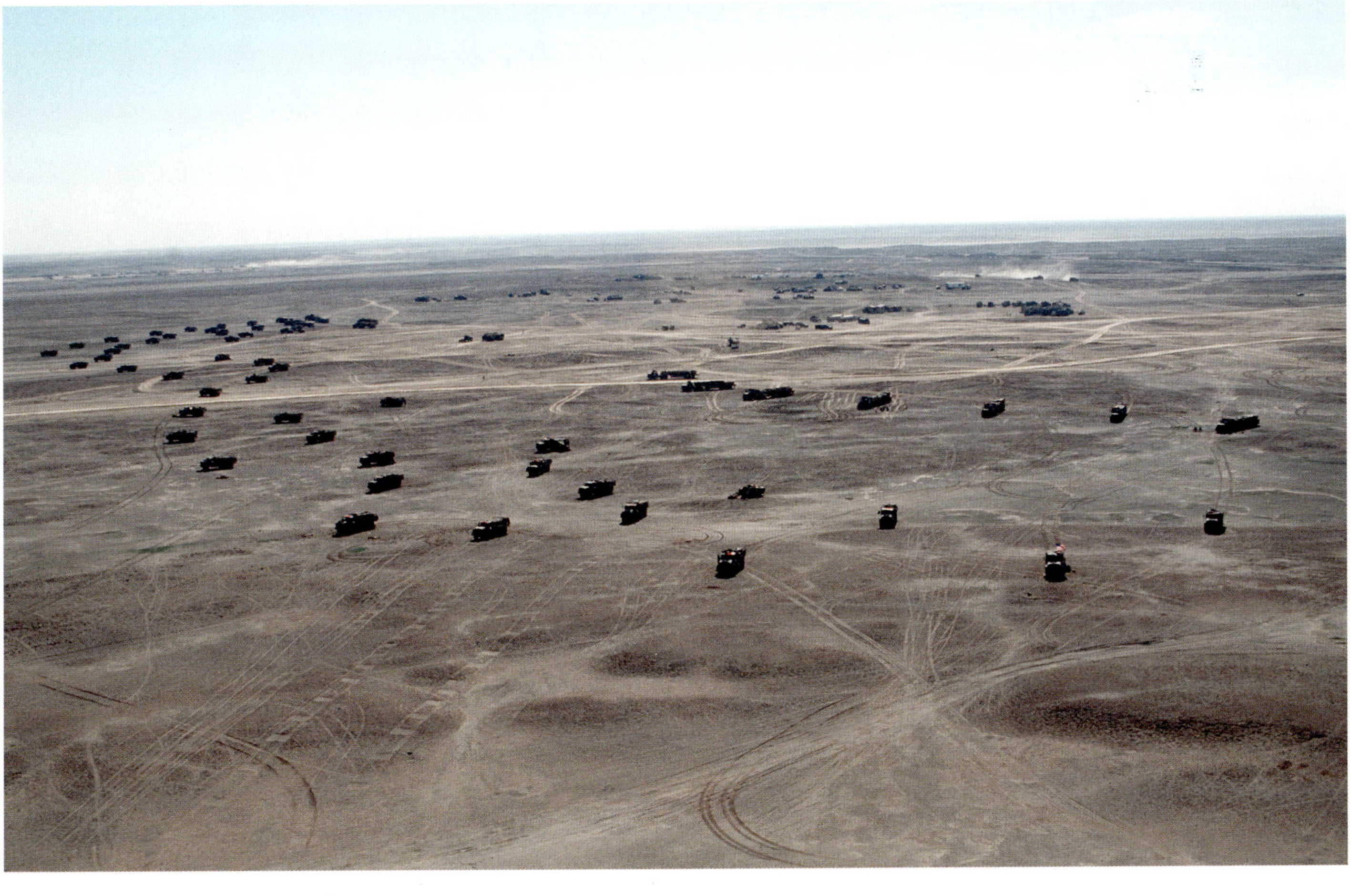

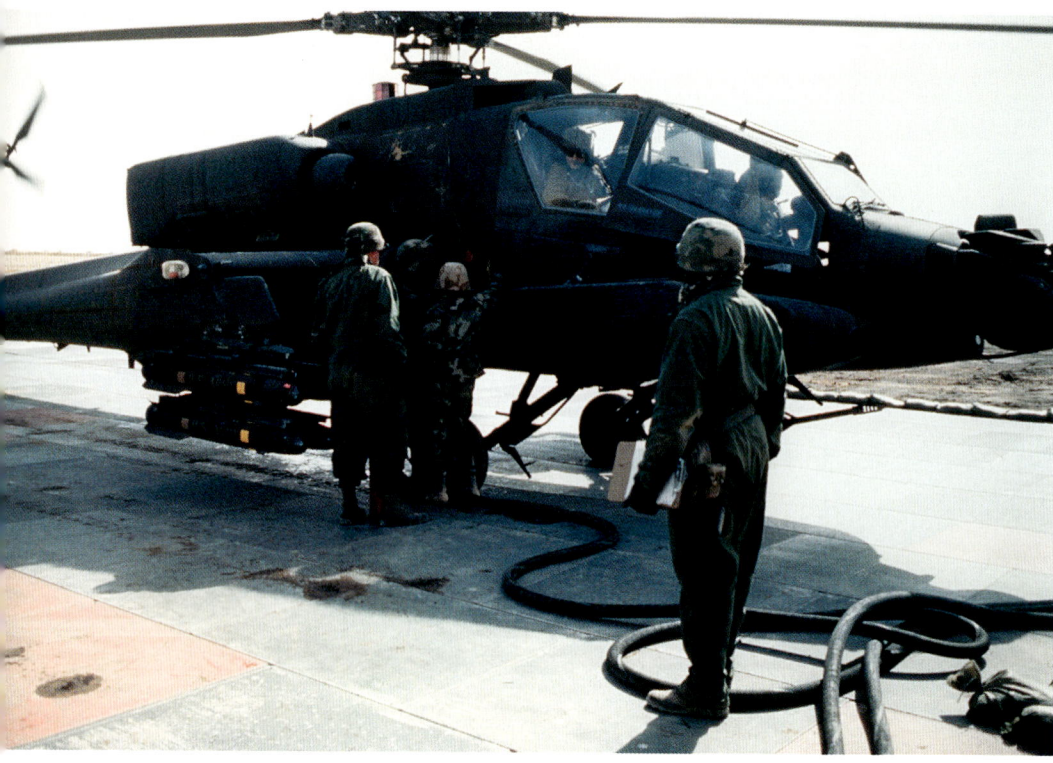

ABOVE: Fuel tankers moved close behind VII Corps armoured spearheads to keep the tanks of AH-64As fully topped up. (US DOD/COMBAT CAMERA)

joined the battle against the Medina Division's reserve units. An attack by the 2nd Battalion, 1st Aviation Regiment destroyed 30 tanks, 11 armoured personnel carriers and 12 other vehicles. By evening, the Medina Division had effectively been destroyed, with Apaches and air force strike jets accounting for 186 tanks and 137 other armoured vehicles.

At 5.15am on February 28, VII Corps rolled forward to engage the Hammurabi Division, which US intelligence believed was the last formation of the Republican Guard that was still able to fight. For three hours until the calling of the ceasefire at 8.00am the Apaches of 1st Regiment hit scores of the Iraqi division's tanks and other vehicles.

As the final battle with the Republican Guard was unfolding, USAF Northrop Grumman E-8A Joint STARS airborne stand-off radar aircraft were tracking Iraqi units retreating from Kuwait up the main road to Basra. The 11th Brigade's Apaches were alerted to strike the retreating Iraqi columns near the Safwan border crossing, but at the last minute the mission was switched to the attack helicopters from the 1st Division. By the time Apaches were on station the ceasefire had come into effect and attack helicopters were ordered to cease fire.

VII Corps' right flank, during its advance on the Republican Guard, was protected by the troops of the 1st (UK) Armoured Division. Its advance was screened by Westland Gazelle AH1 scout helicopters and TOW missile- »

more Iraqi positions in front of the 3rd Division. The Apache brigade hit 33 tanks, 18 armoured personnel carriers and 35 other vehicles. During the attacks, the American aviators reported that large numbers of Iraqi tank crews appeared to have abandoned their vehicles and fled on foot.

To keep the Apaches in the fight, US supply convoys had pushed forward to set up FARPs just behind the main line of American tanks. The battle was so dynamic that the FARPs had to continue moving to keep up. On

occasions US helicopter crews had to land next to Abrams tanks to ask their crews for directions to the nearest FARP.

As dawn broke on February 27, the 1st Armored Division closed on the Medina Division, resulting in the last big tank battle of the war. Abrams tanks went head-to-head with Iraqi T-72s for several hours. US commanders first probed the Iraqi positions with helicopter patrols that accounted for several hits from Hellfire missiles. In the afternoon, more Apaches and A-10s

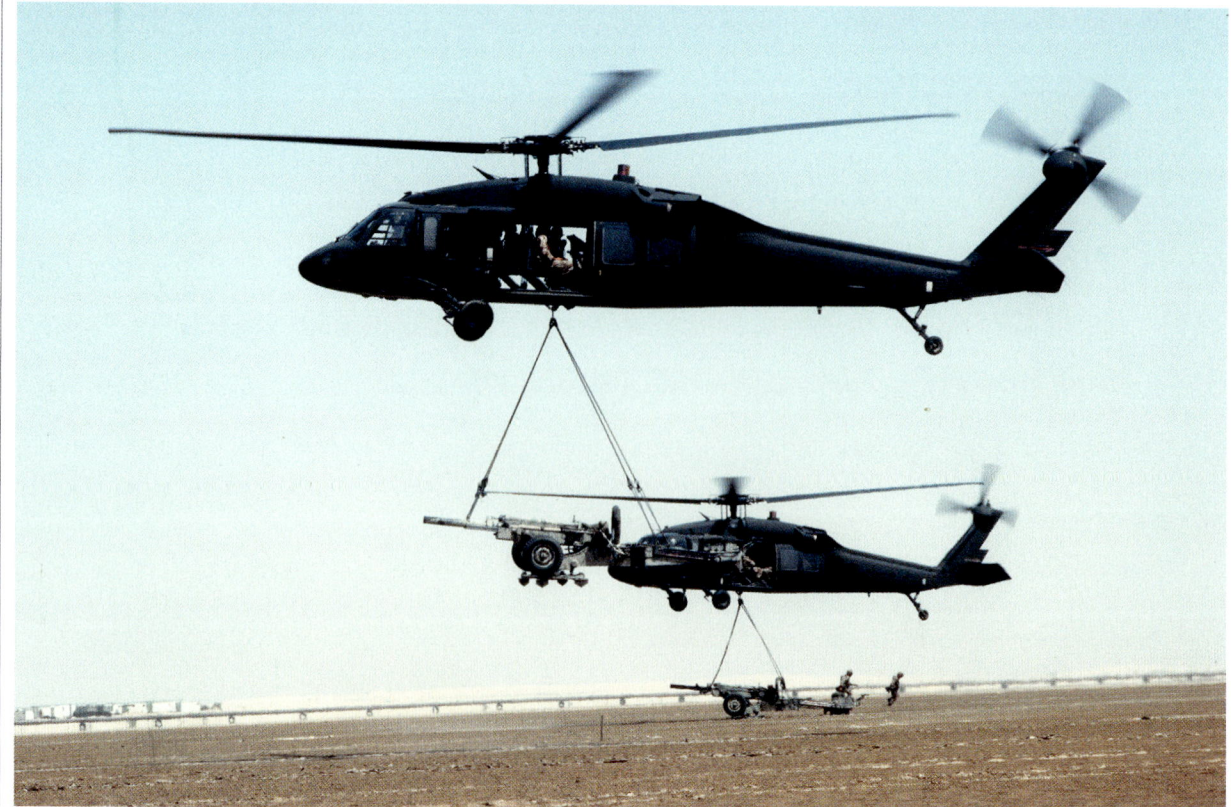

RIGHT: As VII Corps advanced, XVIII Airborne Corps moved deeper into the Euphrates valley to block the escape routes of the Iraqi Republican Guard. (US DOD/COMBAT CAMERA)

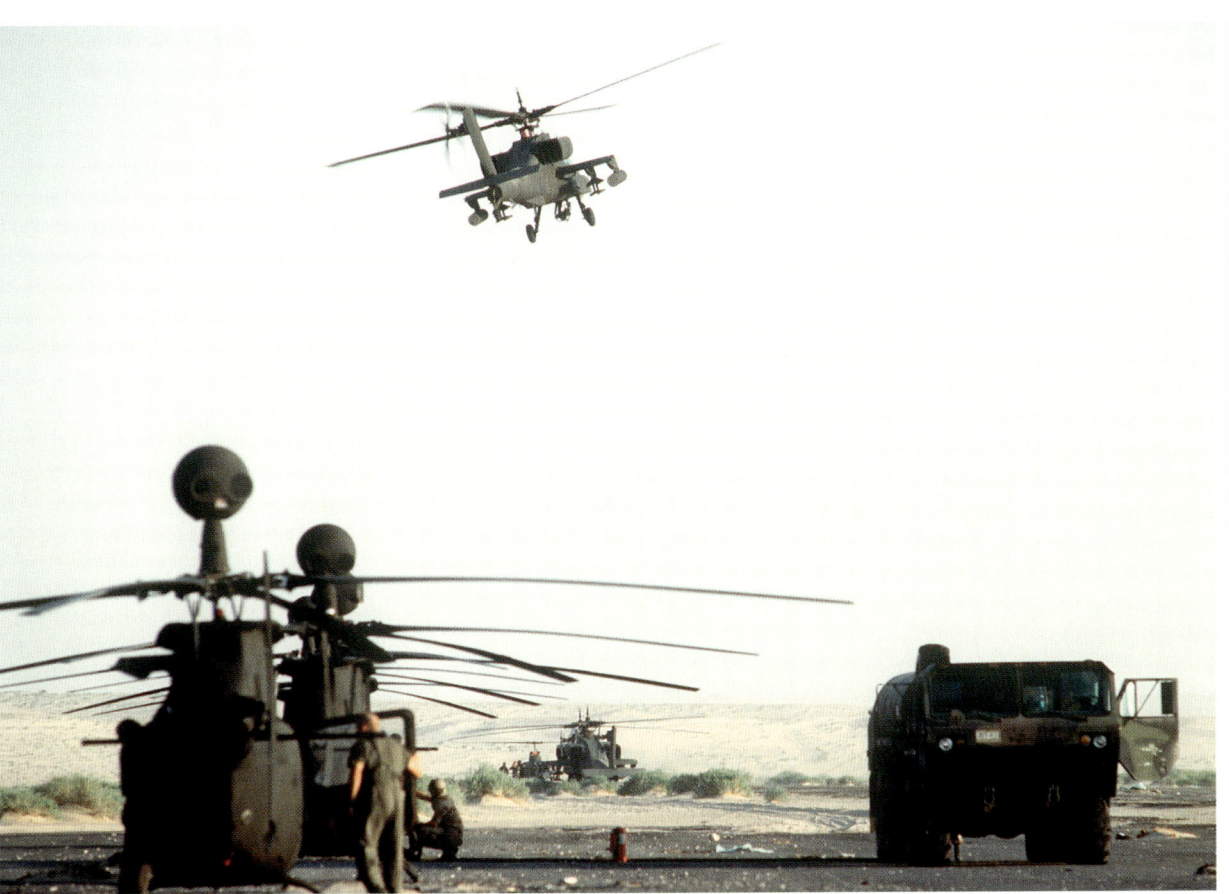

LEFT: Apache units of VII Corps flew around the clock to strike at Iraqi tank positions.
(US DOD/COMBAT CAMERA)

BELOW: Bridges across the Euphrates had been dropped by US air strikes, cutting off the Republican Guard as VII Corps approached.
(US DOD/COMBAT CAMERA)

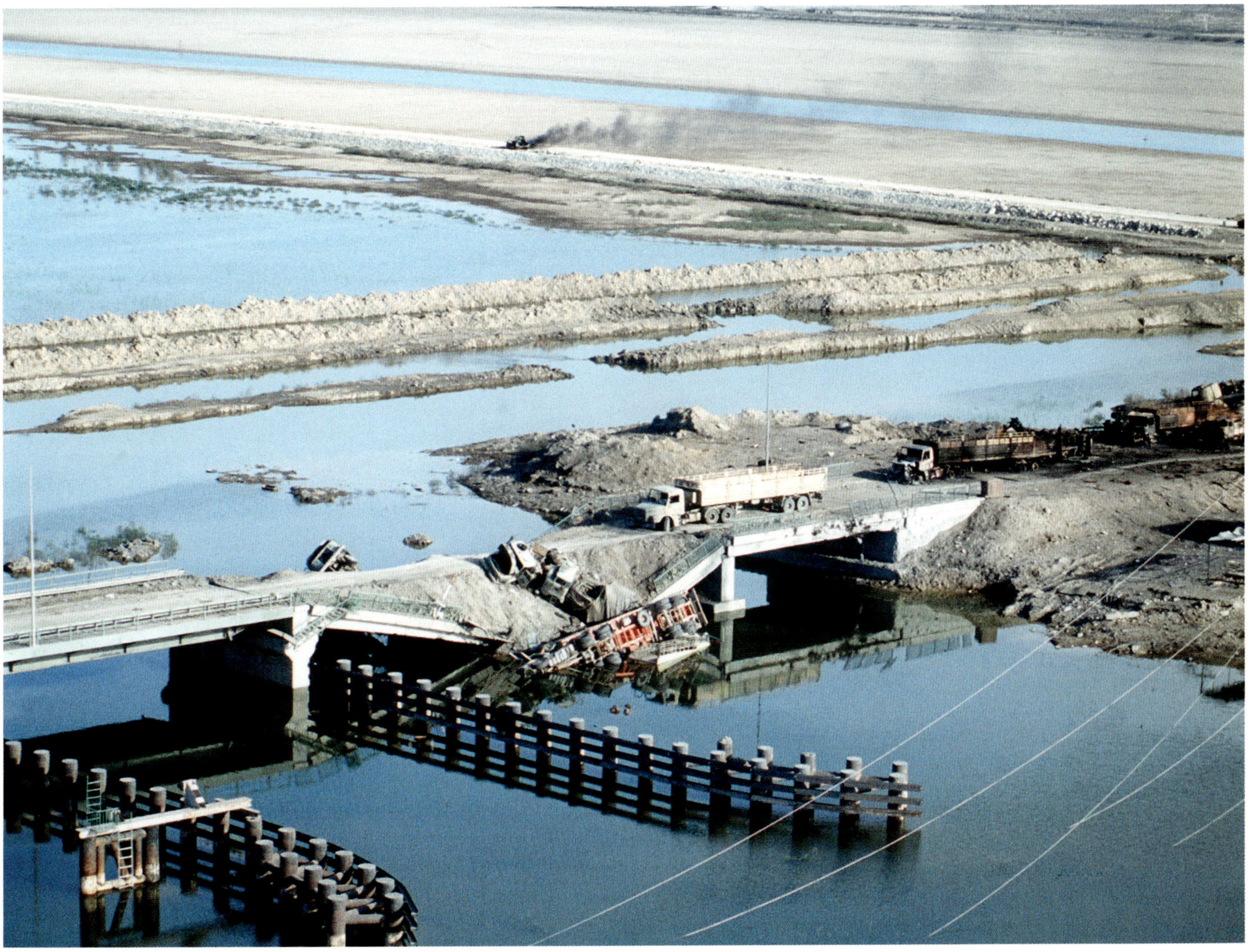

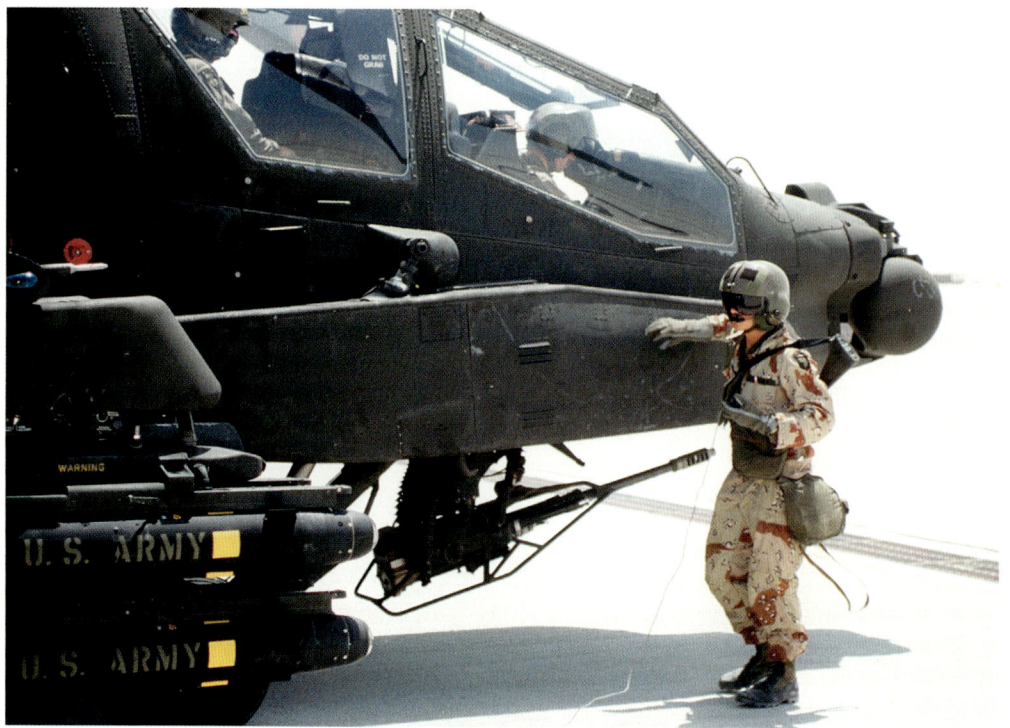

Apaches and Cobras to strike the Iraqi armoured column. By the time the engagement was over, 23 T-72, seven T-55, 65 armoured personnel carriers, 34 artillery pieces and more than 400 trucks were burning wrecks.

Operation Desert Storm was the first combat test of the AH-64A and the US AirLand Battle concept. In the aftermath of the war the US Army heaped praise on the Apache, crediting its AH-64A crews with the destruction of more than 500 tanks, 120 armoured personnel carriers, 30 air defence systems, 120 artillery pieces, 325 other vehicles 10 radar sites, 50 bunkers, 10 helicopters and other aircraft on the ground. Thanks to the AH-64A video recording systems these claims could be analysed extensively and were generally considered accurate. Overall, the coalition claimed to have destroyed or captured 3,000 Iraqi tanks, so the Apache's contribution to the victory was considerable.

The Hellfire missile combined with the TADS/PNVS night vision system on the AH-64A proved to be a winning combination. Apache crews could see and hit Iraqi tanks at ranges in excess of 5km. At these ranges Iraqi tank crews could not hear or see their attackers. The first sign they would have of the presence of American attack helicopters would be when the first Hellfire missile knocked out a nearby tank.

While US Army helicopters were undoubtedly superior to anything in the Iraqi arsenal, a key factor in the success of the Apaches and other

armed Westland Lynx AH1 attack helicopters of 4 Regiment Army Air Corps. Operating in co-operation with armoured reconnaissance units, it scouted ahead of the British division. On February 26, a Lynx of 654 Squadron AAC destroyed two MTLB armoured personnel carriers and four T-55 tanks using TOW missiles. That engagement was the first recorded combat use of that missile from a British helicopter.

With the calling of the ceasefire on the morning of February 28, US and coalition units halted their advance. The Iraqi army had been devastated by the coalition air offensive and the lighting advance during the '100 Hour' ground war. Iraq was now engulfed in revolution and Saddam Hussein tried to re-organise his shattered army to protect his regime. One Iraqi armoured unit tried to move along Highway 8 in the Euphrates valley on March 3 but it found the road blocked by the US 24th Division. This escalated into a major battle and the divisional commander called up his

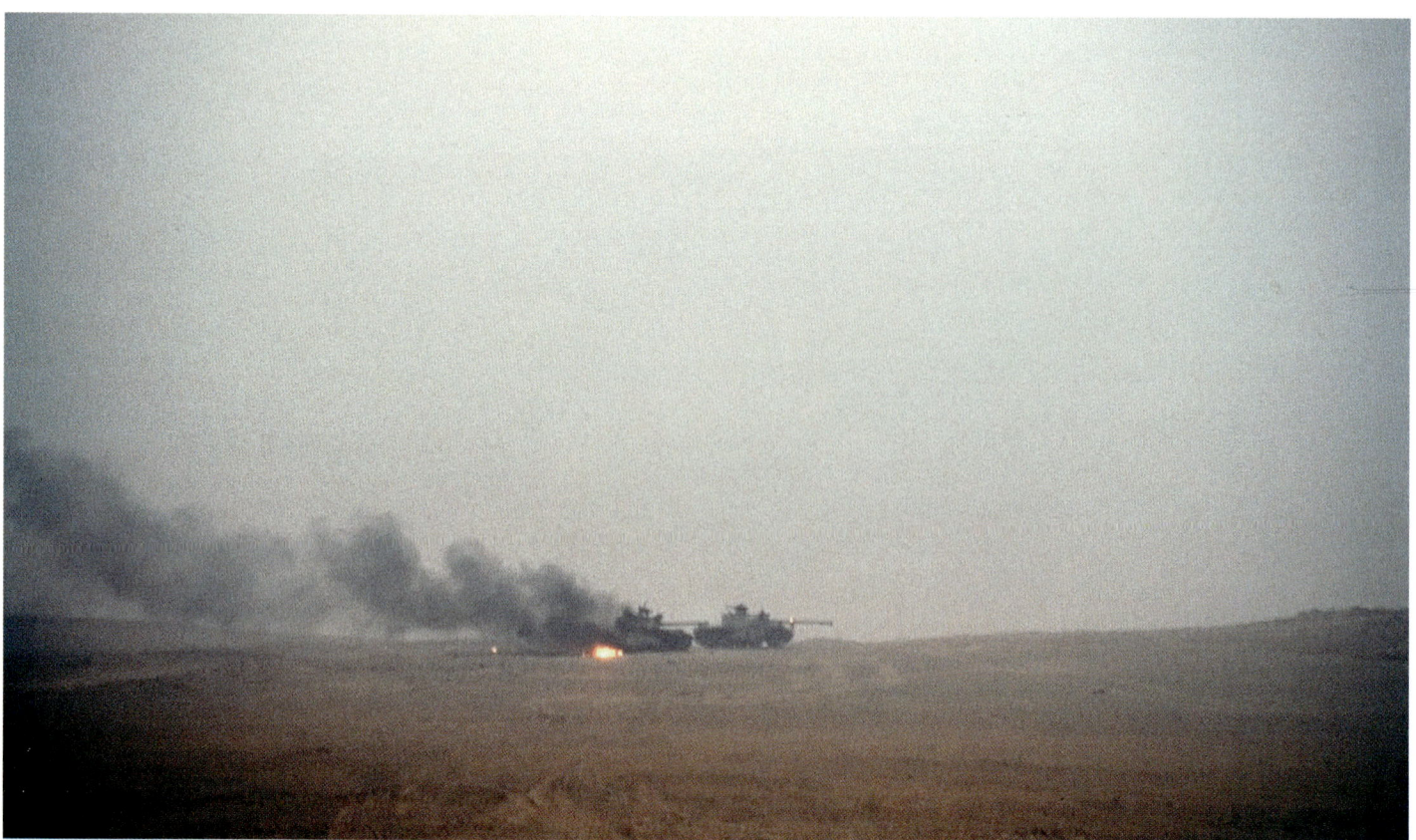

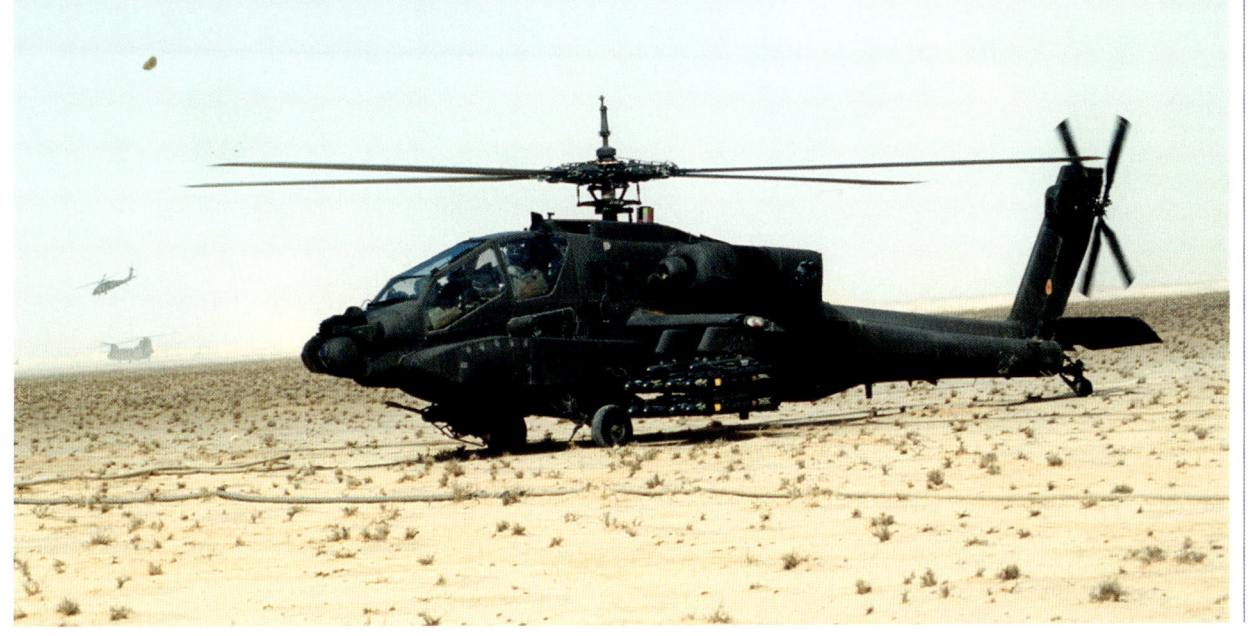

helicopters was the experience and expertise of the US Army's pilots and maintainers. Their ability to keep helicopters flying in dust storms at remote FOBs cannot be underestimated.

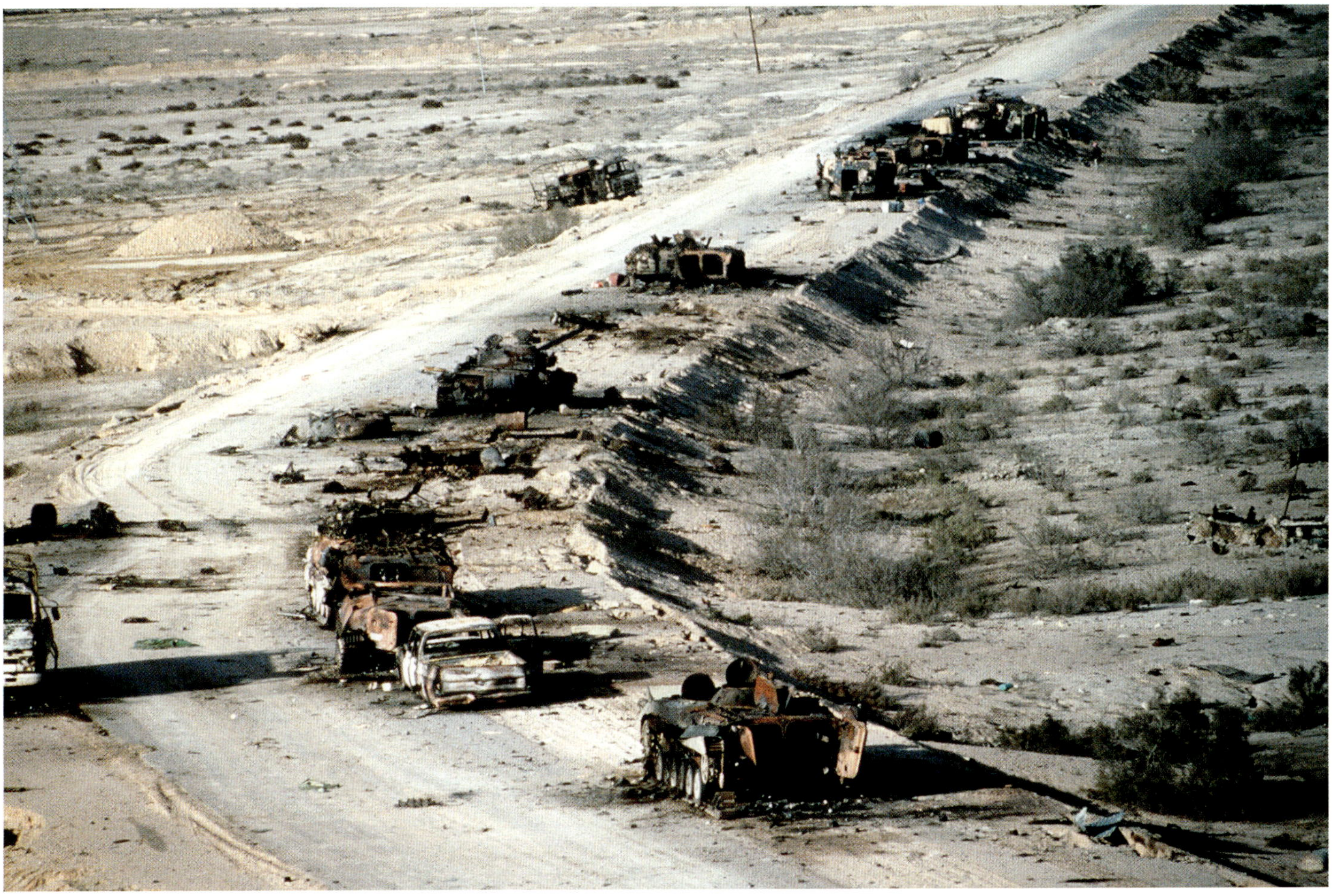

The US helicopters also proved remarkably robust, and they kept flying through terrible weather, as well as surviving enemy fire. Although dozens of US helicopters were hit by enemy fire, fewer than half a dozen were shot down and

destroyed. Almost all the damaged helicopters were returned to service. The US crews pushed their helicopters to the limit, and, after the war, the US Army had to launch a $276 million effort to repair and deep-clean more than 990 AH-64As, OH-58Ds, UH-60s and CH-47Ds.

In the wake of Operation Desert Storm, the US Army also launched major programmes to improve and upgrade all its helicopters. Several other armies started or accelerated

programmes to buy new attack helicopters. However, US Army aviators were very aware that the one-sided nature of the victory against the Iraqis did not mean that the Apache was an all-conquering wonder weapon. The coalition rapidly achieved air supremacy, the Iraqi ground-based air defence was poorly equipped and organised, and the open desert terrain made tank units very vulnerable. America's next enemy might not make victory so easy.

ABOVE: When a Republican Guard column tried to break through a roadblock of the US 24th Infantry Division it was devastated by AH-64A strikes. (US DOD/COMBAT CAMERA)

LEFT: AH-64As destroyed more than 500 Iraqi tanks and opened the road to victory by coalition forces. (US DOD/COMBAT CAMERA)

Whiskey Cobra Action

US Marine Aviators Strike Saddam's Army

RIGHT: Guns ready. A pair of AH-1W Cobras head for the action during the Battle of Khafji.
(US DOD/COMBAT CAMERA)

The Gulf War's Battle for Khafji in January 1991 saw the combat debut of the US Marine Corps' advanced version of the classic Cobra gunship, the AH-1W or Whiskey Cobra. This modernised version of the attack helicopter was vastly different from its Vietnam War-era predecessor and could fire more modern weapons, as well as featuring advanced sensors and avionics.

In response to Iraq's occupation of Kuwait in August 1990, the US mobilised an international coalition to protect Saudi Arabia. The US Marine Corps was in the forefront of the American response and deployed a powerful aviation contingent to provide the 1st Marine Expeditionary Force (1 MEF) with aerial firepower, battlefield mobility and surveillance.

Operating under the command of the 3rd Marine Air Wing (3 MAW), the USMC aviators were based ashore in Saudi Arabia with the assault troops, on the island of Bahrain and on US Navy warships in the northern Arabian Gulf.

Three USMC Cobra squadrons were part of this deployment, including the active-duty Marine Light Attack Helicopter Squadrons (HMLA) 367 and 369 with the new AH-1W and the legacy AH-1T/Js that were taken to

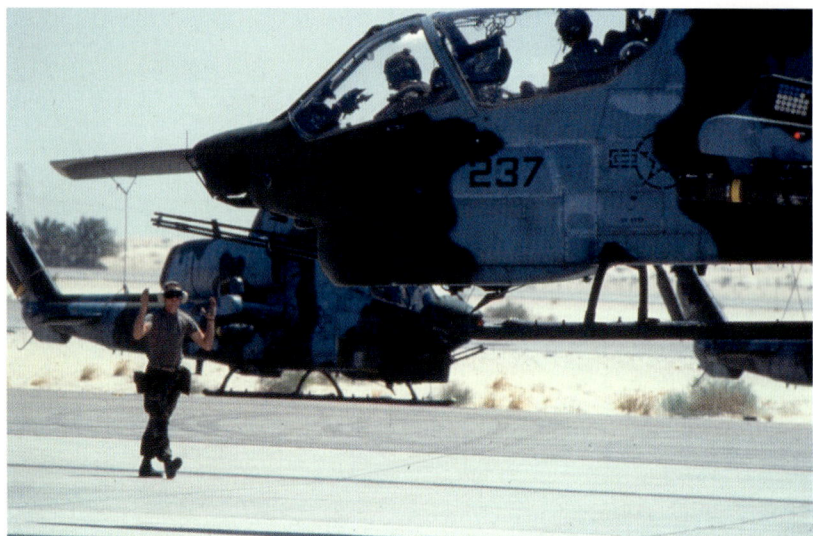

the Middle East by the reserve unit, Marine Attack Helicopter Squadron (HMA) 77.

The Cobra force was split between units operating ashore and others designated to support the operation from amphibious landing ships in the Arabian Gulf. These afloat forces were meant to divert Iraqi attention from US Army operations to build up its armoured forces and flank the main Iraqi force inside Kuwait. They also functioned as reserve that could reinforce the ashore forces of the 1st Marine Division.

To provide close air support, 39 AH-1W/T/Js Cobra helicopter gunships were available to 3 MAW from shore bases. Troop transport ashore in Saudi Arabia was conducted by 60 CH-46E Sea Knights, or Frogs, and there were 30 utility UH-1N Hueys and 53 CH-53D/Es Sea Stallions on hand to move heavy cargo. Operating on US Navy warships in the Gulf were a further 18 AH-1W/T/Js, 20 UH-1Ns, 60 CH-46Es and 22 CH-53Es.

USMC Cobra gunships got their first taste of action during the Battle

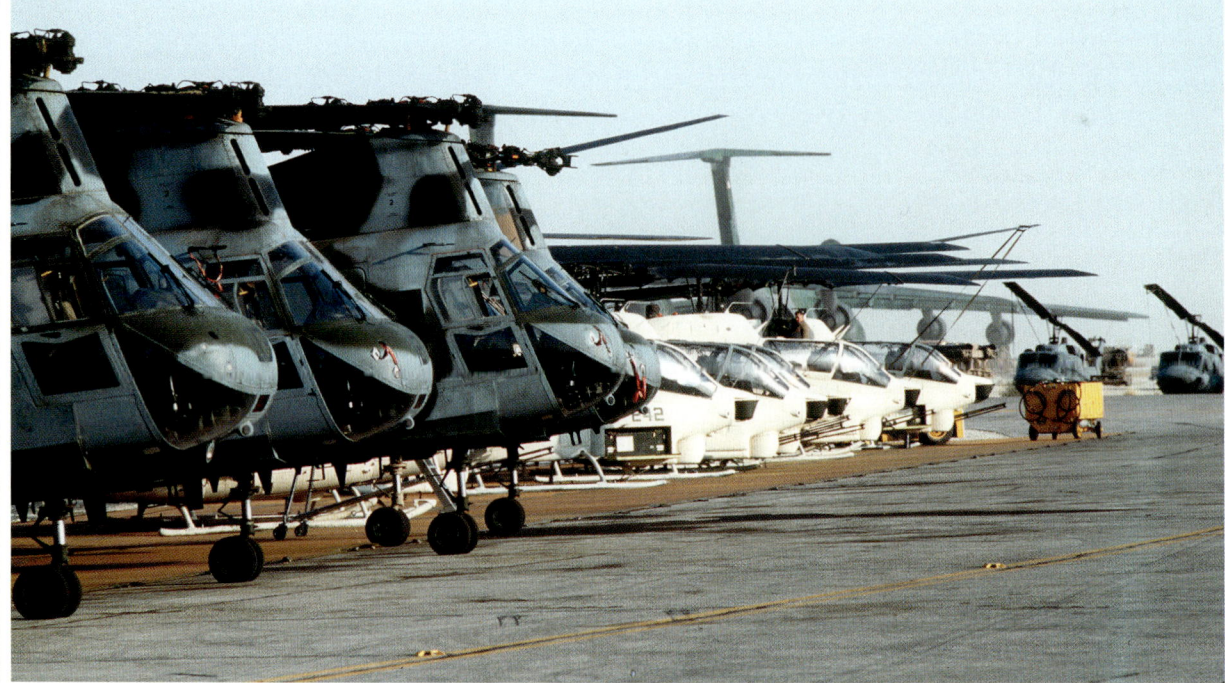

RIGHT: US Marine Corps CH-46E Sea Knights, AH-1W Cobras and UH-1Ns being unloaded from USAF transport aircraft at Dhahran air base during the Desert Shield build up.
(US DOD/COMBAT CAMERA)

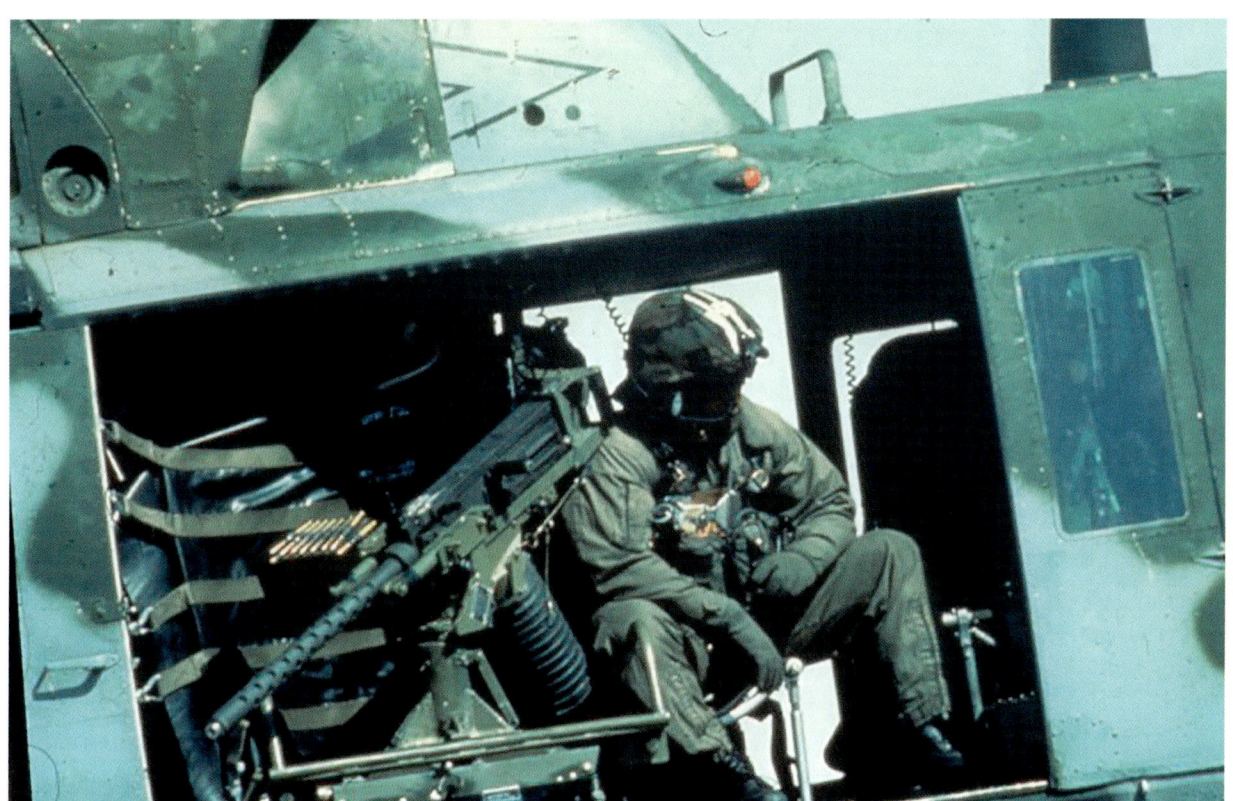

for Khafji when they were sent to confront Iraqi tank units. The Saudi town of Khafji was just south of the border with Kuwait and in January 1991 a garrison of Saudi troops was positioned to protect it and a nearby oil refinery from Iraqi attack. After the start of the coalition air offensive on January 17, the Saudi troops were on high alert and the USMC sent forward small air-naval gunfire liaison teams to co-ordinate the provision of artillery and air support in case the Iraqis moved south. Other USMC ground reconnaissance units in light armoured vehicles patrolled out in the desert along the border with Kuwait.

US Marine air support for Khafji fell on the Cobras of HMLA 369, commanded by Lieutenant Colonel Michael Kurth, and HMLA 367, commanded by Lieutenant Colonel Terry Frerker. Due to special arrangements with the US Air Component Command, the USMC helicopters were assigned to exclusively support I MEF so its Cobras were able to respond rapidly to the Iraqi offensive.

Eight AH-1W Cobras based at a forward operating site at al-Mishab responded to initial calls from the US Marines, ensuring that the Iraqi advance into Khafji, which kicked off on January 29, did not go.

According to the official USMC history of the battle, not long after 1.00am on January 30, a flight of four Cobras from Kurth's squadron, led by Major Michael L Steele, engaged in a gun duel with six Iraqi armoured »

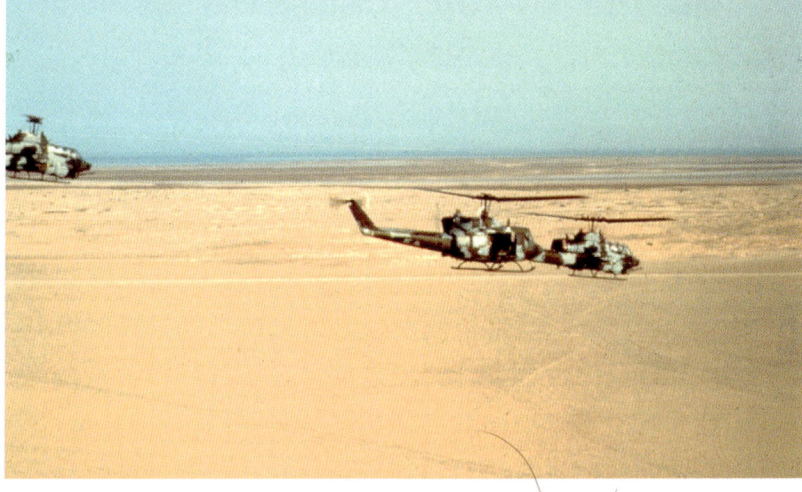

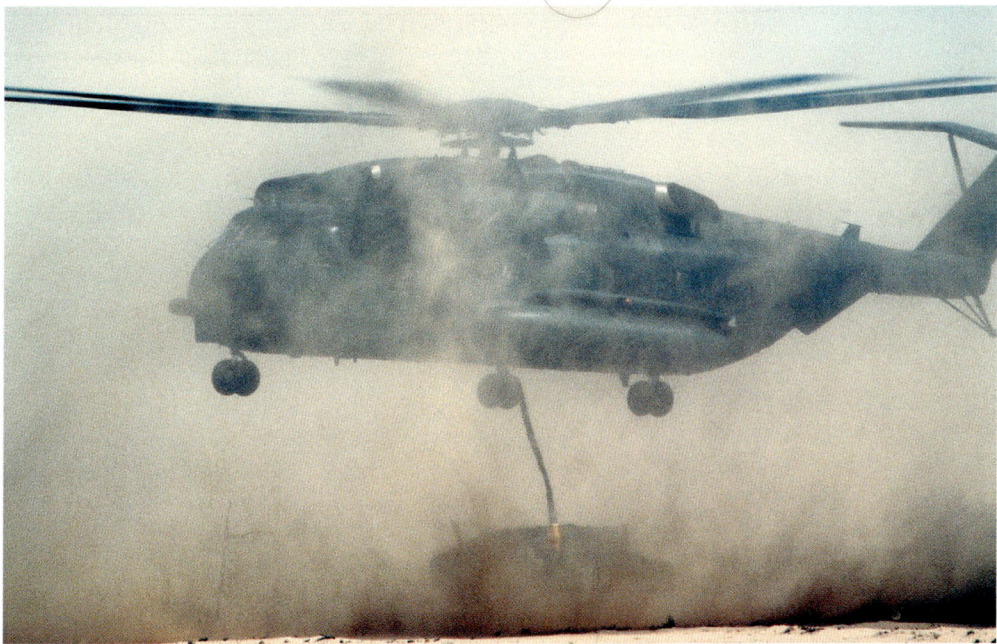

RIGHT: Desert Storm air assault – marine style. An air assault rehearsal in December 1990. The 3rd Marine Air Wing conducted one large scale air assault into Kuwait during the 100-hour ground war to deliver a US Marine Corps battalion behind Iraqi lines. (US DOD/COMBAT CAMERA)

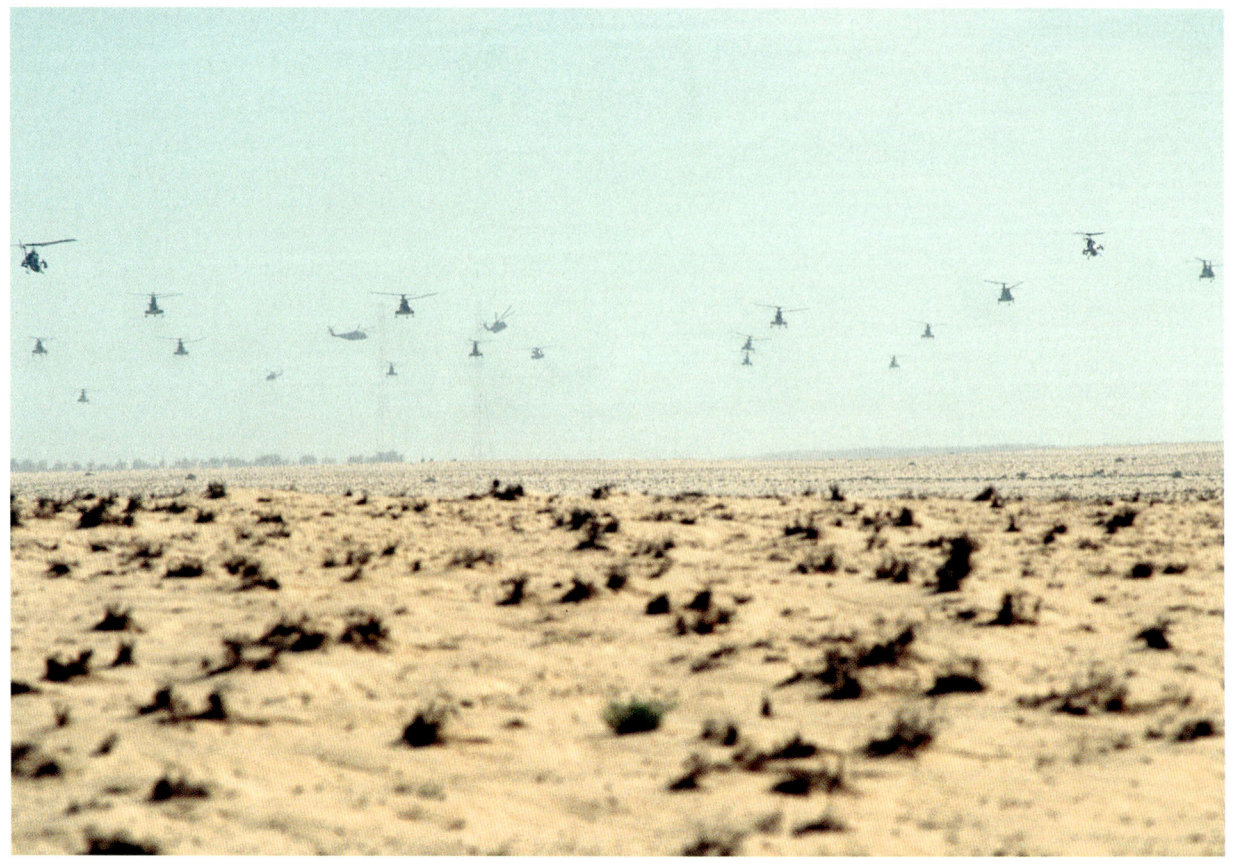

BELOW LEFT: US Marine Corps helicopter units set up forward operating bases in towns in northern Saudi Arabia to be ready to react to any Iraqi incursions. (US DOD/COMBAT CAMERA)

BELOW RIGHT: Extended-range border patrols were flown by the AH-1W with CH-53E Sea Stallions providing deployable refuelling support. (US DOD/COMBAT CAMERA)

personnel carriers on the coast road, pitting the helicopters' 20mm Gatling guns and 2.75mm rockets against the armoured personnel carriers' 73mm main guns.

Two AH-1Ws from Frerker's squadron, led by Major Gary Shaw, had an even more hair-raising experience. Launching from al-Mishab to provide air support to a Saudi army observation post on the border, the USMC helicopters found themselves circling and waiting for a forward air controller to provide them with targets. Eager to support the Marines on the ground, they overstayed their fuel limits and had to attempt to reach the US logistics base at Kibrit, only to find themselves flying over an Iraqi armoured column which fired on them. They then attempted to

divert back to al-Mishab, but their navigation equipment malfunctioned and they landed instead at the al-Khafji oil refinery. This was a stroke of luck. They refuelled their aircraft from the refinery's supplies as the Iraqis marched into the city. This unconventional refuelling worked well and they were able to return to their home base.

Another flight of Cobras, led by Captain Randall Hammond, engaged, and destroyed four T-62 tanks during the battle. When nine Iraqi soldiers waved white flags and indicated they wished to surrender, the pilots used their helicopters to "round 'em up like cattle" until US Marines on the ground could secure the prisoners. Iraqi artillery fire forced the two Cobras to withdraw but not before one Cobra destroyed

a final T-62 with a wire-guided missile. The explosion caused "its turret to flip upside down and land on the open hole like a tiddlywink," Captain Hammond later recalled.

During January 30, Saudi forces, and their supporting US Marines' Cobras of HMLA 367 continued to try to contain the Iraqi tank units along the frontier and in Khafji, with the helicopter squadron reporting one tank, seven armoured personnel carriers, one jeep and one truck destroyed by TOW missiles.

The next battle raged through the southern half of Khafji on January 31, as Saudi troops backed by US airpower launched a counter-attack. USMC McDonnell Douglas AV-8B Harriers and AH-1Ws provided direct support to the Saudi and Qatari troops, with the air-naval

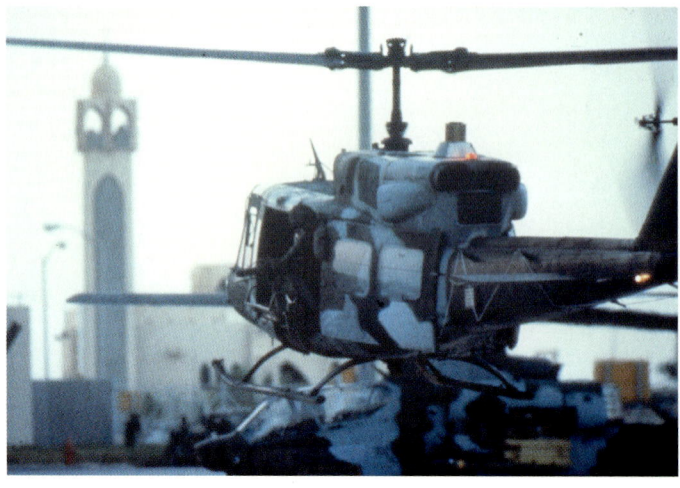

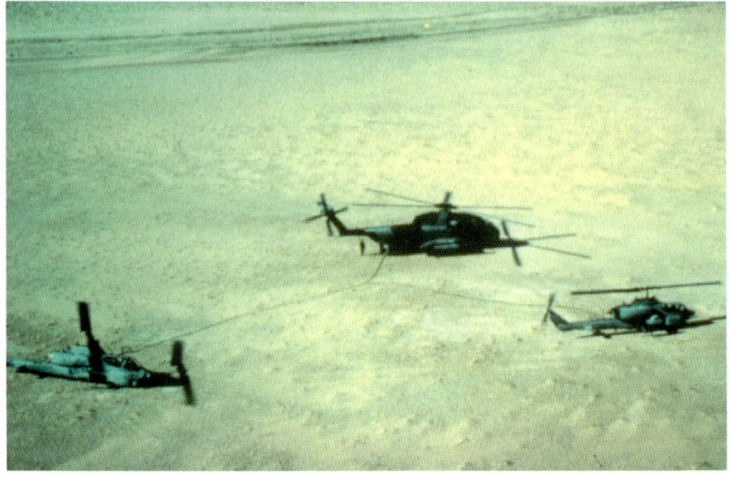

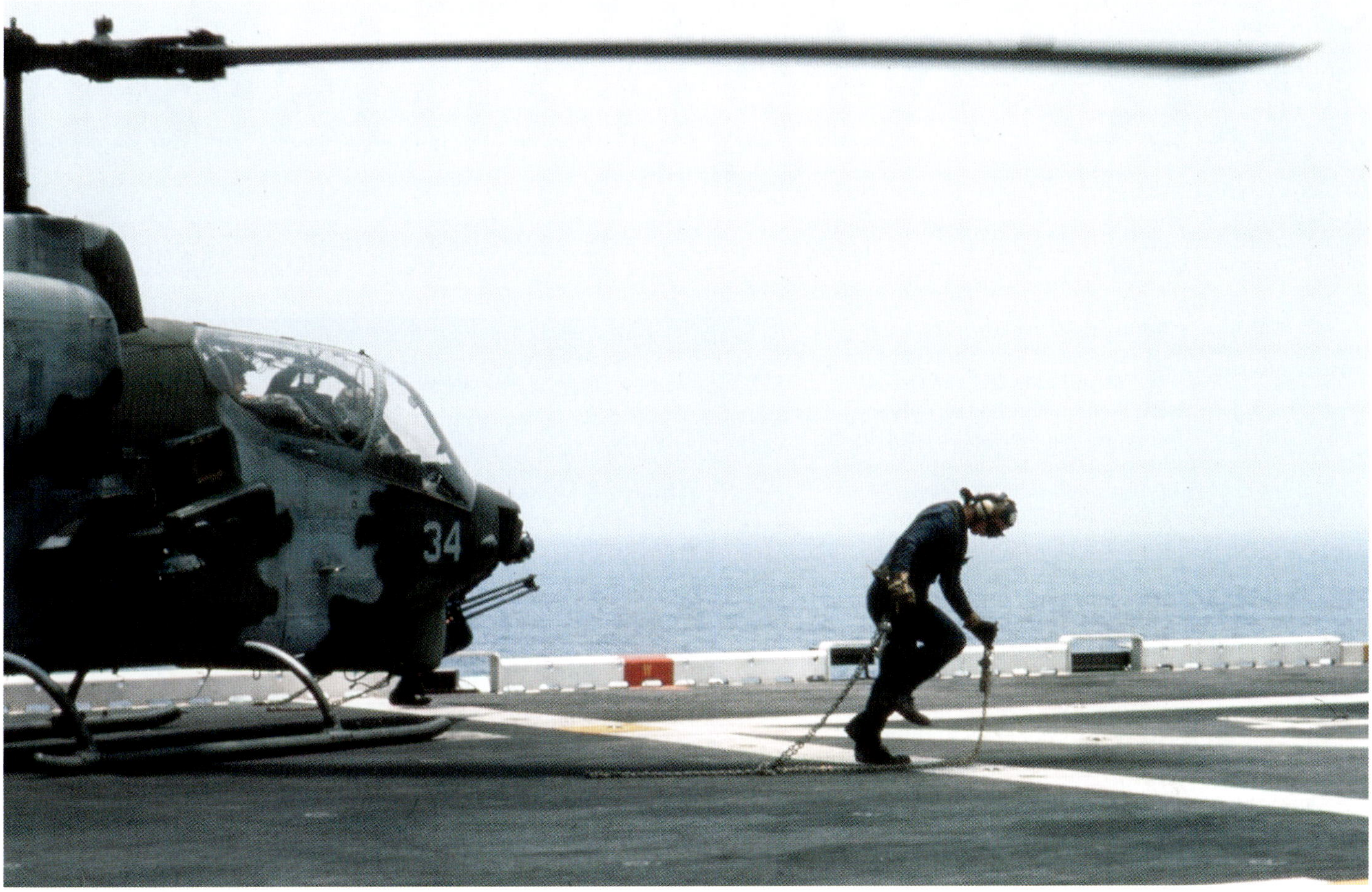

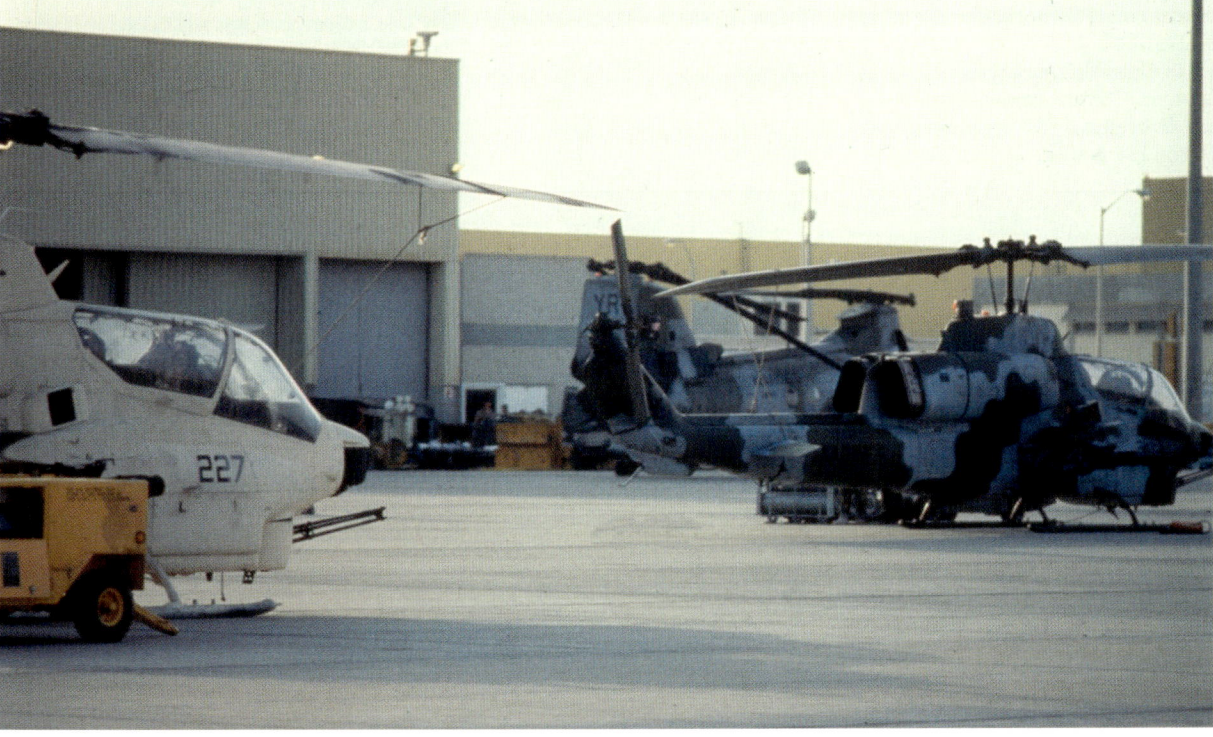

ABOVE: Cobras operated from the USS *Nassau* in the Arabian Gulf as part of the coalition deception plan to make the Iraqis think a massive amphibious landing would take place in Kuwait. This kept the Iraqis guessing where the main US land assault would actually take place.
(US DOD/COMBAT CAMERA)

LEFT: The AH-1W proved to be robust and highly effective in multiple engagements during Operation Desert Storm.
(US DOD/COMBAT CAMERA)

gunfire teams directing the Cobras in a strafing run against the town's water tower. Harriers destroyed Iraqi vehicles at the major road intersection in one quarter of the city.

By the following afternoon the Iraqis had been pushed back to Kuwait. US airpower had been decisive in breaking the Iraqi resistance and the AH-1W had passed its first combat test with flying colours, engaging Iraqi tanks at long range with TOW missiles.

When the 1 MEF started its offensive into Kuwait on February 24, the Cobras flew top cover for the advancing US Marines. The Iraqis were soon in full retreat. By the time the 100-hour ground war was over, the AH-1Ws had flown 1,273 sorties with no losses. In Operation Desert Storm, the AH-1W was credited with destroying 97 tanks, 104 armoured personnel carriers and other vehicles and two anti-aircraft artillery positions.

Into Afghanistan

Operation Enduring Freedom 2001

RIGHT: AH-1Ws fly top cover for a USMC convoy heading out of FOB Rhino. (US DOD/COMBAT CAMERA)

In the aftermath of the 9/11 attacks on New York and Washington DC, the United States unleashed its military power on Afghanistan to hunt down the mastermind of the atrocities, Osama bin Laden and his Al Qaeda organisation. Before the man hunt could begin in earnest, the US military had to defeat Afghanistan's Taliban regime, which was giving sanctuary to the terrorist mastermind. After several weeks of air and cruise missile strikes, by November 2001 the US military was poised to put boots on the ground in the central Asian country to establish the first American base on Afghan soil. Small groups of US Army Special Forces had previously entered Afghanistan to mobilise rebel fighters against the Taliban, but it was only a matter of time before large combat forces would be needed to complete the victory.

US Central Command chief, General Tommy Franks, had massed a contingent of US Marines, dubbed Naval Expeditionary Task Force 58, off the coast of Pakistan on board the amphibious warships USS *Peleliu* and USS *Bataan,* to be ready to pounce should an opportunity arise.

With the military situation in southern Afghanistan appearing to be moving more favourably in the last week of November, General Franks decided the time was ripe to introduce US combat forces into the region. Task Force 58's mission commenced with Objective Rhino operations to seize Camp Rhino, an old dirt airstrip in the desert to the east of the Taliban capital, Kandahar. Six US Marine Corps

CH-53Es – three each from the 15th and 26th Marine Expeditionary Units (MEUs) – carrying more than 200 US Marines, launched from the USS *Peleliu.* The first three helicopters conducted night aerial refuelling with USMC Lockheed KC-130R Hercules tankers en route to the objective, 350 nautical miles away from the ships in the northern Arabian Sea. The three helicopters in the second wave had difficulty conducting aerial refuelling but pressed on. The first CH-53Es flown by crews from Marine Medium Helicopter Squadron (HMM) 163 were the first aircraft in the landing zone and delivered the first US conventional troops safely onto Afghan soil.

According to the USMC official history of the operation, the first flight of aircraft lifted from the USS *Peleliu* around 4.15pm on November 25 and headed inland. Led by Major William Bufkin II, the escort force included four Bell AH-1W Cobras and three Bell UH-1N Huey helicopters.

As the first assault division was exiting their fuelling track, just

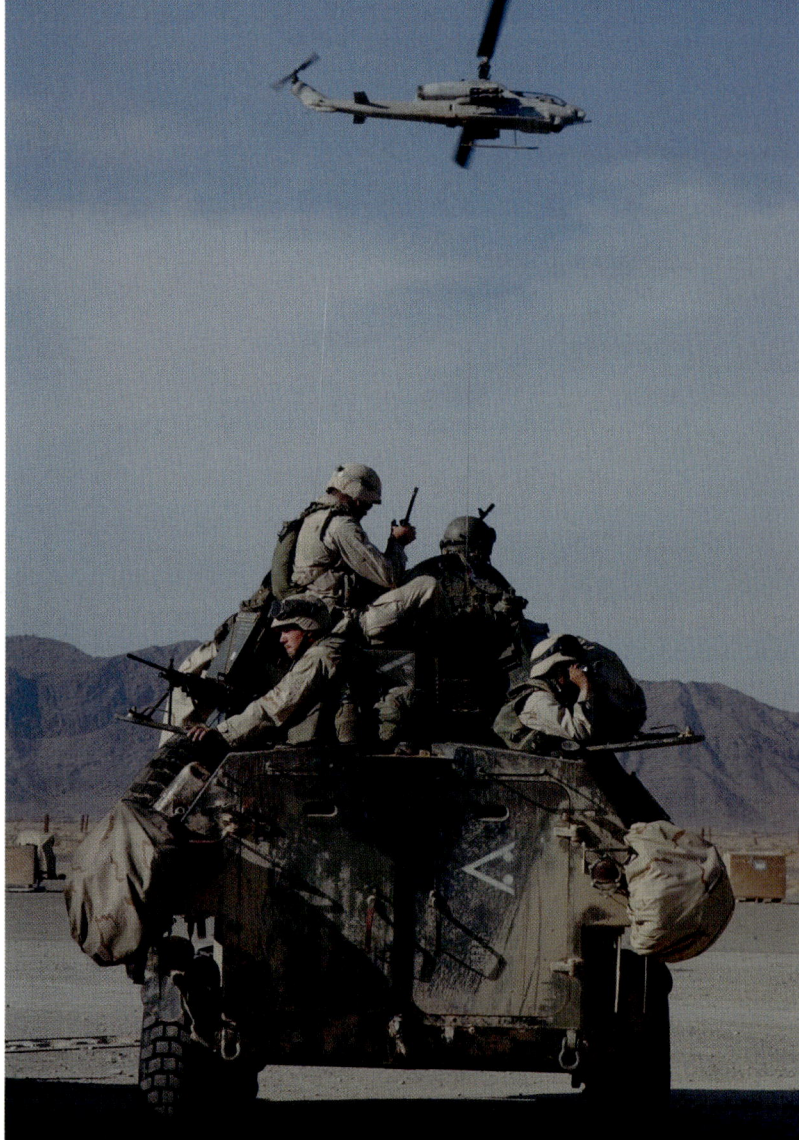

BELOW: The devastating 9/11 attacks on New York and Washington DC prompted President George W Bush to order US troops to strike Afghanistan and hunt down the Al Qaeda network's bases. (US DOD/COMBAT CAMERA)

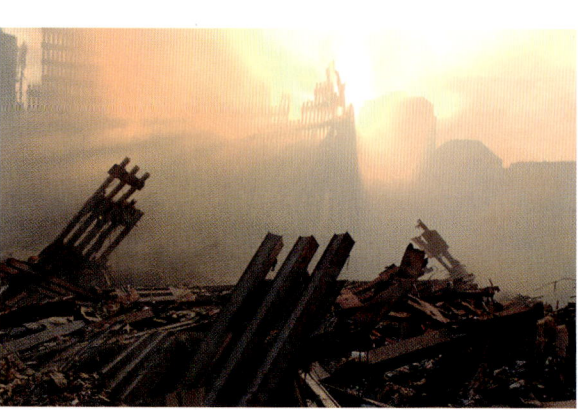

five miles south of the border, the escort force were flying in formation. They flew in staggered waves – two Cobras, three Hueys and then two more Cobras clearing the remaining 92-mile path into Camp Rhino. The escort force had first headed toward Shamsi in Pakistan to refuel at a US-controlled airstrip, before continuing toward the objective area. The assault force headed toward a 57-mile long helicopter aerial refuelling track established just south of the Afghan border to take on fuel from USMC Lockheed KC-130K Hercules tankers.

As the assault force crossed the border behind the Cobras, the moonlit terrain shifted from low mountains to flat desert, and the speeding aircraft rose from 75 to 200 feet above sea level to compensate for the decrease in visual contrast. The crews also conducted penetration checks, switching off unnecessary devices that produced illumination or emitted an electronic signature, to decrease the likelihood of premature detection during the final leg of their journey. As the assault element approached the abandoned airfield, visible two miles in the distance, the escort flight leader relayed confirmation that the runway remained clear of hostile forces by passing the radio code word 'Winter'.

After more than four hours in the air, the first flight of CH-53 helicopters and their Cobra escorts began to descend towards the landing zone at

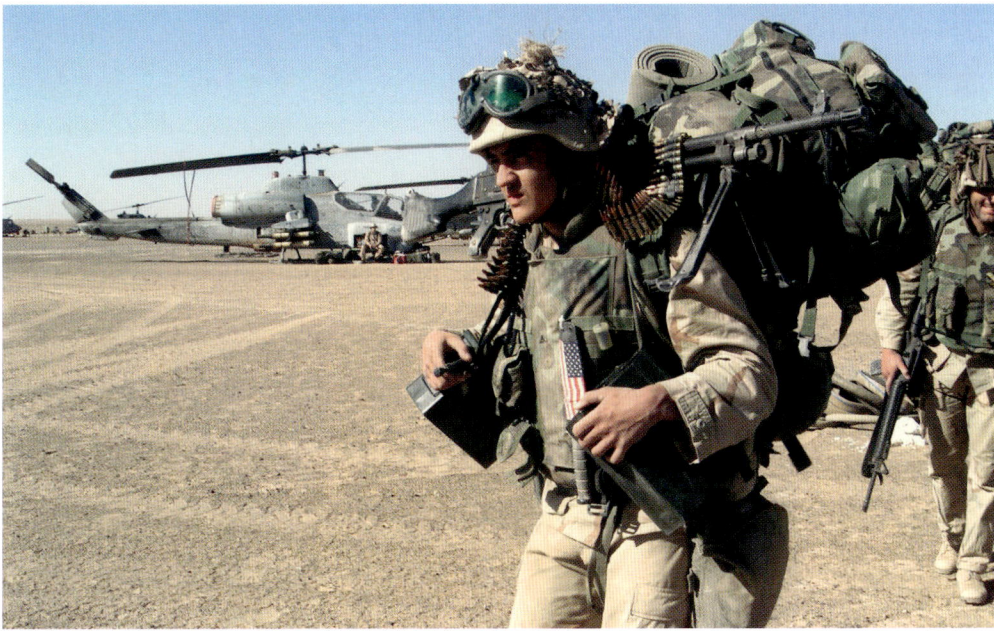

10 minute intervals, guided to their destination by flashing infrared strobe lights that the SEALs had placed in the middle of the dirt runway. Due to severe brownout conditions – thick, towering dust clouds stirred up by the aircrafts' spinning rotor blades – several of the pilots were forced to approach the runway several times before successfully landing. The Huey and Cobra helicopters began to take up positions along the airfield where they remained on a 15-minute strip alert. In a classic case of understatement, a

Captain Fallon later remarked, "It was a fairly busy 30, 40 minutes until the second wave hit the deck".

The helicopters were met by a US Navy SEAL reconnaissance team that had been inserted on November 21 to keep the airstrip under surveillance. A US Navy Lockheed P-3C Orion AIP aircraft provided continual Intelligence, Surveillance and Reconnaissance (ISR) coverage around the US Marines throughout the night and on all subsequent nights. At the same time, a USAF Northrop Grumman E-8C Joint ❯❯

ABOVE: US Marines escorted by AH-1Ws arrived at FOB Rhino to establish the first US base in Afghanistan. (US DOD/COMBAT CAMERA)

BELOW: CH-53E Sea Stallions were refuelled in mid-air as they transported the first wave of US Marines to Objective Rhino. (US DOD/COMBAT CAMERA)

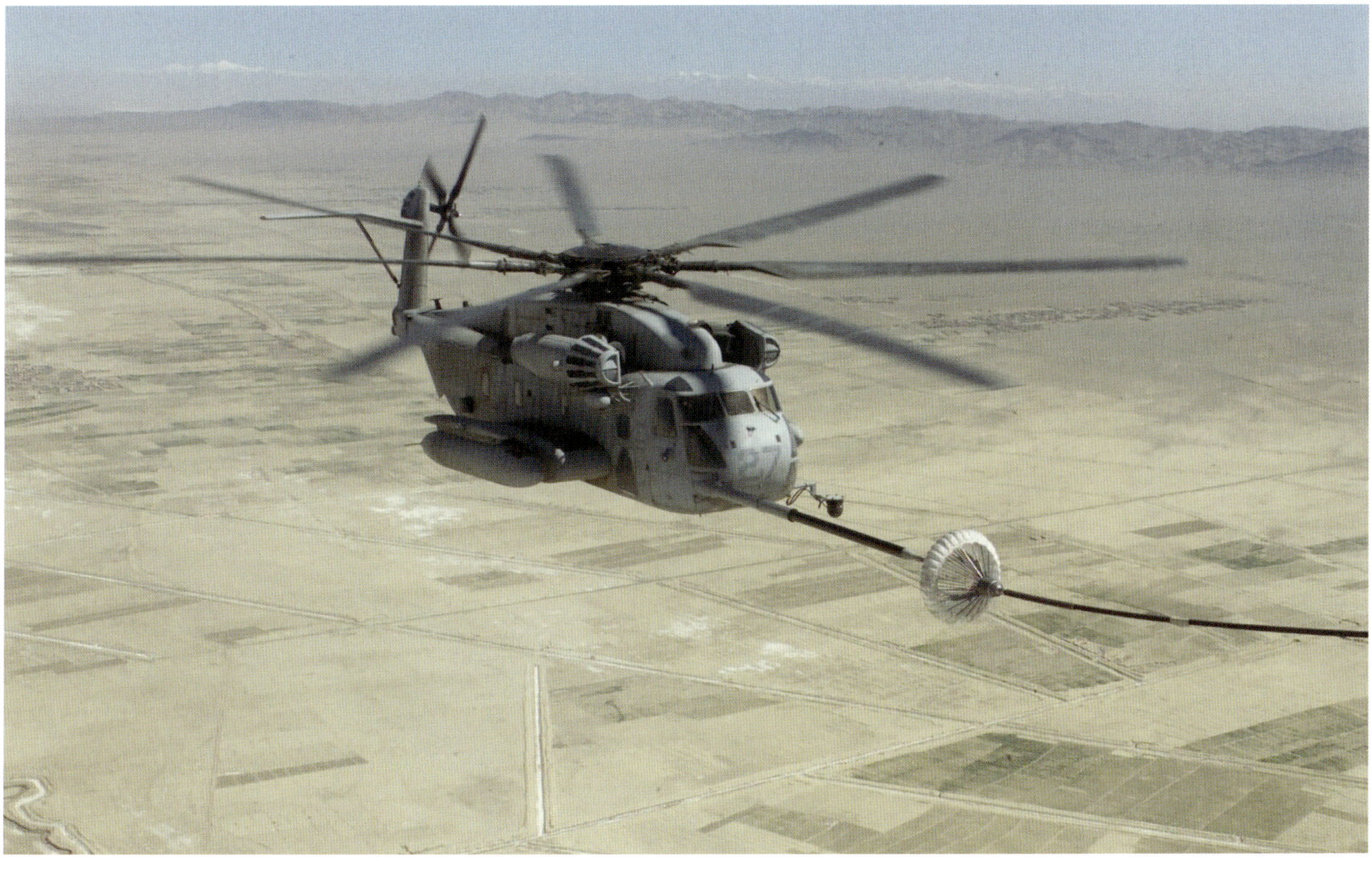

RIGHT: AH-1Ws launched from the USS *Peleliu* were the first US attack helicopters to operate over Afghanistan.
(US DOD/COMBAT CAMERA)

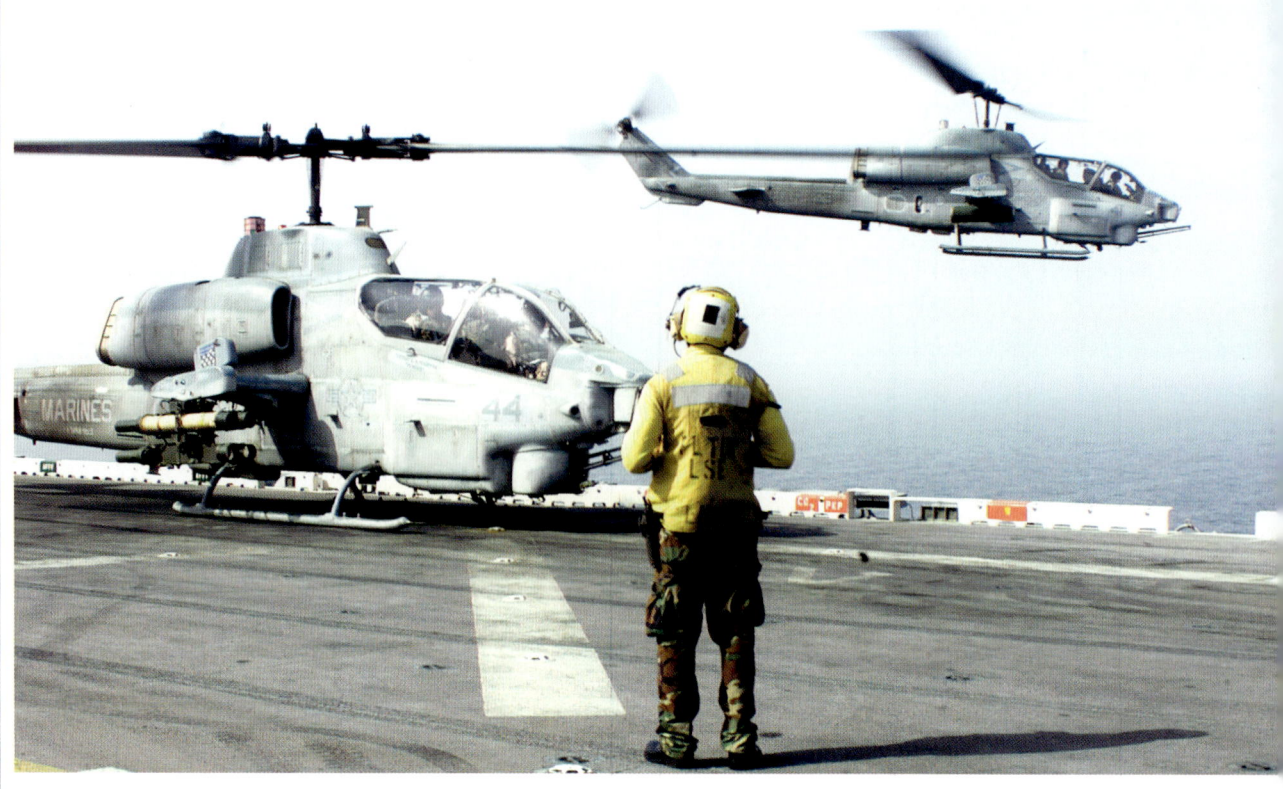

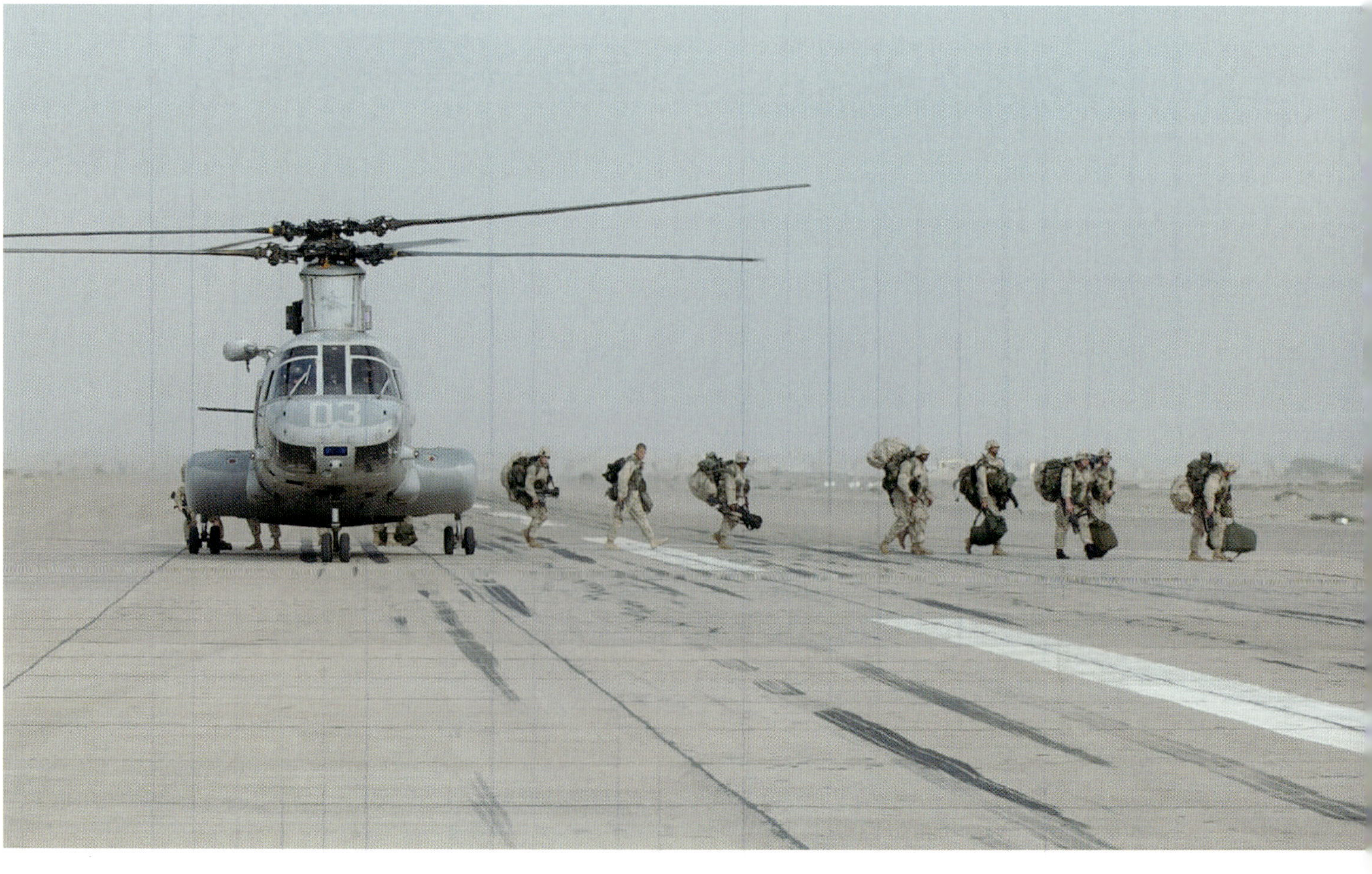

BELOW: More waves of US Marines followed on CH-46E Sea Knights in the days after the establishment of FOB Rhino.
(US DOD/COMBAT CAMERA)

STARS surveillance aircraft provided wide-area surveillance with its radars, which could detect vehicle movement over hundreds of square miles of desert.

The operation was a tour de force of power projection operations. Once Camp Rhino's runway was lit by USAF Special Tactics Squadron (STS) personnel and declared KC-130 capable, additional troops flew in on USMC KC-130s from the US air base at Jacobabad in Pakistan, where they had been pre-positioned. The first KC-130 to land on the dirt airstrip was flown by a VMGR-352 detachment aircrew, landing an hour and a half after the insert of the assault force.

The following day a Northrop Grumman E-8A JSTARS radar surveillance aircraft detected several Taliban armoured vehicles to the northwest of Camp Rhino. After Airborne-Forward Air Controllers in

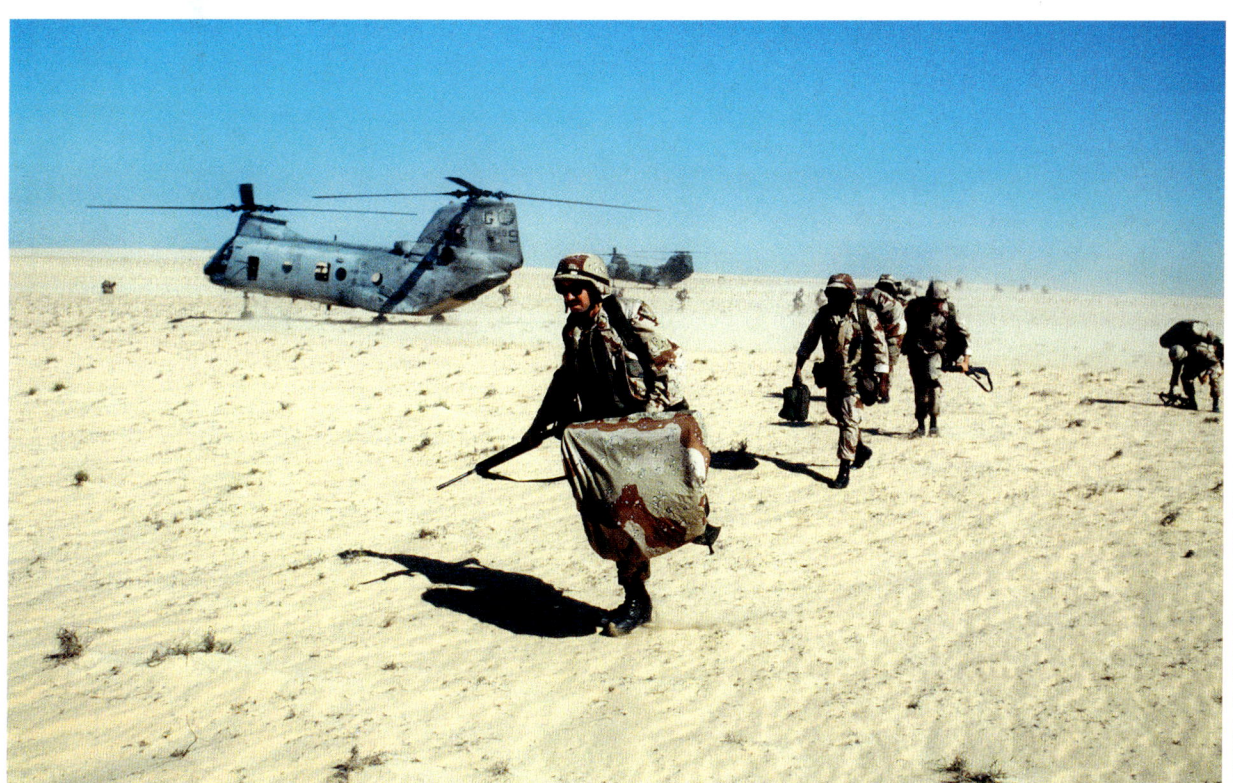

Grumman F-14 Tomcat fighter jets had confirmed their identity, more F-14s from the USS *Theodore Roosevelt* and AH-1Ws flying from the newly renamed Forward Operating Base (FOB) Rhino, were called to attack the column.

The Marine aircrews included Captains John Barranco and David Steele, who were piloting the first aircraft with the call sign Evil Eye 34, and Captains Kristian Pfeiffer and Richard Lawson, who were piloting the second Cobra call signed Evil Eye 35. The Cobras headed toward the convoy and at the E-8As' request helped coordinate the attack, watching as the Tomcats engaged the armoured personnel carriers. After the US Navy fighters had completed their bombing run, striking just in front of the lead armoured personnel carrier and disabling it, the Marines took their turn. Emerging from behind a nearby ridge the Cobras used their 20mm cannon and rockets to engage the two armoured vehicles and eight to ten dismounted personnel.

Captain Barranco later described the attack, saying: "At least some of the Taliban were out of the vehicles. I'm guessing they thought they hit a mine since the F-14s were so high. They heard us and some of them started firing wildly in the air toward the sound of the Cobras – the rest started running. We made several passes destroying the vehicles and killing the squad. Passing back over the convoy, the pilots used their night-vision goggles and infrared sensors to assess the battle damage but

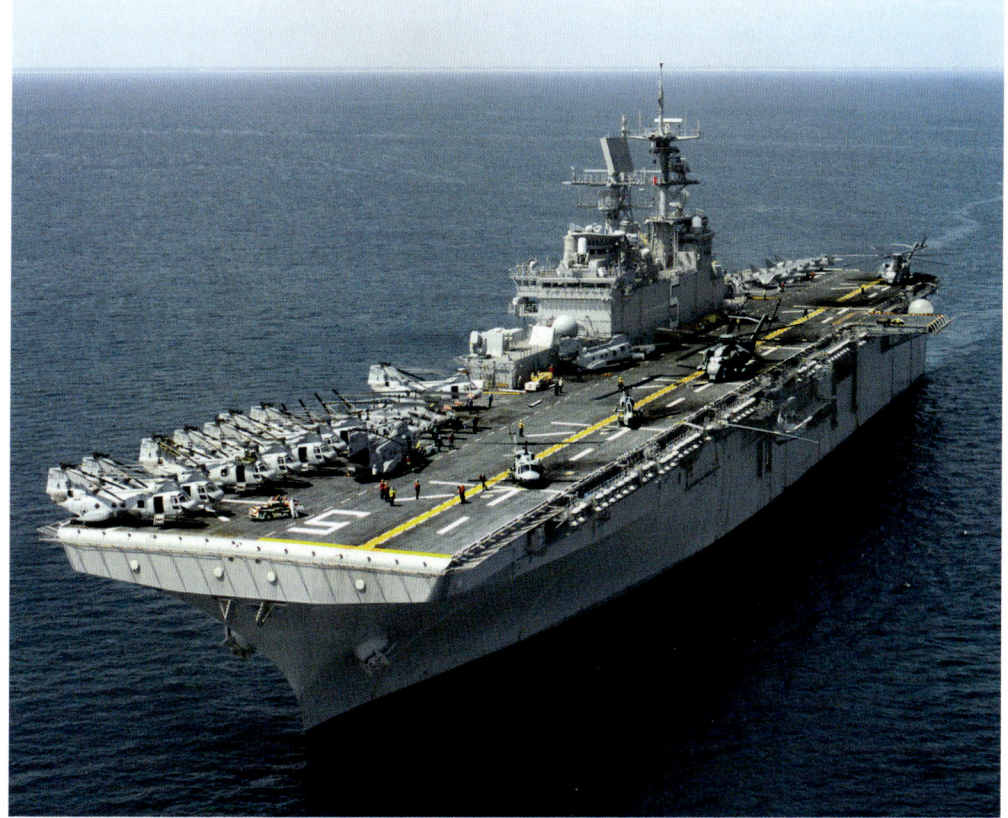

determined that nothing of military value was left."

The first wave of Boeing C-17 Globemaster aircraft arrived at FOB Rhino on 28th November, transporting SEABEES from Naval Mobile Construction Battalion (NMCB) 133 to begin improving the condition of the airstrip to allow it take sustained air operations. By this point over 1,000 US Marines were ashore in Afghanistan and were ready to start offensive operations.

Naval Expeditionary Task Force 58

USS *Peleliu* Amphibious Ready Group [*Peleliu* ARG]
15th Marine Expeditionary Unit Special Operations Capable [15th MEU SOC]
 • Battalion Landing Team 1/1 [BLT 1/1]
 • Marine Medium Helicopter Squadron 163 [HMM-163]
 • MEU Service Support Group 15 [MSSG 15]

USS *Bataan* Amphibious Ready Group [*Bataan* ARG]
 • 26th Marine Expeditionary Unit Special Operations Capable [26th MEU SOC]
 • Battalion Landing Team 3/6 [BLT 3/6]
 • Marine Medium Helicopter Squadron 365 [HMM-365]
 • MEU Service Support Group 26 [MSSG 26]

KC-130K Tanker Support
Marine Aerial Refueler Transport Squadron 252 and 352 [VMGR-252 and VMGR-352]

Apache Strike in Afghanistan

Operation Anaconda

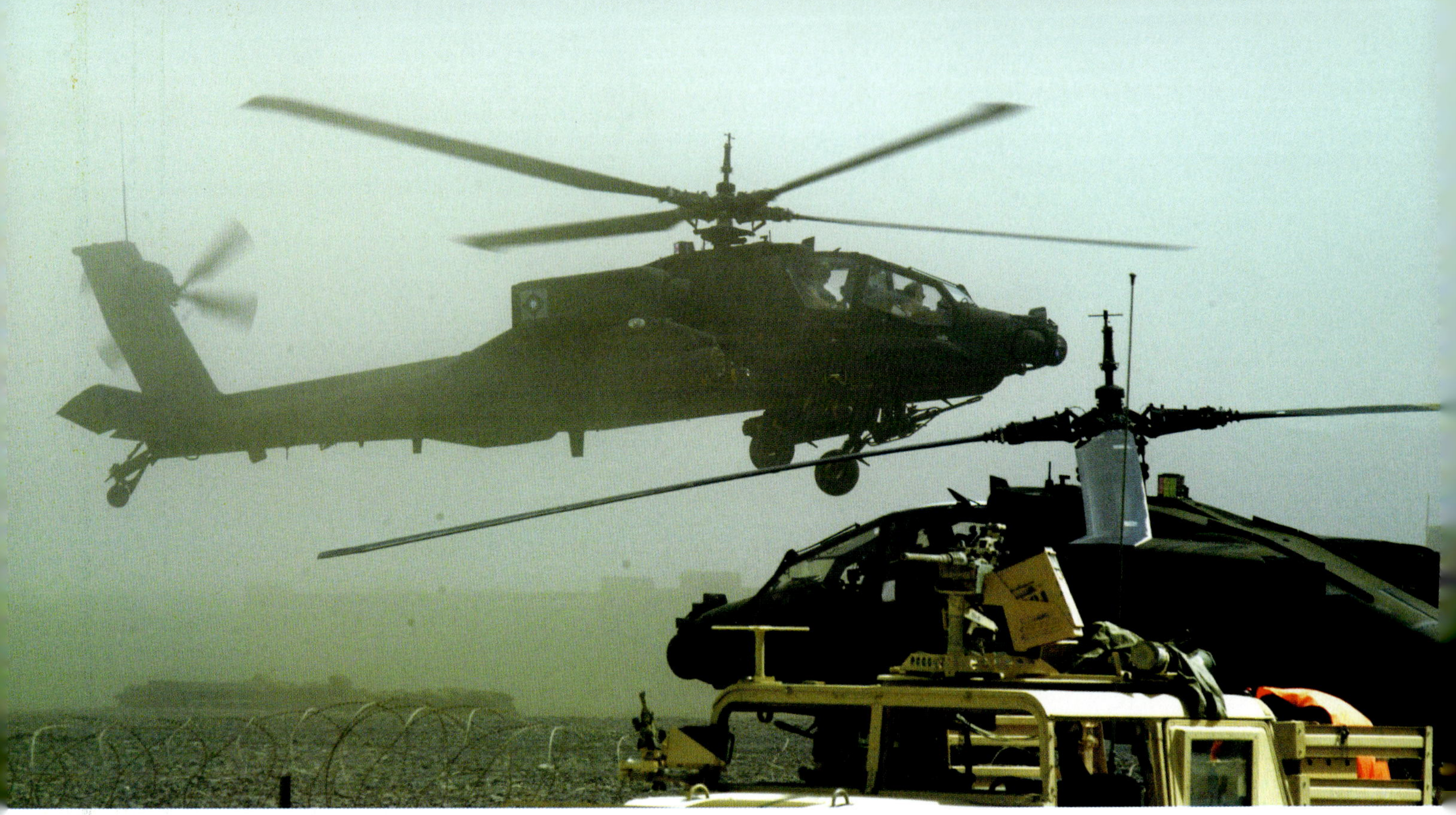

ABOVE: AH-64As were the main fire support available to the 101st Airborne troopers during the first day of Operation Anaconda.
(US DOD/COMBAT CAMERA)

During December 2001 the US had some 28,000 military personnel committed to Operation Enduring Freedom, of which around 7,000 were on the ground in Afghanistan.

The US Marines of Task Force 58 were repairing Kandahar airfield to transform it into the main US base in southern Afghanistan. They had been replaced by a brigade combat team of the 101st Airborne Division (Air Assault) by the middle of January 2002.

US Defense Secretary Donald Rumsfeld was determined to keep troop numbers to an absolute minimum to avoid getting the US sucked into what he described in a derisory fashion as "nation building". The big fear held by Rumsfeld and many senior US military officers was that if the Afghan people saw large numbers of American troops in their country they would regard them as invaders and turn on them, as they had on the Soviets back in the 1980s. This was a quick way to a Vietnam-style 'quagmire' said Rumsfeld. Every aspect of the troop rotation was

RIGHT: Once on the ground, the 101st Airborne troopers found themselves facing heavy resistance from dug-in Al Qaeda fighters.
(US DOD/COMBAT CAMERA)

scrutinised intensely by the Defense Secretary, who even initially vetoed the 101st Airborne taking any of its McDonnell Douglas AH-64A Apache gunships with it to Afghanistan. Requests to deploy artillery were rejected.

As US intelligence analysts got to work on all the leads their troops were collecting around Afghanistan,

indications were growing that there was a large concentration of several hundred Al Qaeda fighters, including many senior commanders, in the Shah-i-Kot valley in Paktia province, near the mountainous border with Pakistan. US Central Command chief General Tommy Franks decided that a large-scale offensive was needed to trap and destroy the enemy fighters.

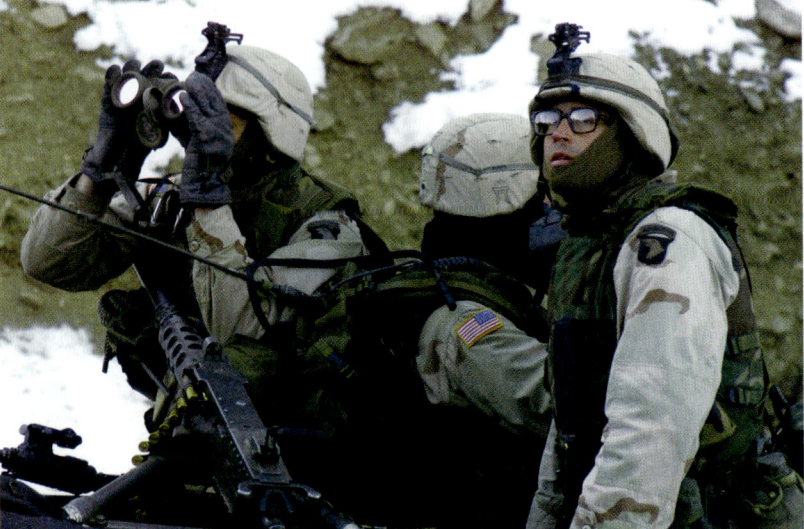

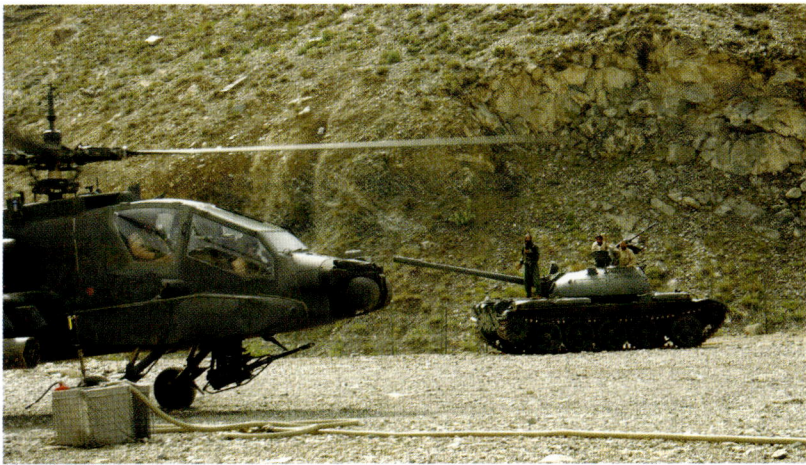

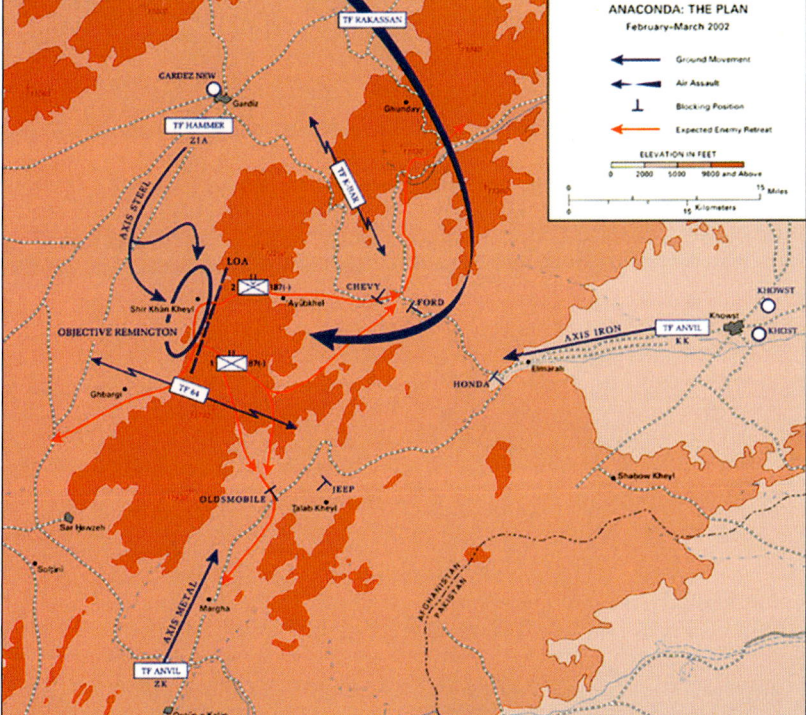

ANACONDA: THE PLAN
February-March 2002

Afghan militia force, led by US Army Special Forces teams, was to launch a direct attack to drive the enemy fighters towards a cordon of US soldiers from the 101st Airborne and 10th Mountain Divisions, who were to be simultaneously dropped by Chinook helicopters in the hills on the eastern side of the valley. Escaping Al Qaeda fighters would either be picked off in the open by Apache attack helicopters, killed by fast jets called in by US forward air controllers or be caught by the guns of the US troops.

The operation kicked off in the early hours of March 2 with the advance up the valley by the Afghan militia force. USAF Rockwell B-1B Lancer heavy bombers and Lockheed AC-130 Spectre gunships were sent ahead to bomb Al Qaeda positions. Things started to go wrong almost immediately. The first B-1B over the valley was supposed to bomb pre-planned targets, including 12.5mm DShK heavy machine guns that were a grave threat to the in-bound CH-47 Chinooks carrying the 101st Airborne troopers. It suffered a technical fault after only six of its bombs had been released and had to call off its attack.

Then disaster struck when a technical fault in an AC-130's navigation system led it to attack the Afghan militia convoy by mistake. Two militia fighters were killed, and more than a dozen injured. Several of their US advisors were also wounded. The incident caused the militia attack to grind to a halt in confusion as the US medics tried to recover the wounded from wrecked trucks. It also meant that the US troops soon to ❯❯

LEFT: Apaches of the 101st Airborne had to support Operation Anaconda from a rudimentary forward operating site. (US DOD/COMBAT CAMERA)

LEFT: The plan for Operation Anaconda soon fell apart as US troops ran into heavy resistance from dug-in and fully alerted Al Qaeda fighters occupying mountain-top positions. (US DOD/COMBAT CAMERA)

BELOW: 101st Airborne Division trooper prepare to board a CH-47 Chinook during the build-up for Operation Anaconda. (US DOD/COMBAT CAMERA)

To avoid a repeat of the problems that had bedevilled the drive to trap Osama bin Laden at Tora Bora in December 2001, the Pentagon wanted US Army infantry troops to be involved in strength.

The plan, for what eventually became known as Operation Anaconda, was complex and involved several military organisations – US, Afghan and allies – that were operating under different chains of command in the same small piece of territory. Airpower was central to the delivery of the assault and cordon forces, as well as providing supporting fire power. The operation soon went badly wrong and afterwards USAF and US Army commanders traded rhetorical blows about the poor performance of the air support.

Covert observation teams were first to be landed by helicopter on three mountain peaks dominating the Shah-i-Kot valley to try to locate the Al Qaeda positions. Then an

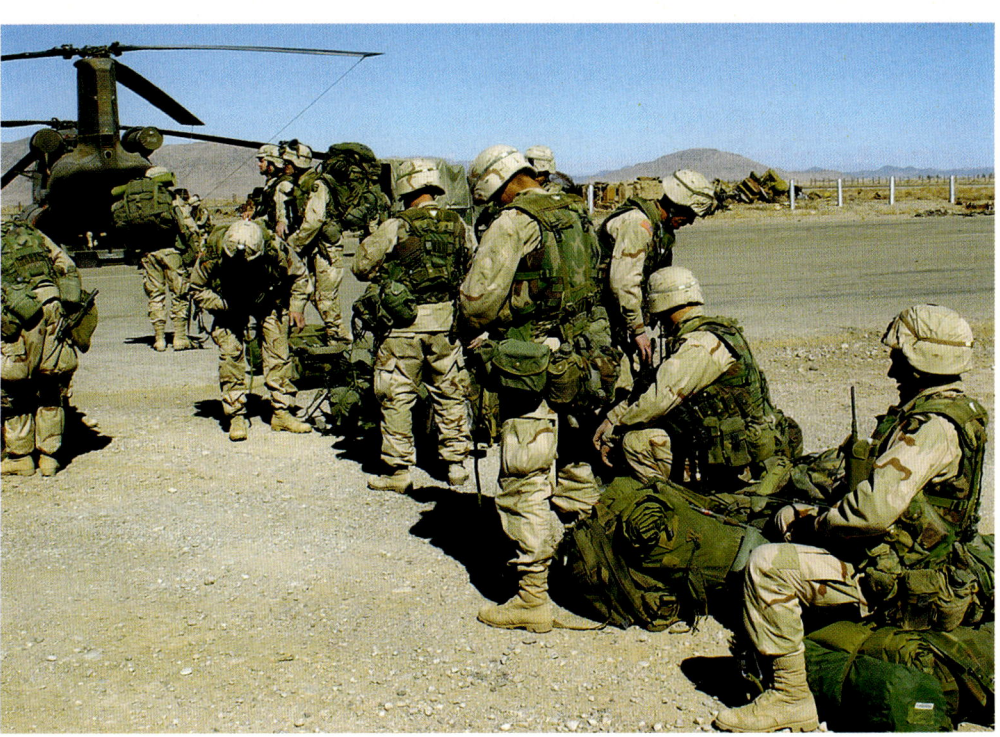

RIGHT: US Army Chinooks played a key part in the battle, landing the first wave of US troops and then bring in ammunition and supplies to keep them fighting.
(US DOD/COMBAT CAMERA)

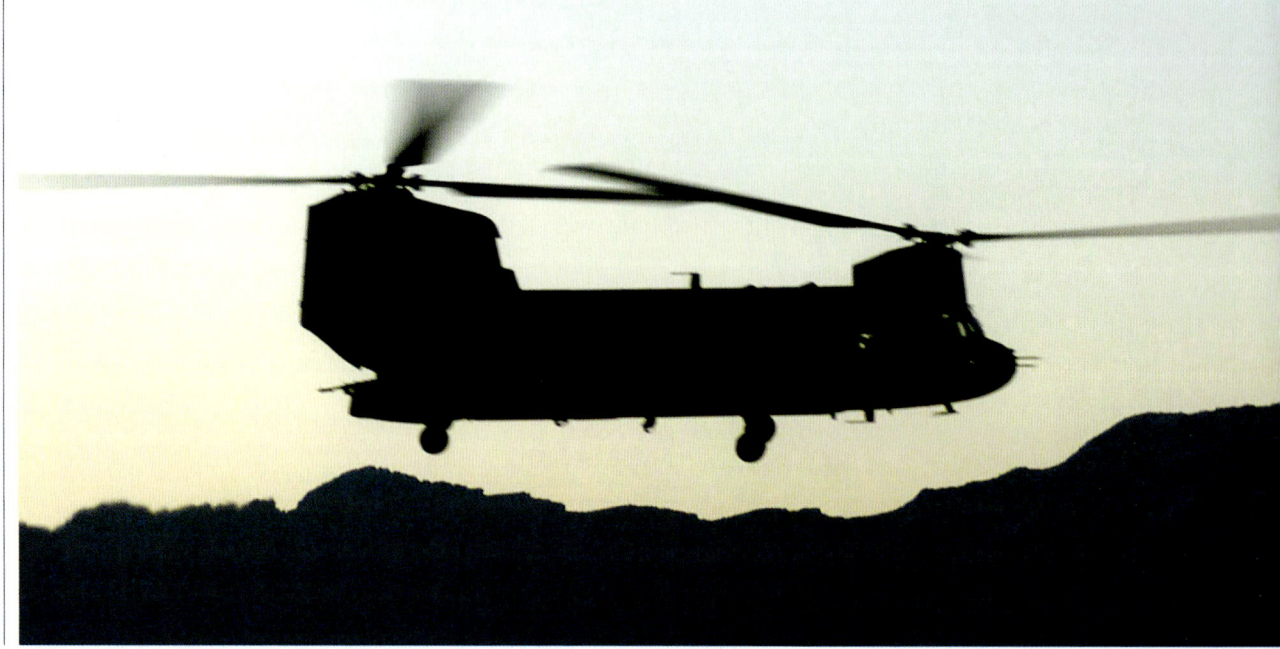

BELOW: A US Special Operations Forces' MH-47 Chinook was shot down on the third day the battle and efforts to rescue the survivors soon took centre stage.
(US DOD/COMBAT CAMERA)

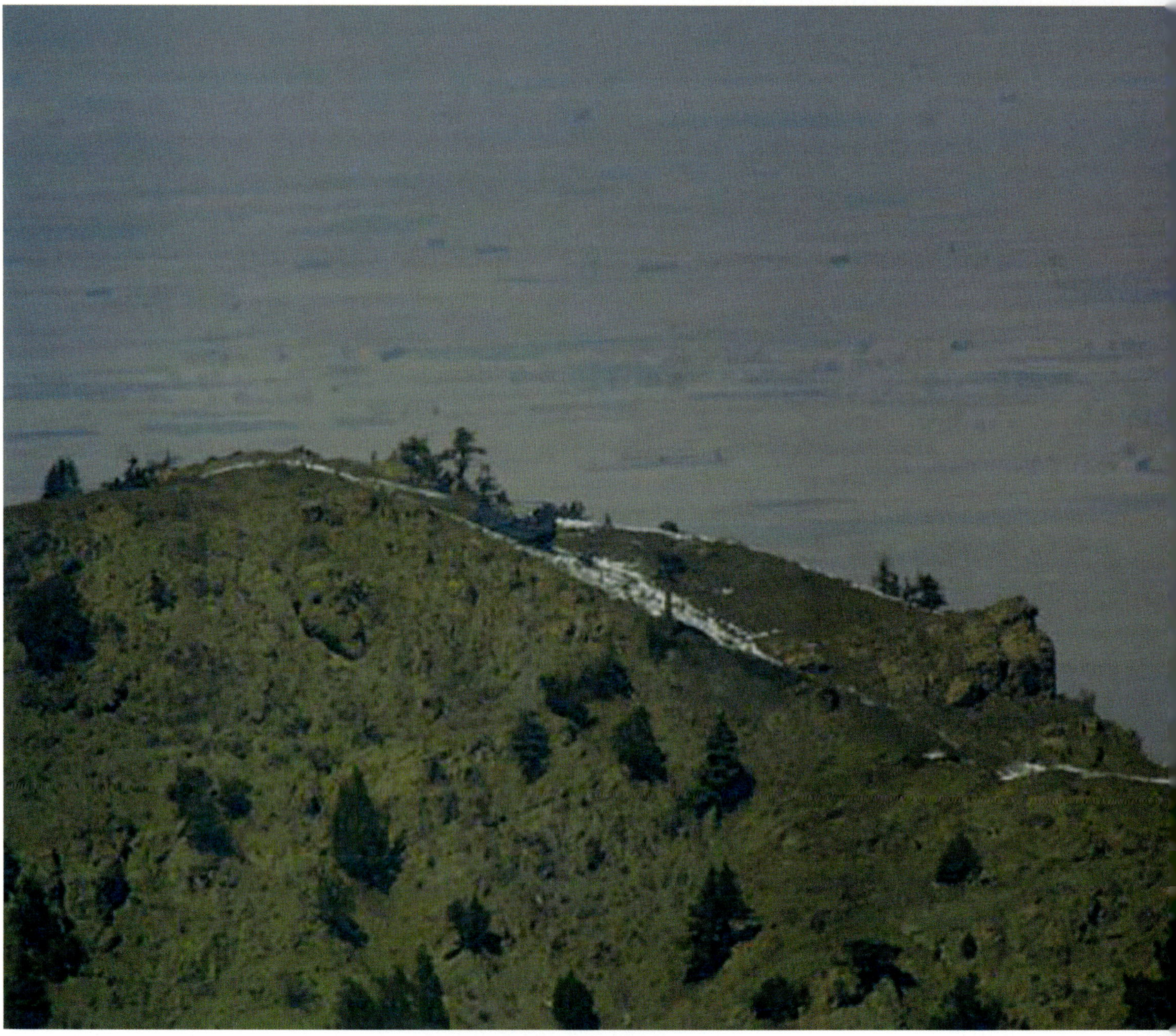

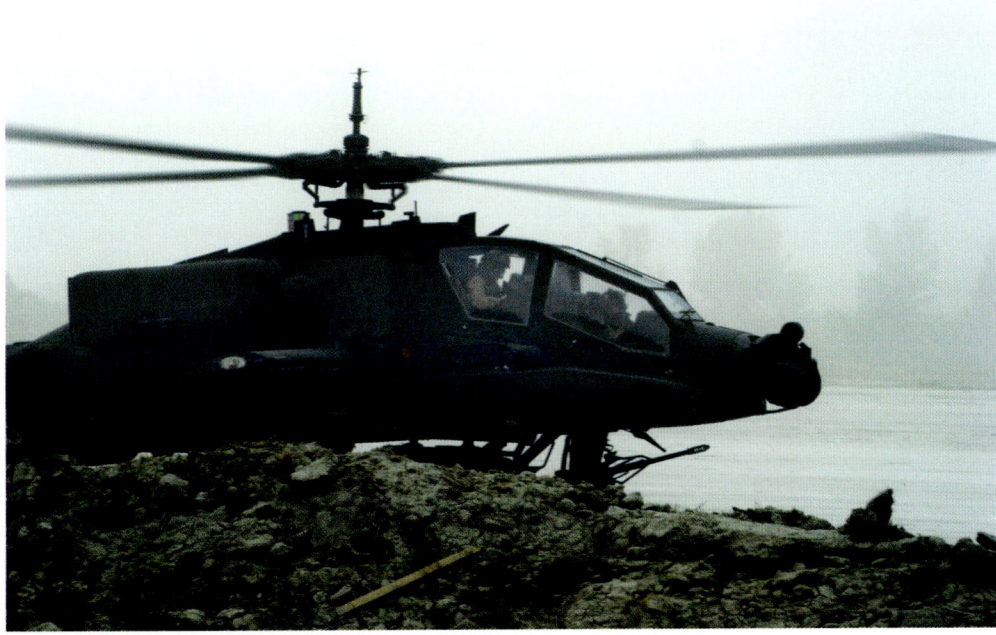

be dropped off in the mountains by waves of Chinooks would be facing a fully alerted and prepared enemy.

The expectation of very limited enemy indirect fire capability meant that only a single 120mm mortar was brought in on the first wave of Chinooks. The primary fire support for the troops was provided by Apaches of the 3rd Battalion, 101st Aviation Regiment.

Just as the 'friendly fire' incident was unfolding, 101st Airborne CH-47Ds were arriving at their landing zones to offload hundreds of American soldiers. As the soldiers ran down the

giant helicopter's ramps they came under unrelenting fire from AK-47s, heavy machine guns, rocket-propelled grenades (RPGs), mortars and light artillery. Fortunately, the escorting Apaches were soon duelling with Al Qaeda machine gun teams at ranges under 200m.

The orbiting Apaches attempted to suppress enemy mortar teams but ran into a wall of RPG and 12.7mm fire, with one Apache losing all of its electronics to an RPG hit. Instead of 150-200 Al Qaeda fighters as had been expected, post assessment held that the area contained

750 to 1,000 fighters dug in on the high ground around the valley. The insurgents used their ZPU-1 anti-aircraft guns, DShKs and small arms fire against the attack helicopters.

The Apaches weaved across the battlefield to dodge heavy fire and re-position themselves to employ their guns, rockets and AGM-114 Hellfire missiles. The presence of the Apaches overhead diverted the attention of the Al Qaeda gunners and allowed most of the American troops to take cover and begin returning fire. Insurgents began intentionally firing their RPG rockets into the air so that when »

ABOVE: All five AH-64A Apaches committed on the first day of Operation Anaconda took heavy damage but kept flying and fighting.
(US DOD/COMBAT CAMERA)

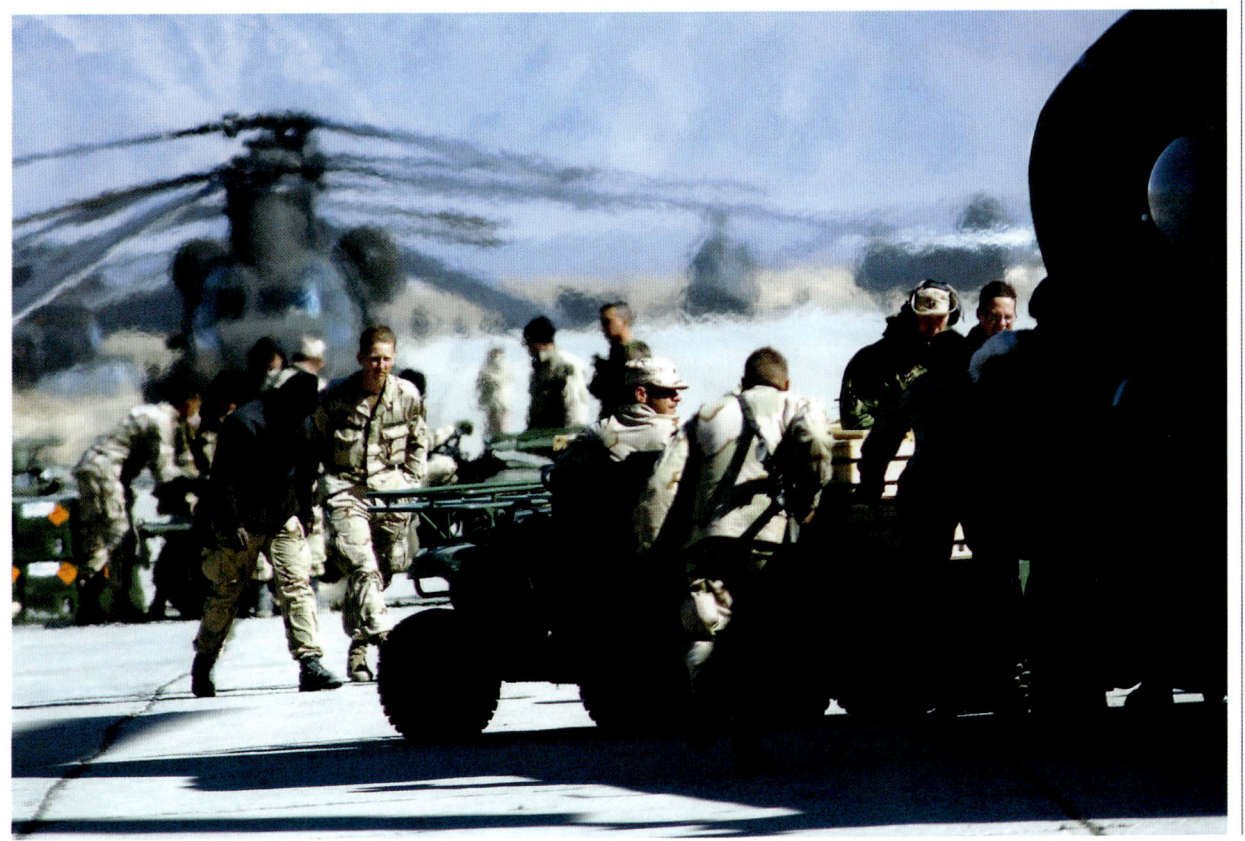

LEFT: Bagram air base was the hub of US helicopter activity during Operation Anaconda.
(US DOD/COMBAT CAMERA)

they automatically detonated at 920m they would catch the helicopters in flak bursts. This was a tactic that had been learned in the Soviet-Afghan War two decades before.

For the rest of the morning, the Apaches were constantly in action over Shah-i-Kot, but as each helicopter ran out of ammunition they peeled off and returned to a forward arming and refuelling point (FARP) 50 miles away from the battlefield. All of the helicopters were riddled with bullet holes or peppered with RPG shrapnel.

Two Apaches were damaged early on in the day, with one Apache forced to return to base when an RPG destroyed its left-side Hellfire mount sending shrapnel through the airframe. It had also been peppered by small arms, further RPG rounds and DShK rounds. One machine gun round penetrated the cockpit, narrowly missing the pilots.

Another Apache took a hit in its transmission and began rapidly losing oil. It was forced to landed within sight of the Al Qaeda fighters. Staying in position until a rescue force arrived

RIGHT: Afghanistan's awesome terrain had a major impact on US helicopter operations, limiting performance and causing flight hazards.
(US DOD/COMBAT CAMERA)

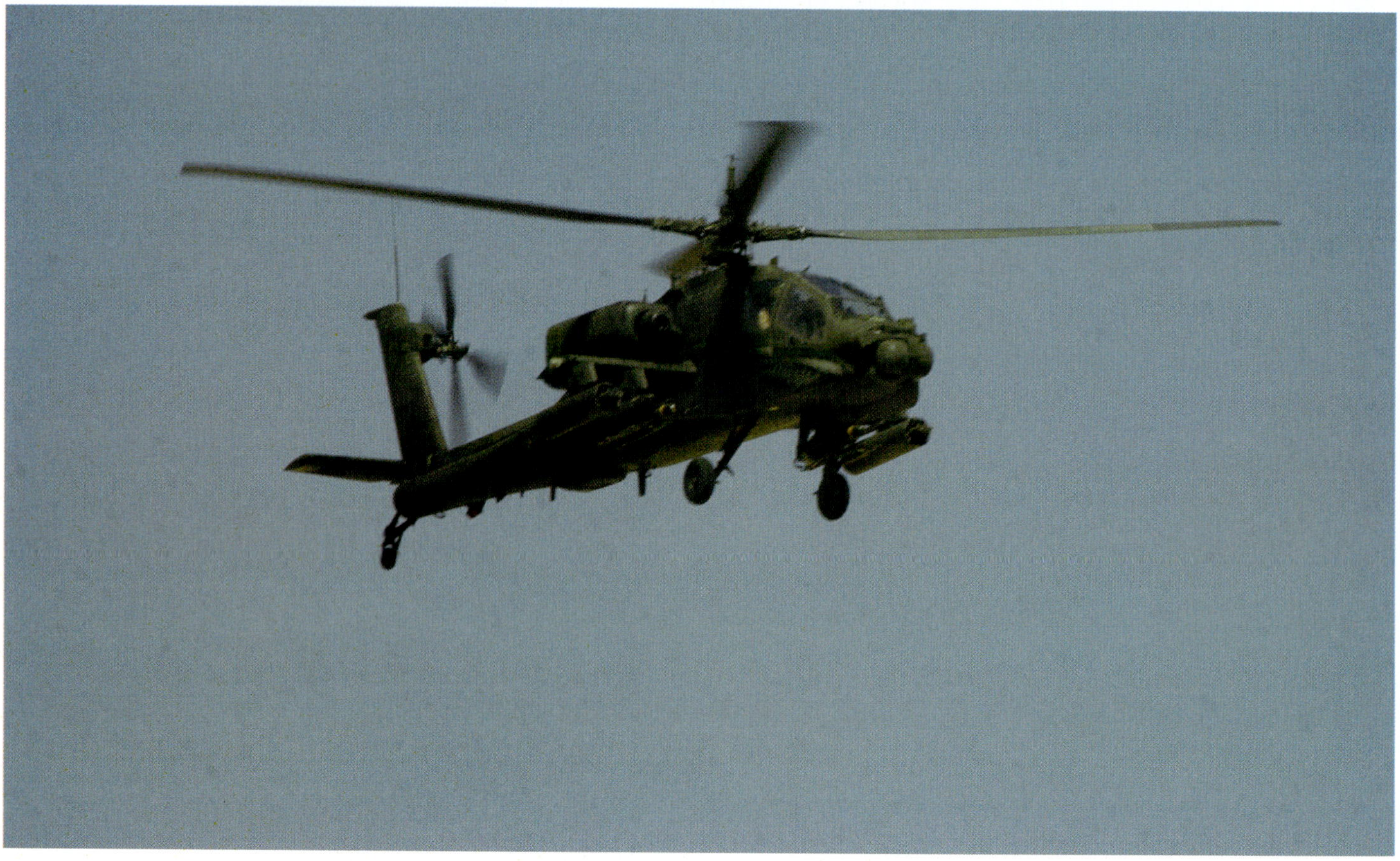

BELOW: Al Qaeda fighters and their Taliban allies soon came to fear the mighty Apache.
(US DOD/COMBAT CAMERA)

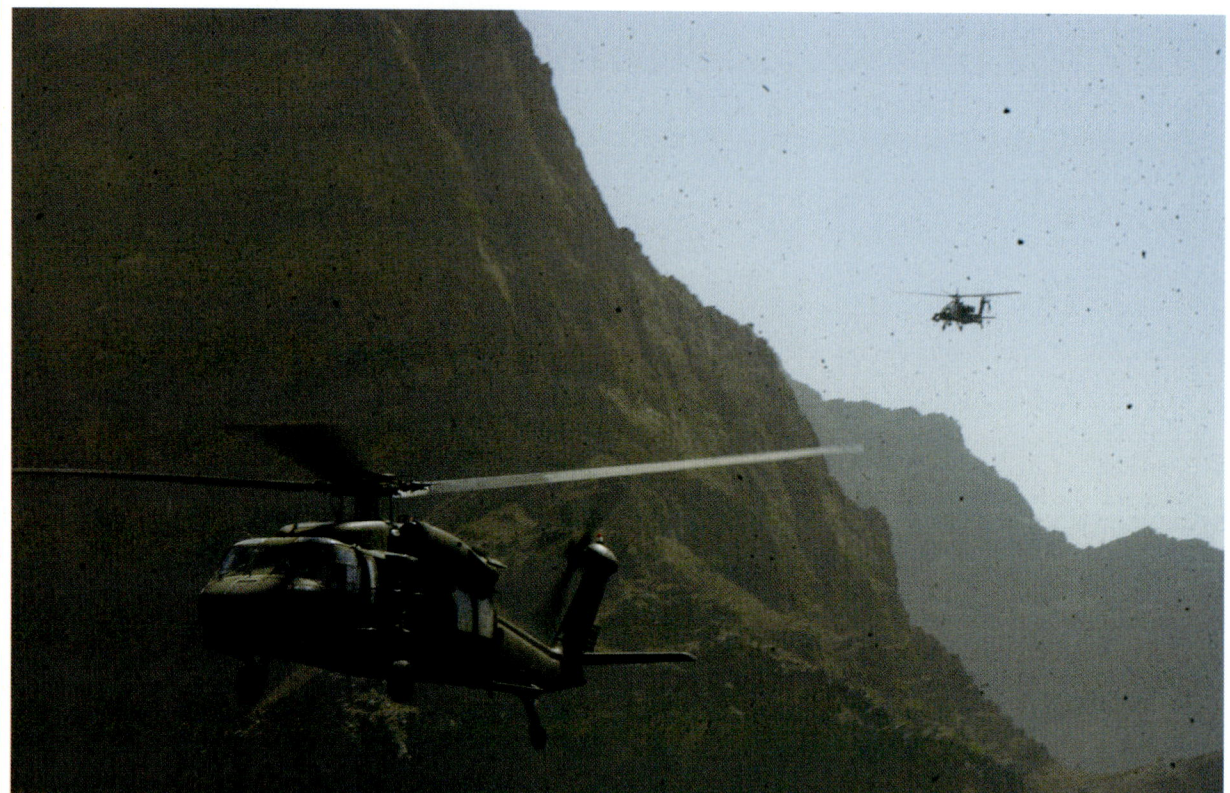

was not an option, so the crew had to dismount from the cockpit to top up their helicopter's transmission with oil. The Apache started up and headed off for the FARP, still leaking oil, but crew miraculously made it. By midday all the Apaches were at the FARP undergoing repairs. Only two were fit to go back into action later that afternoon to make repeated attack runs and stop an Al Qaeda attempt to overrun an exposed US position.

Shah-i-Kot was the scene of the most intense battle involving US forces since the infamous 'Blackhawk Down' incident in Somalia in 1993. Eight Americans died during the confused Battle of Roberts Ridge on Takur Ghar peak in the Shah-i-Kot valley.

US commanders were now aware that they faced determined and skilled opponents so they moved quickly to step up their game, drafting more aircraft into the battle. US Marine Corps Bell AH-1W Cobra gunships were flown to Bagram from amphibious ships sailing in the Arabian Gulf and 16 more Apaches from the 101st Airborne were airlifted from the division's home base in Kentucky.

The fighting in the Shah-i-Kot valley continued for another week after the Battle of Roberts Ridge. By the time the Afghan tanks rolled into the valley on March 12, it was deserted. They found scores of wrecked machine guns, mortars, and several abandoned artillery pieces but fewer than 100 dead fighters were found on the battlefield.

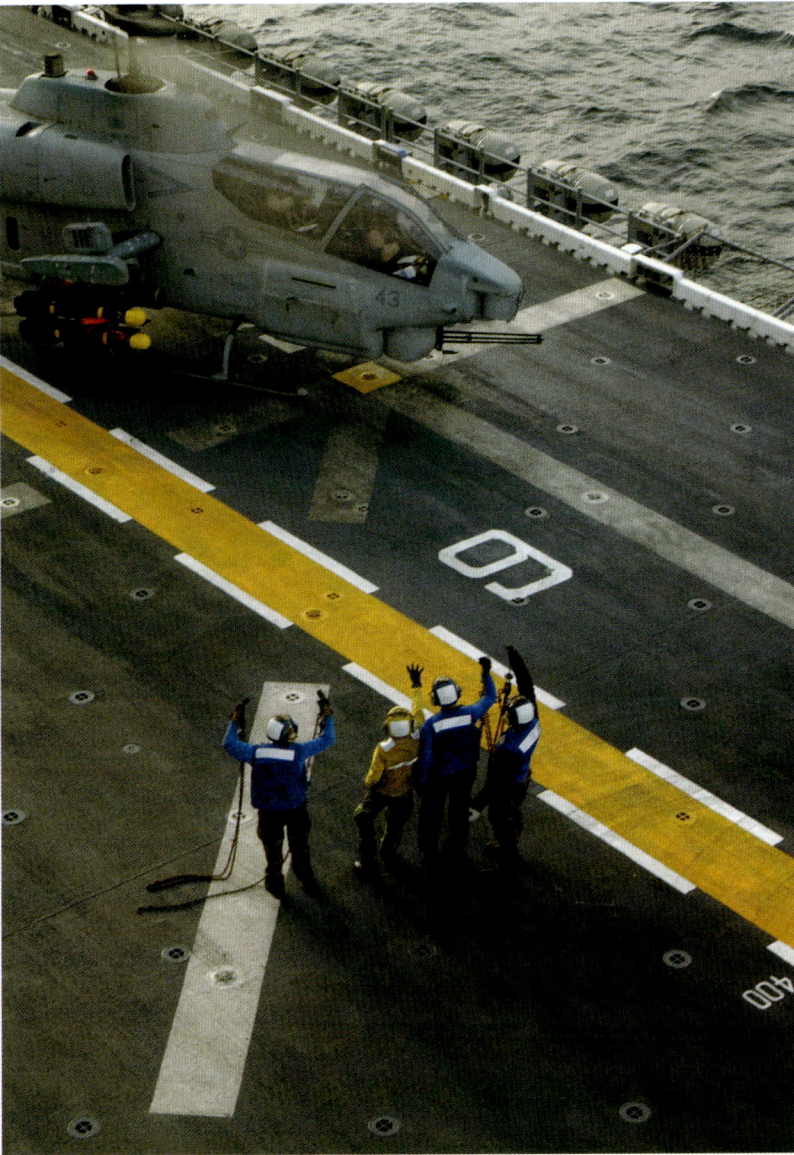

LEFT: US Marine Corps AH-1W Cobras were scrambled from US warships in the North Arabian Sea to reinforce the AH-64As of the 101st Airborne for the final phase of Operation Anaconda. (US DOD/COMBAT CAMERA)

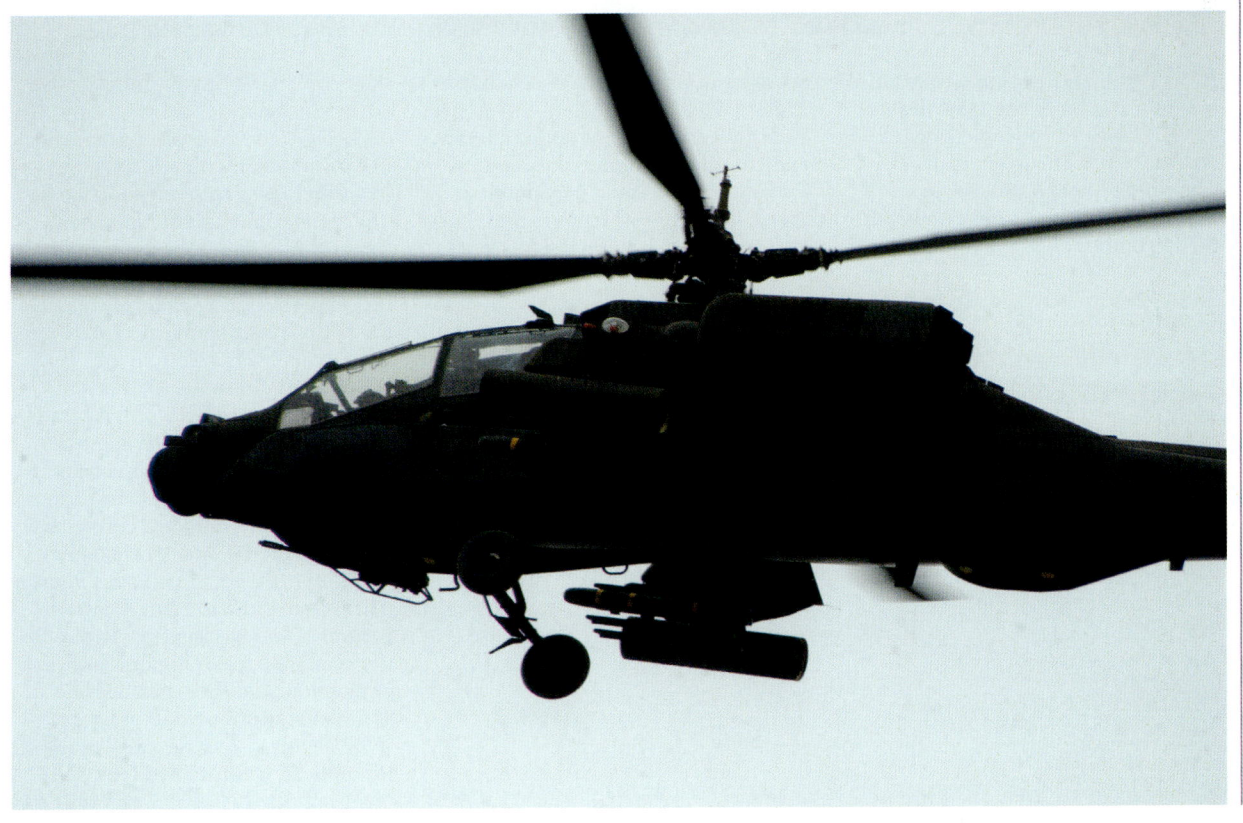

LEFT: US Army AH-64 Apaches remained on duty in Afghanistan until the last US troops pulled out of the country in the summer of 2021. (US DOD/COMBAT CAMERA)

Destroying the Republican Guard

Operation Iraqi Freedom 2003

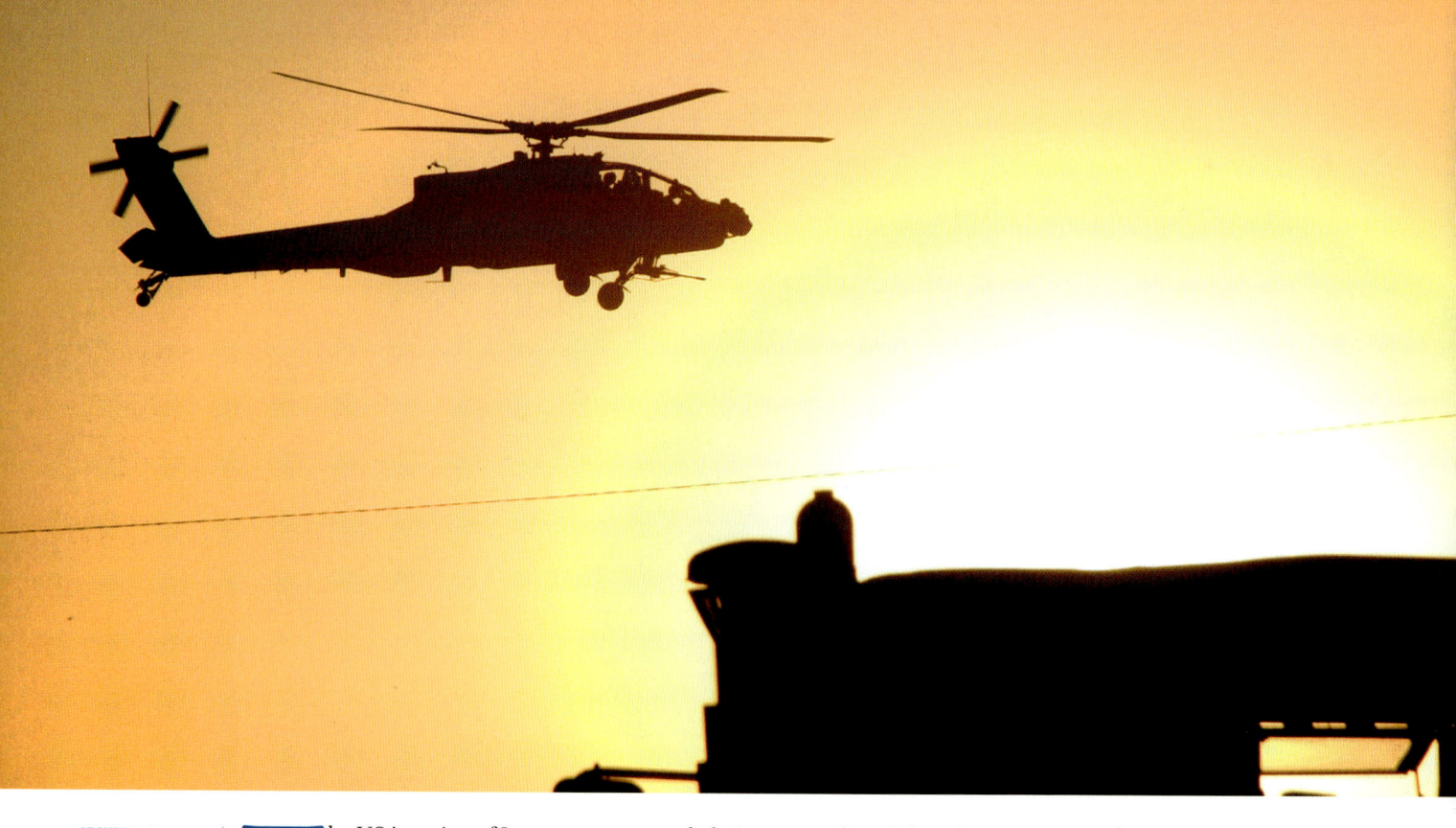

ABOVE: The improved AH-64D was used in action on a large scale for the first time during Operation Iraqi Freedom in 2003.
(US DOD/COMBAT CAMERA)

The US invasion of Iraq in March 2003 saw the biggest concentration of attack helicopters deployed since Operation Desert Storm in 1991. Unlike Desert Storm, however, the US military was not relying on overwhelming strength to defeat the Iraqis. US Defense Secretary Donald Rumsfeld ordered his commanders to focus on precision strikes, special forces raids and rapid movement to knock the Iraqis off balance and allow US troops to drive into the heart of their capital, Baghdad. This was the era of 'Shock and Awe'.

Nearly 150,000 US troops massed in Kuwait and by March 2003 the invasion force was ready to strike under the command of Lieutenant General David McKiernan.

His plan involved US tank columns heading through the desert to engage the main Iraqi Republican Guard force, which was dug-in to the south of Baghdad. En route, McKiernan planned to conduct deep strike raids with McDonnell Douglas AH-64D Apaches against Iraqi rear echelon forces to decimate them before the main US armoured force entered the battle. To get the attack helicopters into range, the 101st Airborne Division (Air Assault) and the 11th Aviation Regiment were to leapfrog across the unpopulated desert region southwest of Baghdad and then establish a series of forward operating bases (FOBs) within striking range of the Republican Guard. The air assault troops of the 101st Airborne were

RIGHT: US helicopter operations come under intense media scrutiny during the opening days of the US invasion.
(US DOD/COMBAT CAMERA)

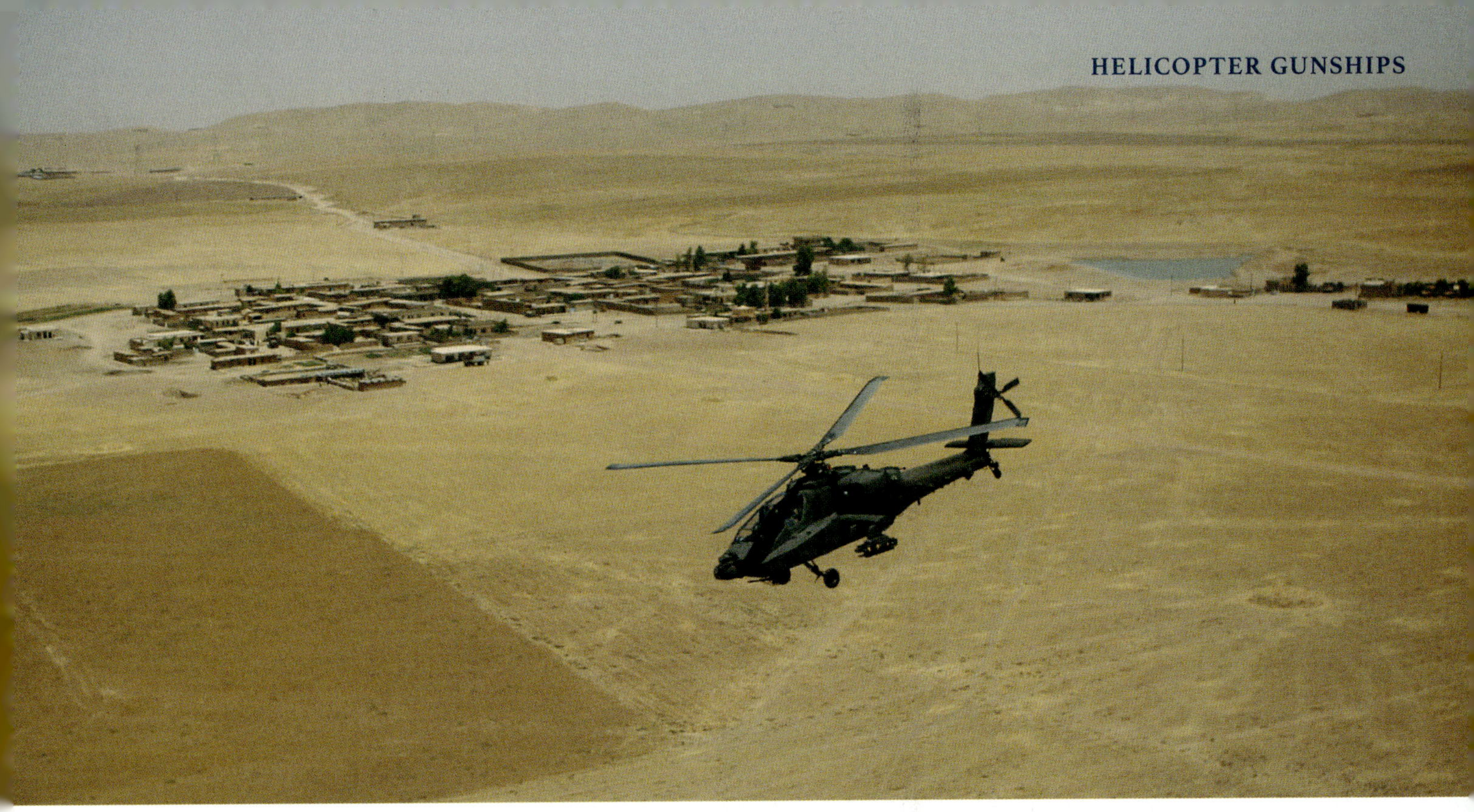

tasked with seizing their future FOBs in helicopter raids and then giant convoys of fuel tankers would link up with them after driving across the desert.

The operation to cross the border got underway on March 20 with minimal resistance from Iraqi troops in the south of the country.

A sandstorm slowed the advance, but once it had lifted McKiernan's troops stepped up their drive on Baghdad where Saddam Hussein had posted six divisions of his supposedly elite Republican Guard Forces Command (RGFC). The first defensive line had been set up between the towns of Karbala and Al-Kut, with the Al Medina Armoured Division in the west, the Al Nida Armoured Division in the centre and the Baghdad Mechanised Division out to the east. Elements of the Nebuchadnezzar and Hammurabi Mechanised Divisions were deployed just south of Baghdad as a second line of defence.

The task given to the US-led air forces was to render these units combat-ineffective before the main elements of the ground forces were committed to action.

Late in the evening of March 23, the US Army's V Corps launched its 11th Aviation Regiment into action. This was the first night-time 'deep strike' raid of the war, designed to hit the Republican Guard's Medina Mechanised Division that was holding the Karbala 'gap', a key route to Baghdad. The Corps' 30 McDonnell Douglas AH-64D Longbow Apache attack helicopters flew into a hornet's nest of anti-aircraft fire.

Just after 1.00am on March 24, the formation of attack helicopters »

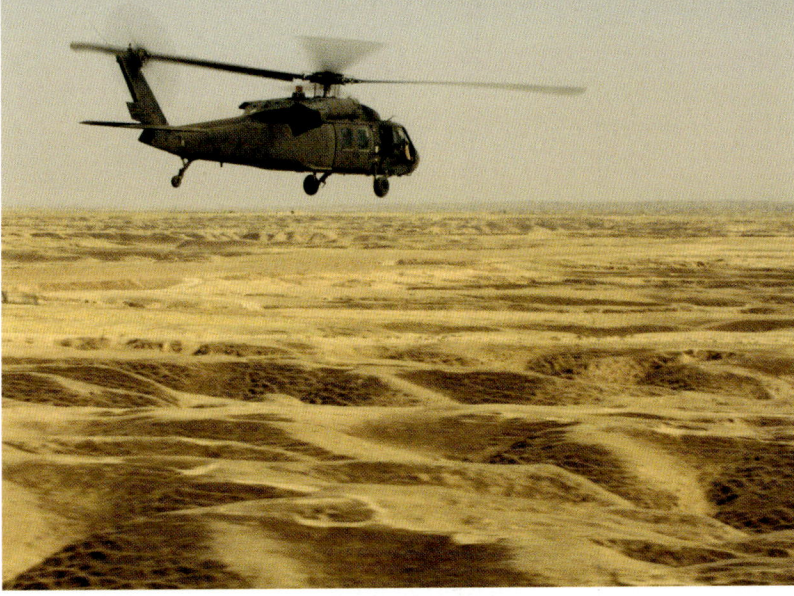

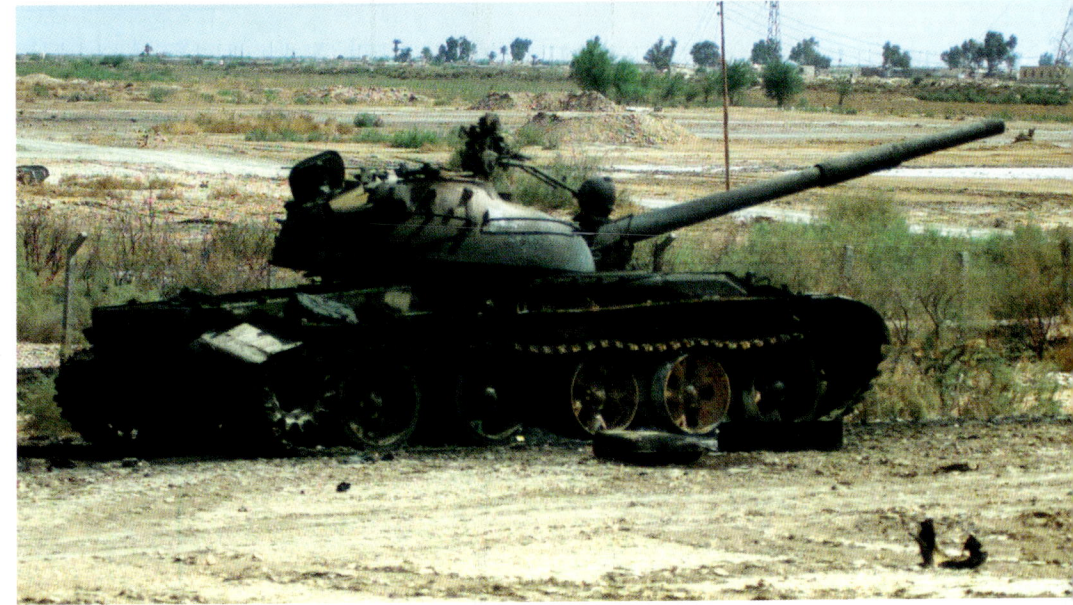

ABOVE: Iraq's desert terrain should have been the perfect environment for US attack helicopter operations, but Saddam Hussein's troops re-orientated their defences into urban areas to neutralise the US advantage in air power. (US DOD/COMBAT CAMERA)

LEFT: US Army aviation units flew over the Iraqi desert to set up forward operating bases within striking distance of the Iraqi capital. (US DOD/COMBAT CAMERA)

BELOW: Saddam Hussein's Republican Guard tank divisions were the main target of US airpower. (US DOD/COMBAT CAMERA)

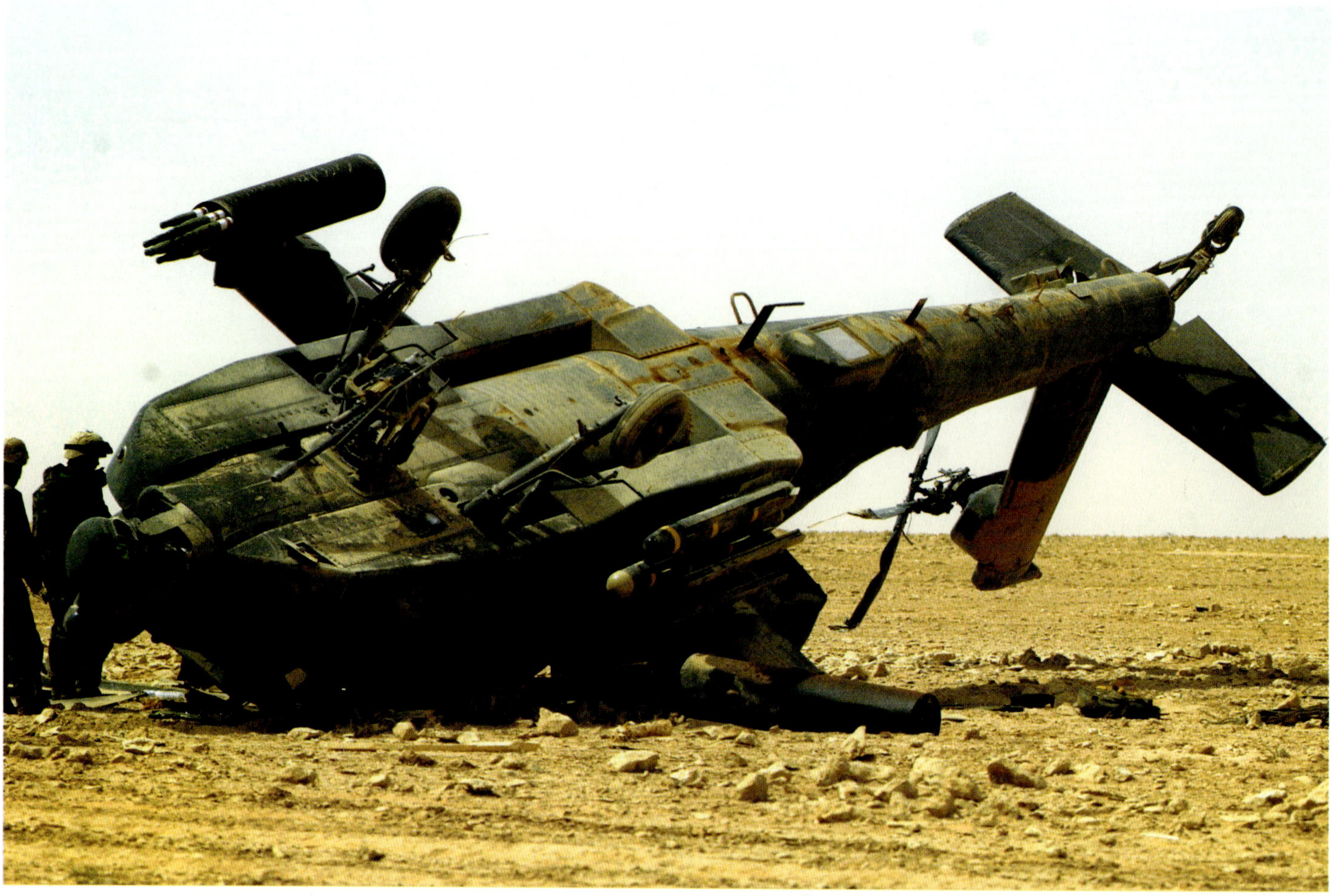

ABOVE: Disaster struck the 11th Attack Helicopter Regiment when it ran into heavy defences during a strike on the Medina Armoured Division.
(US DOD/COMBAT CAMERA)

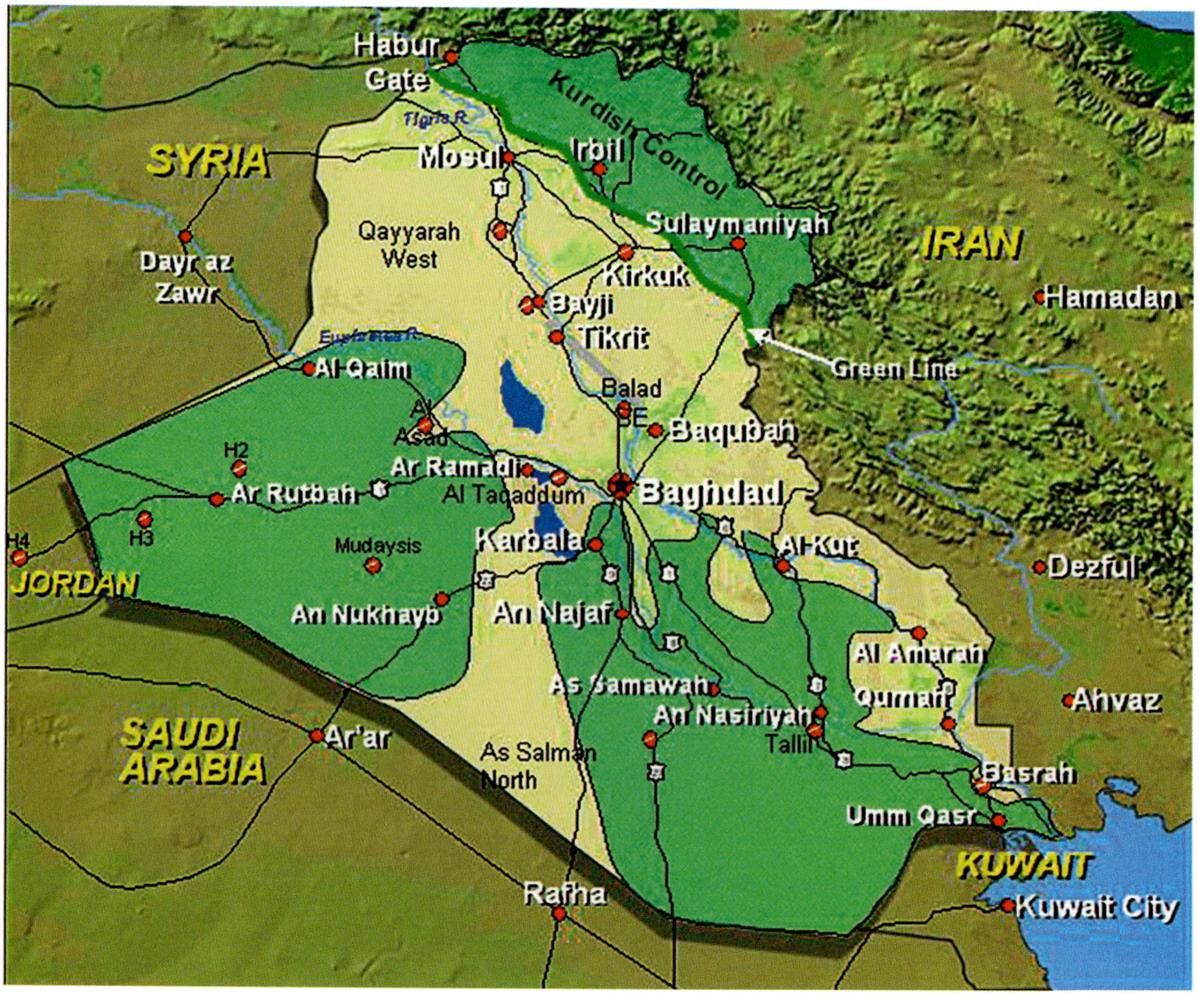

SYRIA

Habur Gate

Tigris R.

Kurdish Control

Mosul

Irbil

Qayyarah West

Sulaymaniyah

IRAN

Kirkuk

Bayji

Hamadan

Tikrit

Dayr az Zawr

Euphrates R.

Al Qaim

Balad

Green Line

BE

Al Asad

Baqubah

H2

Ar Ramadi

Ar Rutbah

Al Taqaddum

Baghdad

Al Kut

Dezful

H4

H3

Mudaysis

Karbala

JORDAN

An Nukhayb

An Najaf

Al Amarah

Qurnah

Ahvaz

As Samawah

An Nasiriyah

Tallil

SAUDI ARABIA

Ar'ar

As Salman North

Basrah

Umm Qasr

KUWAIT

Rafha

Kuwait City

RIGHT: US troops advanced rapidly to the outskirts of the Iraqi capital.
(US DOD/COMBAT CAMERA)

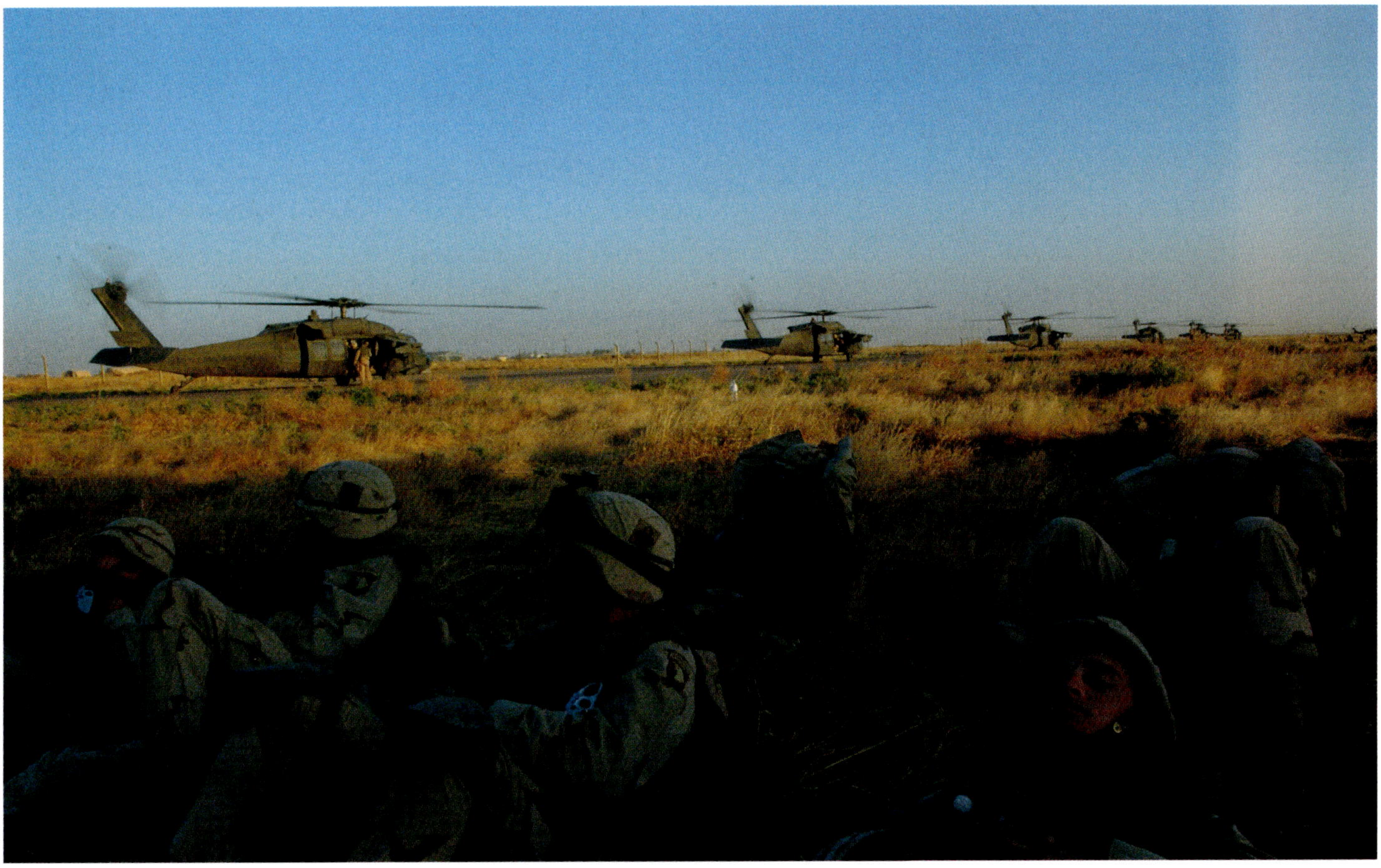

was flying towards their targets at low level above the towns of Al Haswah and Al Iskandariyah. At that point, all the street and house lights in the area blinked out for two seconds. "Immediately thereafter the sky erupted with all manner of ground fire, which was apparent by the red, yellow and white tracers," reported the US Army's official history of Operation Iraqi Freedom. "Initially un-aimed, the fusillade of fire created a 'wall' between the aircraft and their objectives. Although the Apaches were running with lights out, the lights from farms and towns silhouetted the attack helicopters against the night sky. Crews reported damage to their aircraft and difficulty manoeuvring due to the volume of enemy fire."

This was a deliberate trap for the helicopters which the American attack crews could not respond to. Every Iraqi under the 11th Regiment's flight path just let rip with whatever weapon they had, from AK-47s to machine guns and heavy anti-aircraft artillery. There were just too many weapons firing for the Apache crews to be able to pick out a viable target. It was information overload, the crews reported.

"Of the 30 aircraft that departed Objective RAMS for the mission, 29 returned with small arms and some anti-aircraft artillery damage," reported the official history. "One aircraft force-landed due to ground fire and was subsequently destroyed to prevent compromise." The Iraqis captured both pilots. On average, 1st Battalion, 227th Aviation »

ABOVE: The 101st Airborne Division conducted a series of air assault operations to open more forward operating bases deeper inside Iraq. (US DOD/COMBAT CAMERA)

LEFT: OH-58D Kiowa Warriors scouted ahead of US divisions looking for targets for the AH-64Ds to strike. (US DOD/COMBAT CAMERA)

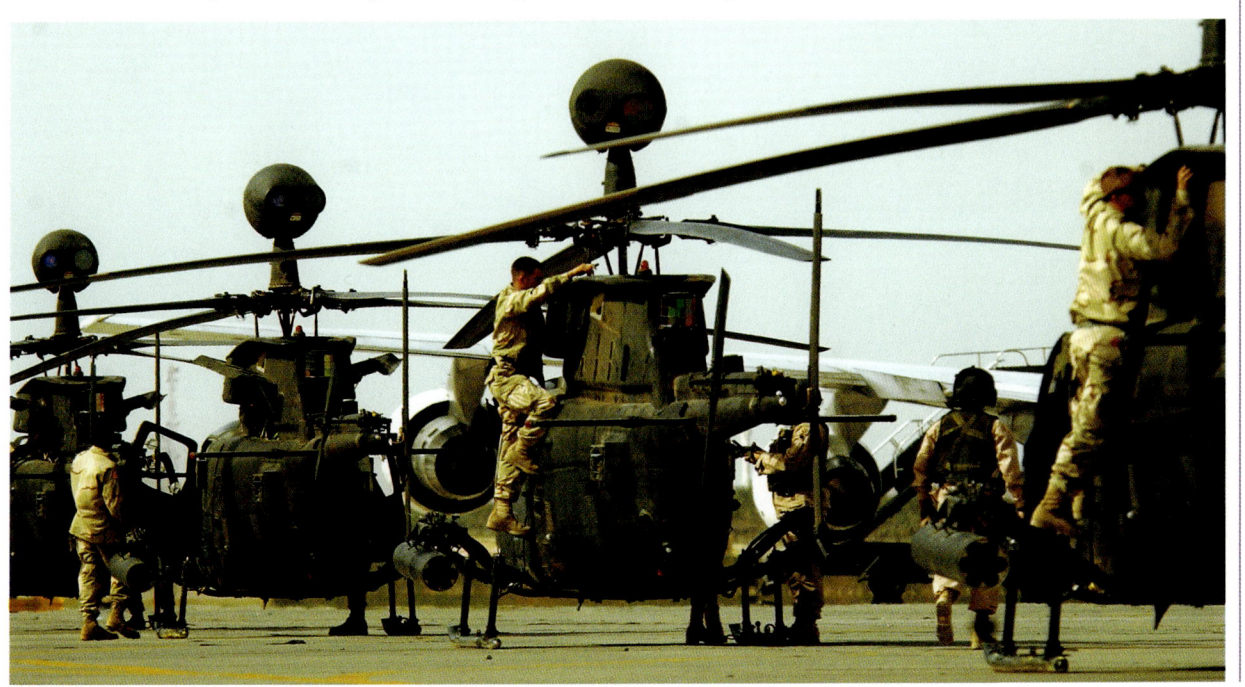

RIGHT: The rugged UH-60 Black Hawk filled many support and logistical roles during Operation Iraqi Freedom. (US DOD/COMBAT CAMERA)

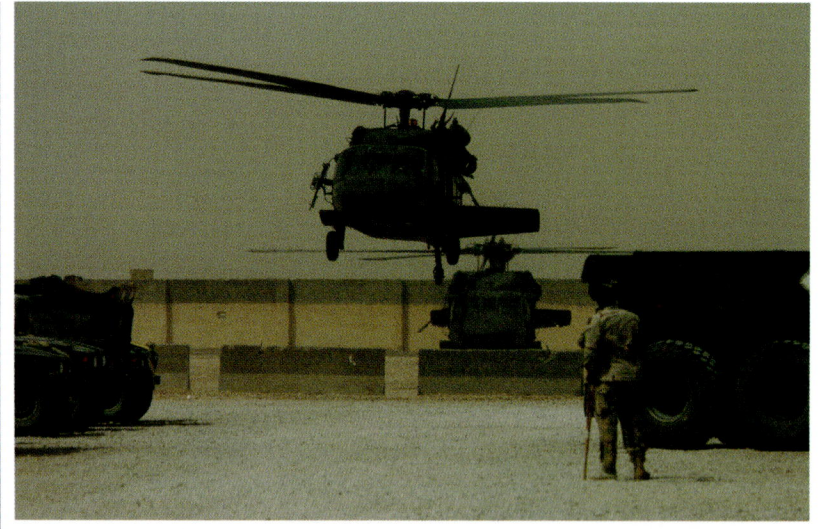

Regiment's aircraft returned sporting 15-20 bullet holes each, and one had a total of 29. If nothing else, the Apache demonstrated how tough an aircraft it is. As one pilot put it, "that airplane is resilient. It is amazing! We got back and looked at all the airplanes and it is incredible that we were able to fly those things home. It is an amazing aircraft."

On the other hand, no one was claiming a victory that night. Assessing battle damage is always difficult and, fundamentally, aside from killing some air defence systems, a few gun trucks and a number of enemy firing small arms, the regiment achieved very little. Only seven of the brigade's Apaches were ready for action a week later, although 11 were reported to be under repair. Two captured Apache crewmen were later paraded on Baghdad TV, although the Pentagon denied the $50 million helicopter had been shot down by an Iraqi farmer.

Four days later, the 101st Aviation Brigade attempted another attack on the Medina Division's positions around Karbala. This time the raid was better organised and the Apache crews were ready for the Iraqis' unorthodox air defence tactics. Fixed-wing air support was co-ordinated to be overhead at the same time.

Lieutenant Colonel Steve Smith, commander of the 2nd Battalion, 101st Aviation Regiment, remembered the operation, stating that "the rest of the night was amazing". He watched tracers coming up, saw fighters dropping 500-pound bombs and listened to one pilot report that people were waving to him from a rooftop. According to Smith a second pilot corrected this misapprehension, saying, "Dude, they ain't waving". Despite receiving groundfire, the Apaches continued to attack tanks and other fighting vehicles along

BELOW: US Marine Corps AH-1W Cobras provided close air support for the I Marine Expeditionary Force as it advanced on Baghdad to the east of the US Army's V Corps. (US DOD/COMBAT CAMERA)

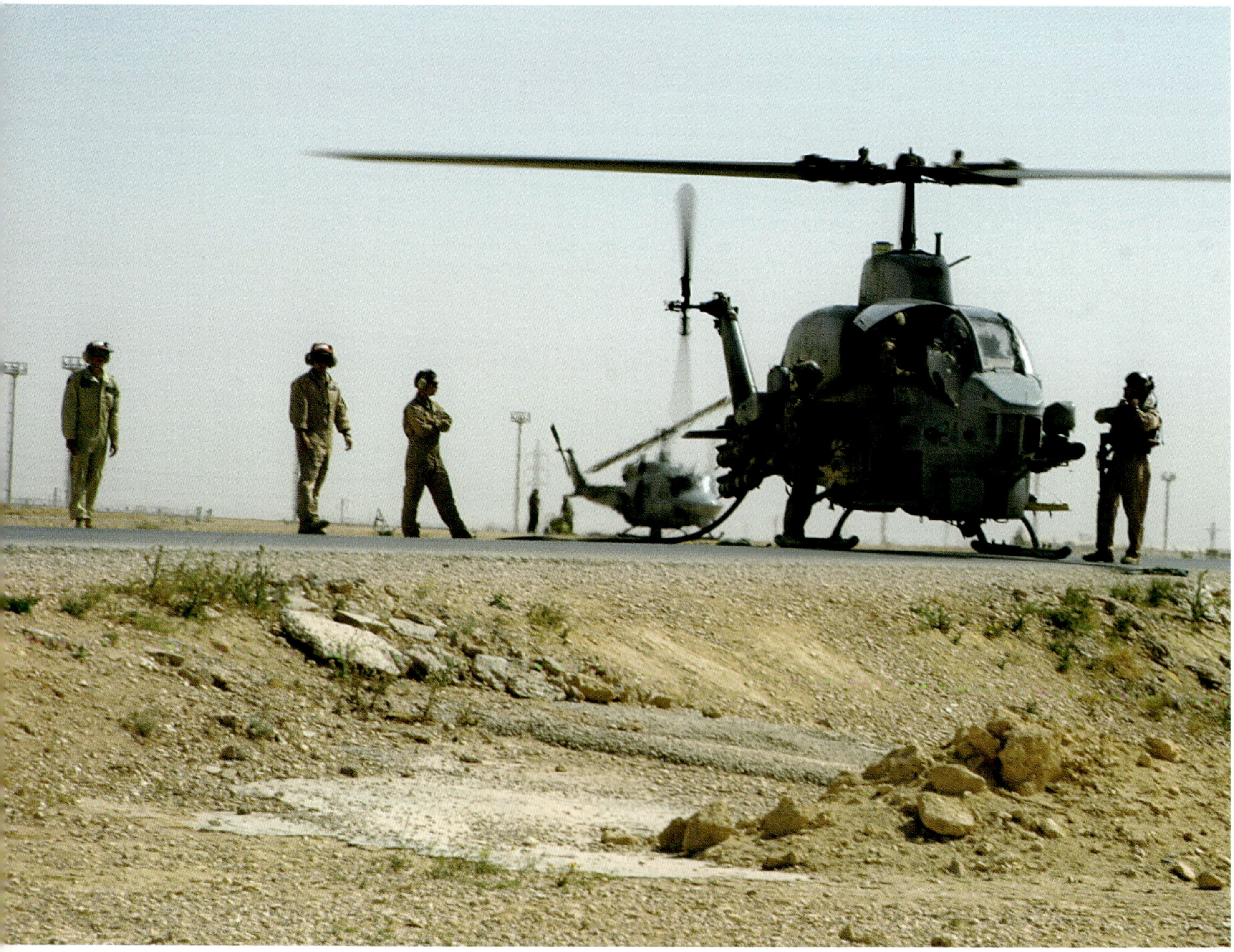

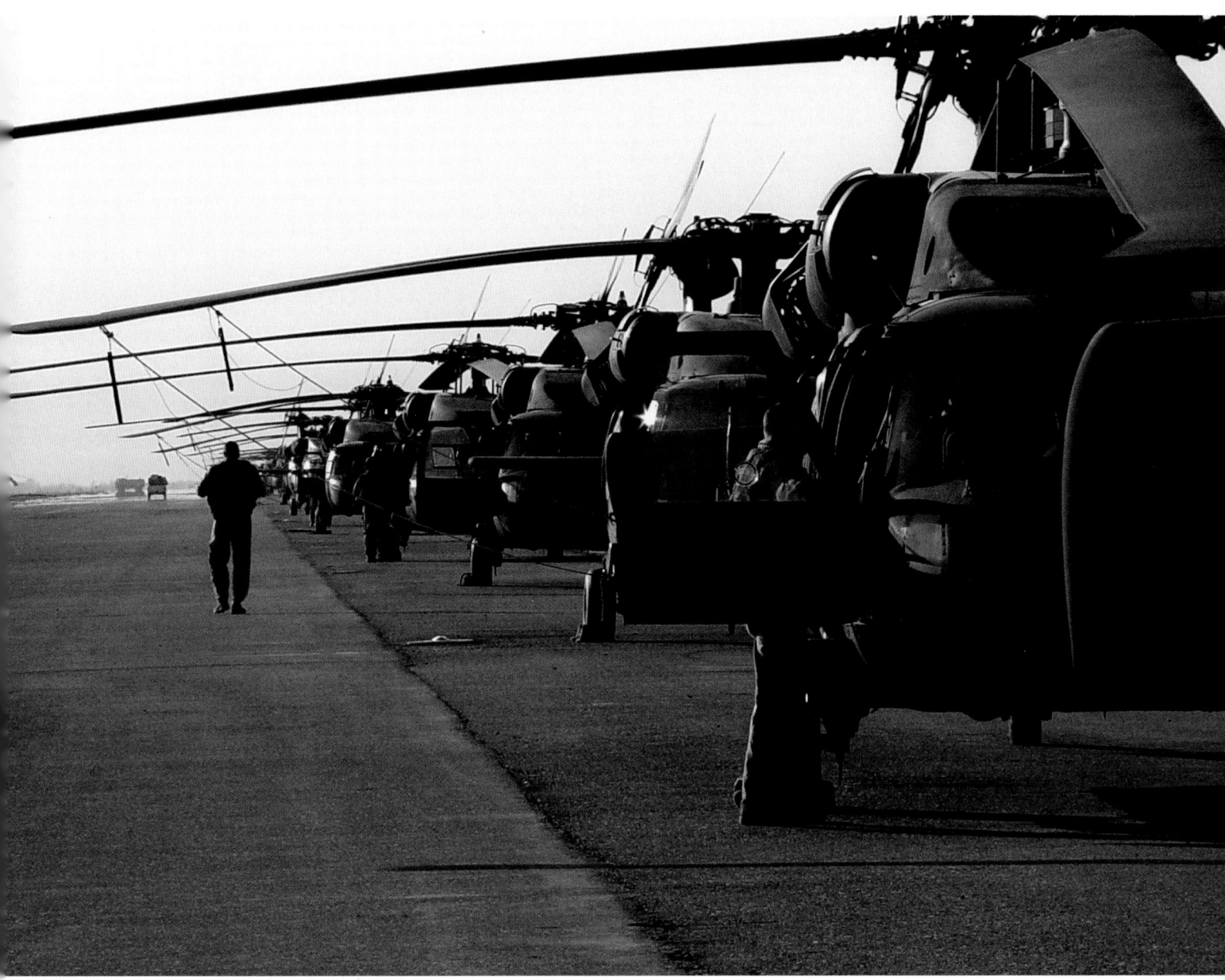

ABOVE: The 101st
Airborne Division waits
for the order to make the
final move on Baghdad.
(US DOD/COMBAT CAMERA)

Highway 9 and anti-aircraft artillery in the open terrain west of the highway. Gun camera tapes verified that the crews engaged the enemy, running in from 5km to 8km. As one aircraft approached the target, its wingman provided overwatch and suppressive fires. Once the lead aircraft had completed the engagement, the wingman would then begin his run in. The fight continued as the attack aviation alternated with CAS to destroy the forces along the highway. US Army, Air Force, and Navy pilots destroyed six armoured personnel carriers, four tanks, five trucks and a fibre-optic facility. They also killed approximately 20 troops. Although not a high count by 'exercise standards', the attack marked an effective use of deep-strike Army attack aviation against a highly adaptive enemy.

In the early hours of April 2 both V Corps and I Marine Expeditionary Force rolled forward to crush what was left of the Republican Guard.

The 3rd Infantry Division bypassed Karbala and raced north towards the Euphrates river with its own Apache gunships flying top cover. Lieutenant Colonel Daniel Williams, the commanding officer of the 1st Battalion (Attack) 3rd Aviation Regiment, described this phase of the war, saying "the mission focus of [my unit] transformed from massed battalion, or phased, attacks against armour and artillery to continuous close combat attacks in support of the [3rd] division's main effort brigade combat team.

"Due to concentrated anti-aircraft and small arms threats all over the Iraqi battlefield, the battalion's aircraft always fought in teams, and we refrained from launching single Apaches in combat operations. The lead aircraft focused eyes and fires out to their point while the wingman provided local security for the team. The battalion commander, operating from an AH-64D, also provided local security behind the attack helicopter company in contact [with the enemy]. In combat, only three [of our aircraft] sustained minor ground fire damage. One was destroyed on take-off due to drown-out conditions. The battalion fired 12,850 rounds of 30mm, 584 rockets, 117 K model 'laser' and 21 'radio frequency' Hellfire missiles."

The 11th Regiment flew extensive flank protection operations during that advance. To avoid the problems encountered during the previous week, those missions were fully integrated with air force suppression of enemy air defence (SEAD) and artillery support.

Two days later, the US Army and US Marines were at the gates of Baghdad, with the 3rd Infantry in control of the city's airport and the 1st Marines pushing into the eastern suburbs.

At the same time as the drive on Baghdad was underway, US and British troops were mopping up towns along the Euphrates that had become centres of resistance. »

RIGHT: OH-58D Kiowa Warriors were armed with rocket pods to mark targets for air strikes.
(US DOD/COMBAT CAMERA)

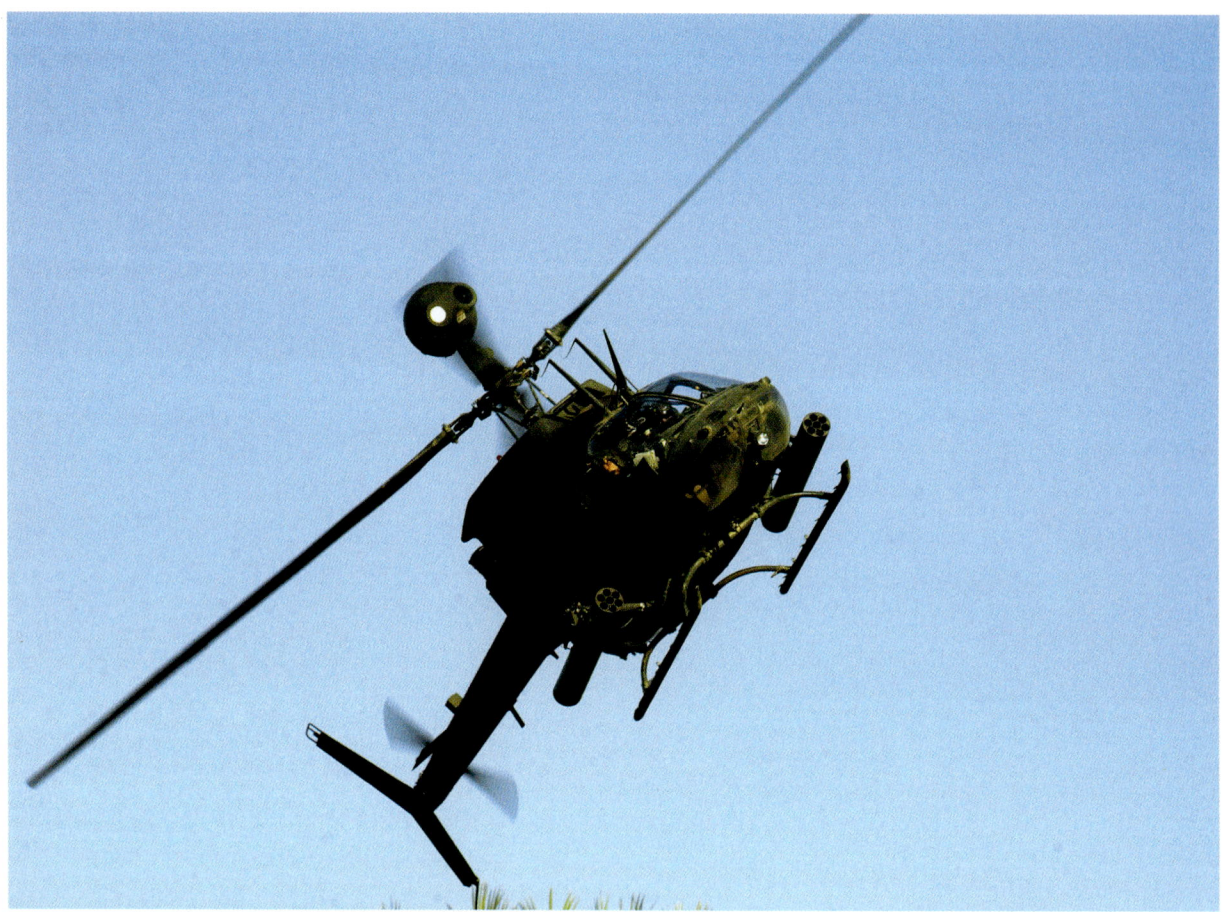

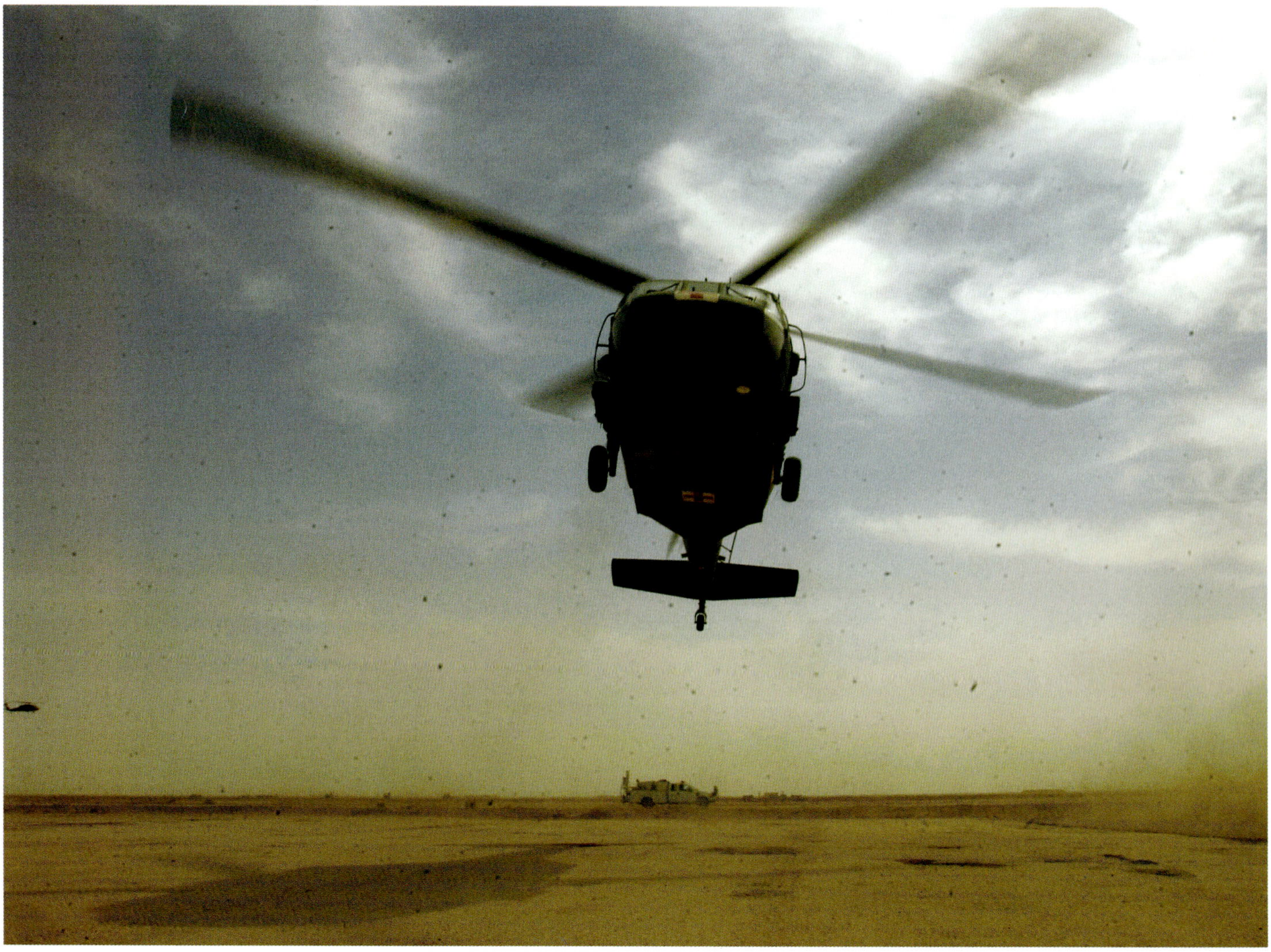

BELOW: UH-60 Black Hawks flew medical evacuation missions to bring US wounded back to field hospitals.
(US DOD/COMBAT CAMERA)

Major US Army Aviation Units – Operation Iraqi Freedom, March-April 2003

V Corps

101st Airborne Division (Air Assault)

101st Aviation Brigade
- 1st Battalion, 101st Aviation Regiment AH-64D)
- 2nd Battalion, 101st Aviation Regiment (AH-64D)
- 3rd Battalion, 101st Aviation Regiment (AH-64D)
- 6th Battalion, 101st Aviation Regiment (UH-60)

159th Aviation Brigade
- 4th Battalion, 101st Aviation Regiment (UH-60)
- 5th Battalion, 101st Aviation Regiment (UH-60)
- 7th Battalion, 101st Aviation Regiment (CH-47)
- 9th Battalion, 101st Aviation Regiment (UH-60)

4th Infantry Division

4th Brigade
- 1st Battalion, 4th Aviation Regiment (AH-64D)
- 2nd Battalion, 4th Aviation Regiment (UH-60)
- 1st Squadron, 10th Cavalry Regiment (OH-58D)

3rd Infantry Division

4th Brigade
- 1st Battalion, 3rd Aviation Regiment (AH-64D)
- A Company, 2nd Battalion, 3rd Aviation Regiment (UH-60)

82nd Airborne Division

TF 1-82nd Aviation
- A Company, 1st Battalion, 82nd Aviation Regiment (OH-58D)
- A Troop, 1st Squadron, 17th Cavalry Regiment (OH-58D)

V Corps Controlled Units

11th Attack Helicopter Regiment
- 2nd Squadron, 6th Cavalry Regiment (AH-64D)
- 6th Squadron, 6th Cavalry Regiment (AH-64D)
- 1st Battalion, 227th Aviation Regiment (AH-64D),
- 5th Battalion, 158th Aviation Regiment (UH-60)

12th Aviation Brigade
- B Company, 3rd Battalion, 158th Aviation Regiment (UH-60)
- B Company, 2nd Battalion, 159th Aviation Regiment (CH-47)
- F Company, 2nd Battalion, 159th Aviation Regiment (CH-47)
- A Company, 5th Battalion, 159th Aviation Regiment (CH-47)
- 1st Battalion, 214th Aviation Regiment (CH-47)
- F Company, 106th Aviation Regiment (CH-47)

Najaf, Karbala, and Hillah were all swept by troops of the 101st Airborne Division who flew by helicopter to secure them. Shayka Mazhar airfield was also captured in a divisional-sized air assault operation.

With Iraqi resistance apparently crumbling, General McKiernan then decided to push his troops forward into the heart of Baghdad to complete the 'psychological fracture' of Saddam Hussein's government.

Co-ordinated Iraqi resistance had all but collapsed, allowing the US Army engineers to clear debris from the runways and taxi-ways of Baghdad airport unhindered by artillery fire. This enabled USAF Lockheed C-130 Hercules transports to fly in on April 6. A battalion of the 101st Airborne Division was flown into the airport by Boeing CH-47D Chinooks and Sikorsky UH-60 Black Hawks to bolster its defence.

By the afternoon of April 9, US troops were in the centre of the Iraqi capital and the leaders of the Iraqi regime were nowhere to be seen. Sporadic fighting continued around the city, with US Army Apaches seeing action to support ground troops.

BELOW: The US Army soon lost control of Baghdad and the city became the epicentre of a six-year long bloody insurgence against the US occupation of Iraq. (US DOD/COMBAT CAMERA)

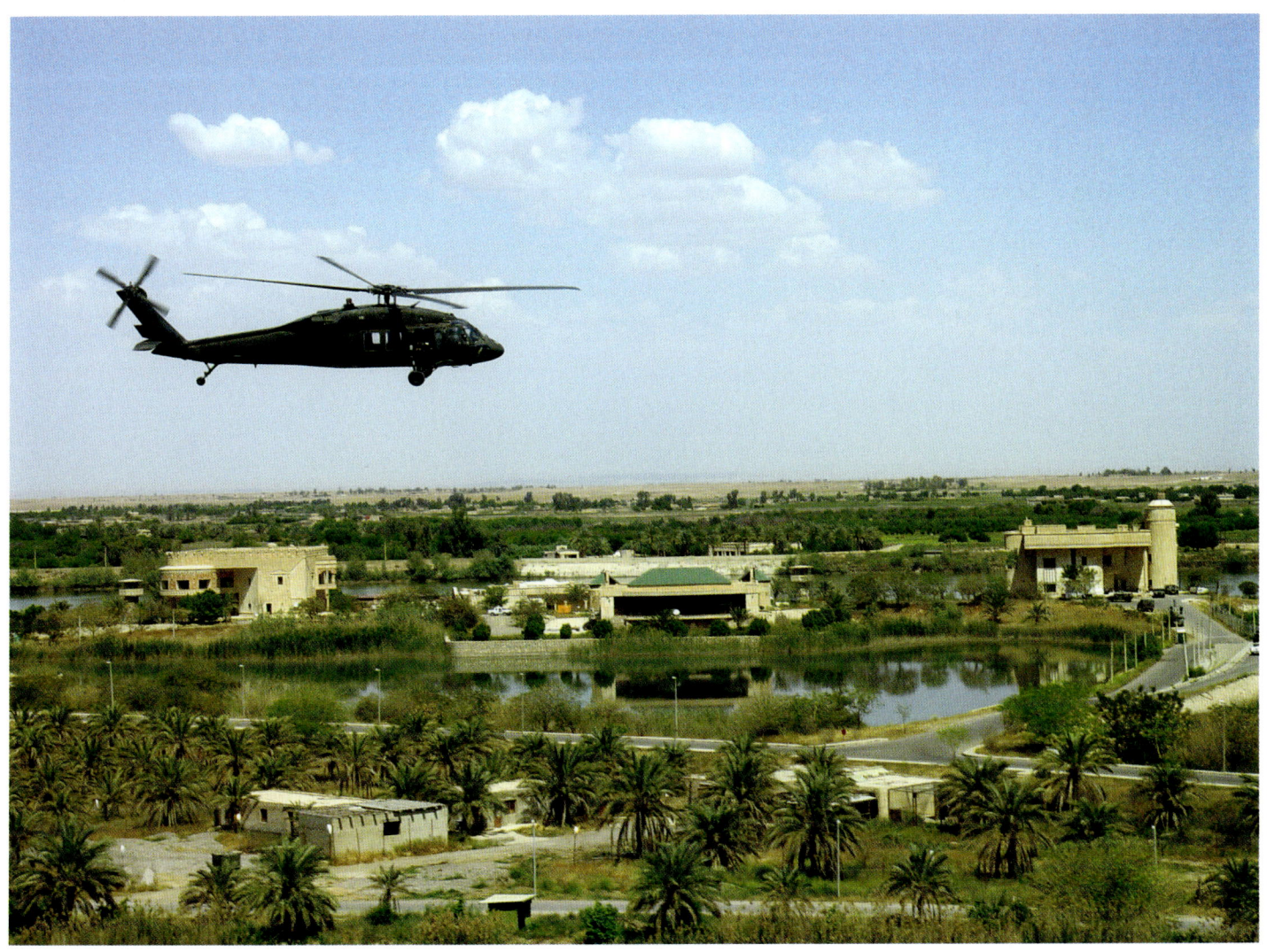

Operation Telic

Army Air Corps Over Iraq 2003

For a month in the spring of 2003, the army aviators of 3 Regiment Army Air Corps (AAC) duelled with Iraqi tanks and artillery gunners. Although the battle appeared to be hopelessly one-sided, as the men and women of 3 Regiment took to the skies over southern Iraq in March and April their enemies were far from beaten.

Operation Telic, as the British participation in the US-led invasion of Iraq was code-named, saw the first and only time to date that an AAC aviation battlegroup has been committed to high intensity combat operations against enemy armour.

In January 2003, at its Wattisham Flying Station home, 3 Regiment was in overdrive getting ready to go to war. Helicopters fitted with the latest secure radios, sand filters for the engine intakes and radar warning receivers, had to be gathered from across the AAC's fleet.

The UK was to deploy an armoured division of 28,000 troops to Kuwait to

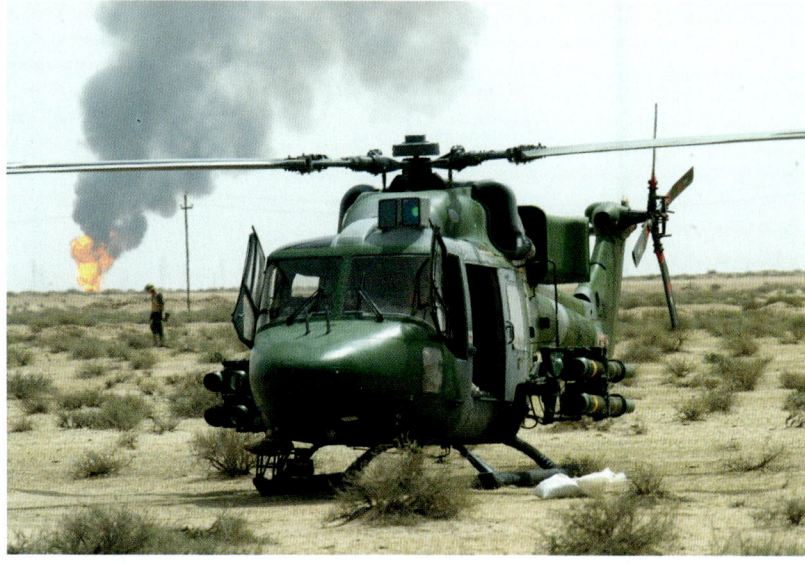

support the southern axis of advance to the Iraqi capital Baghdad. US plans called for the I Marine Expeditionary Force (I MEF) to storm across the border from Kuwait to capture the Rumaila oil field complex and then

turn east to screen Basra, allowing the US Army's V Corps to start its drive on Baghdad. In the wake of I MEF, 1 (UK) Armoured Division would move into southern Iraq and secure it, to release US troops to head north. The

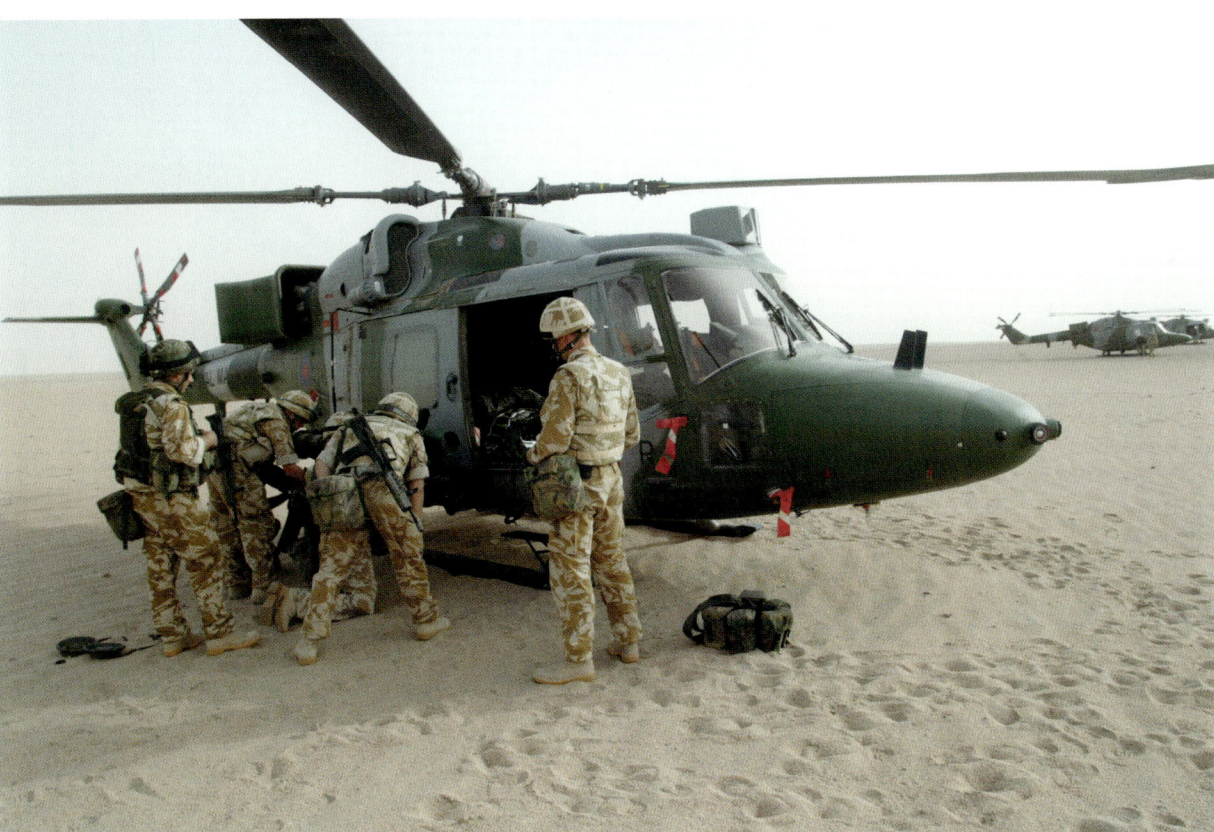

British 7 Armoured Brigade, known as the Desert Rats, were to take on Basra and 16 Brigade was tasked with taking over security of the Rumaila oil field, which contained the majority of Iraq's oil reserves.

A key role in this operation was assigned to 3 Regiment, which took two sub-units with it to the Middle East, 662 and 663 Squadrons, equipped with 10 Lynx AH7, two Lynx AH9 and 10 Gazelle AH1 helicopters.

3 Regiment was designated as an aviation battlegroup for the upcoming operation. It contained a mix of Lynx AH7s armed with TOW wired-guided missiles, two Lynx AH9 liaison helicopters, which were used as airborne command posts, and Gazelle AH1 scout helicopters. The battlegroup had self-contained mobile logistics vehicles and refuelling tanks, as well as infantry from the Royal Irish and Parachute Regiments to protect its ground positions.

When the ships carrying 3 Regiment's equipment arrived in Kuwait, the docks were full of US and British ships unloading cargo only days before the invasion was due to start. The regiment's helicopters were rebuilt on the dockside of Kuwait's main port and then flown out to the main base of 16 Brigade in the desert a few miles from the Iraqi border.

At 3.00am on March 20, US Army and Marine Corps columns started bulldozing lanes through the sand rampart, or berm, along the Iraq-Kuwait border to open routes northwards. By dawn, thousands of US armoured vehicles were heading towards Basra and Baghdad.

Orders were issued for 16 Brigade to move into Iraq in the early hours of March 21. Its infantry regiments began to enter the country in the backs of trucks. 3 Regiment's crews had flown their Lynxes and Gazelles to a tactical assembly area just south of the Iraqi border to be ready to fly deep into Iraq.

As this was happening, 3 Regiment was preparing to dispatch aviation reconnaissance patrols (ARPs) northwards to the Rumaila bridge over the al-Hammar canal to try to give warning of a counterattack by the Iraqi 6th Armoured Division, which was based to north of the canal. The first reconnaissance mission was flown by 662 Squadron on the morning of March 22 and at first there was little sign of enemy activity. These patrols involved a pair of helicopters, a Lynx, and a Gazelle, working as a team. The unarmed Gazelles functioned »

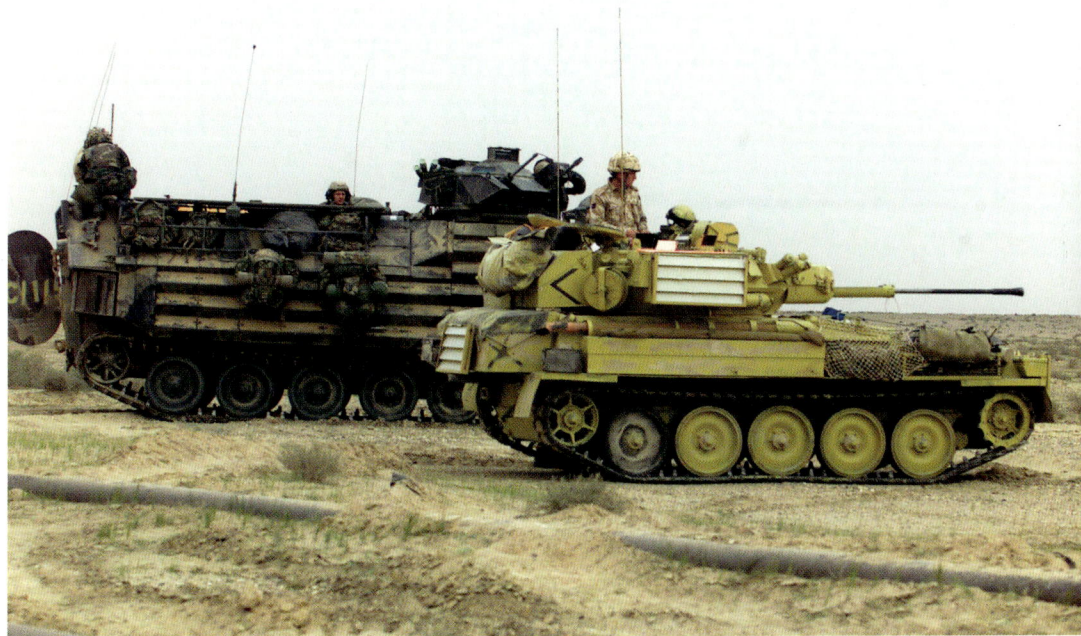

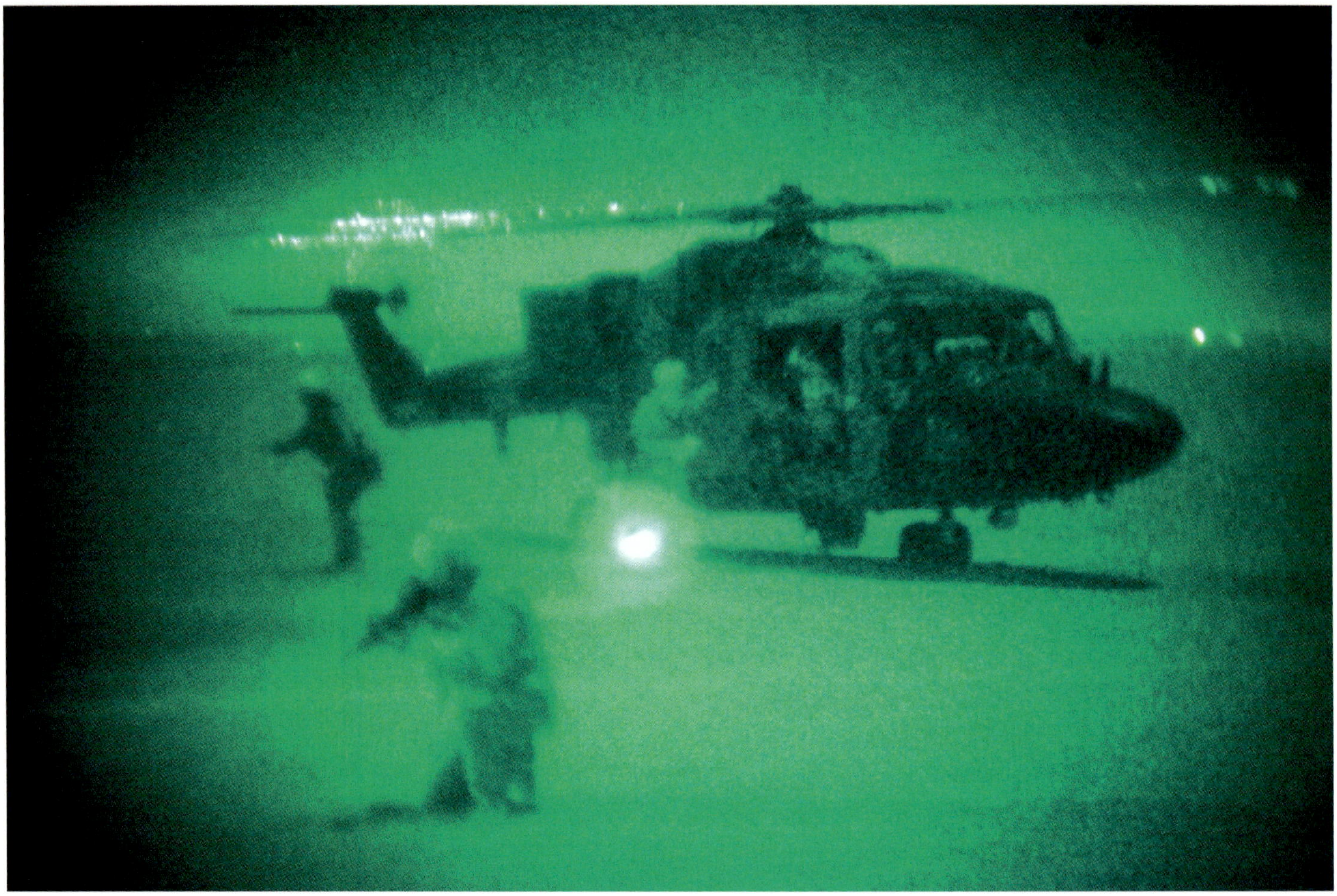

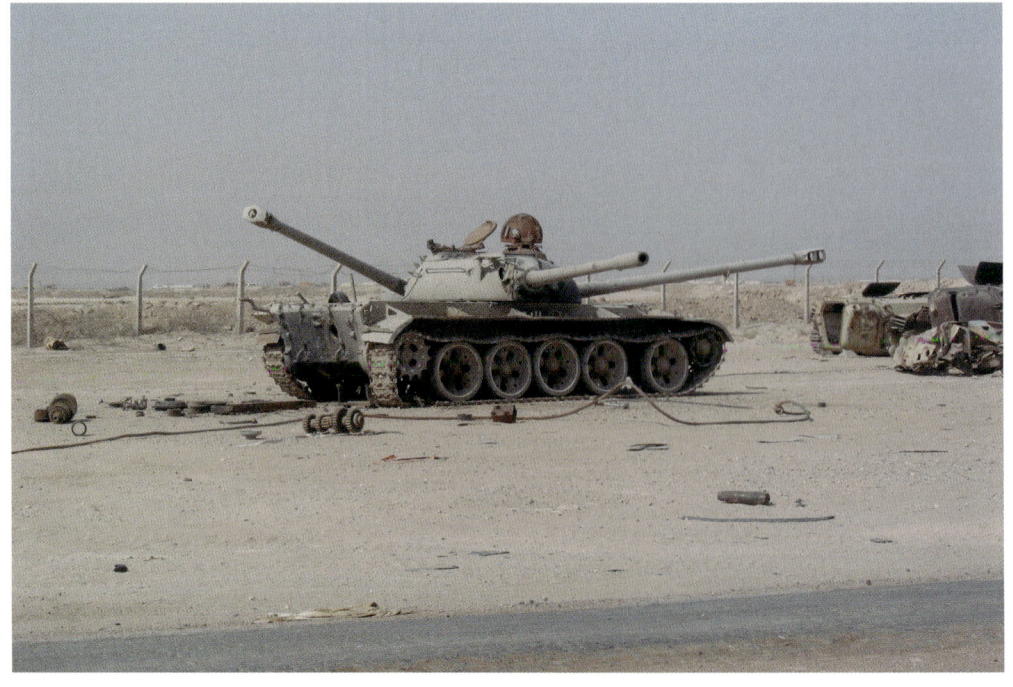

ABOVE: A 3 Regiment Lynx AH9 drops off a patrol of British soldiers during a night-time security operation to intercept sabotage teams threatening the oil infrastructure in southern Iraq. (MOD/CROWN COPYRIGHT)

BELOW: Iraqi tanks were the main target of 3 Regiment's TOW-armed Lynx AH7s during Operation Telic. (TIM RIPLEY)

as the eyes and ears for the TOW-armed Lynxes. This was necessary because the TOW missile requires the Lynx to hover or fly in a straight line as it fires its weapons, making it very vulnerable to enemy fire. By using the Gazelle as a scout, the ARP concept was meant to minimise the time the Lynx had to show itself in order to engage targets.

The size of 16 Brigade's security zone was so big helicopter patrols by 3 Regiment were the only way to monitor it and give any kind of early warning of any Iraqi forces massing nearby.

Major General Robin Brims, the commander of the British division, was not yet ready to assault the city but he wanted to stage a series of operations to specifically target centres of resistance. A series of very violent skirmishes between Iraqi and British troops broke out on the

outer fringes of Basra. To help in these engagements, on March 25 General Brims called forward two Gazelles and three Lynxes from 662 Squadron. They set up a forward operating base at the disused Shaibah airfield to the southwest of Basra. In the early hours of the following morning, the Lynxes staged a raid on Iraqi troops occupying a factory complex, destroying four buildings, an ammunition dump, and a water tower with TOW missiles. The 662 Squadron detachment remained at Shaibah for several more days and was increasingly drawn into the battle for Basra. On March 28, two of its Lynxes discovered and destroyed two heavily armed Iraqi militia 'technical' vehicles with two TOW missiles. This was a major achievement because 3 Regiment was finding that the TOW missile had several limitations. These included a tendency for the missile to 'hang-up' when its rocket motors failed to fire and drop down below the helicopter, spooling out the guidance wire. Unless the wires were immediately cut they could become entangled in the helicopter's tail rotors.

16 Brigade was ordered to focus on containing the Iraqi 6th Armoured Division north of the al-Hammer canal. ARPs of 3 Regiment were ordered to probe along the canal to find the centre of Iraqi resistance

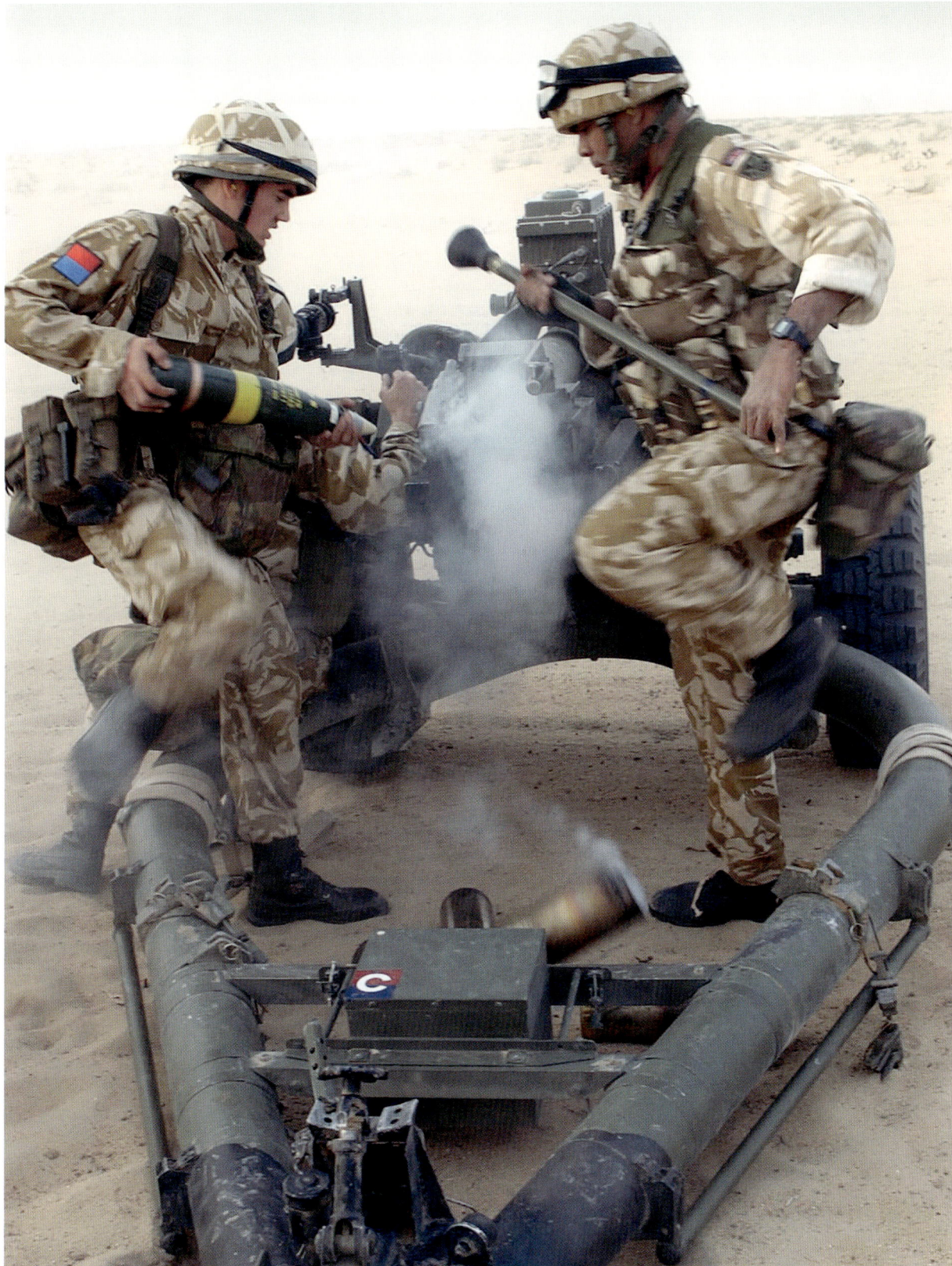

and call down artillery fire and air strikes. At dawn on March 28, a Lynx and Gazelle from 663 Squadron made the first-ever ARP over the forward line of British troops and into enemy territory.

3 Regiment's Lynxes joined the battle, hitting targets with TOW missiles or calling in artillery fire. Iraqi armour was engaged for the first time by 663 Squadron at 8.25am on March 28. An hour later the squadron attacked more Iraqi tanks with a barrage of 12 TOW missiles, destroying two T-55s. Later in the day the squadron also destroyed a BMP armoured personnel carrier.

For over a week the battle grew in intensity as 16 Brigade pushed its reconnaissance forces further north from the al-Hammer canal towards the Euphrates river and the main defensive positions of the Iraqi division. The terrain between the canal and the Euphrates alternated between palm groves and marshy ground, so there was plenty of opportunity for the Iraqis to hide their positions. This was by no means a one-sided battle, with the Iraqis making extensive use of their target location systems to control their return artillery fire. On an hourly basis, British Lynx pilots had to dodge Iraqi tanks, artillery, and mortar fire aimed at their helicopters. If they　»

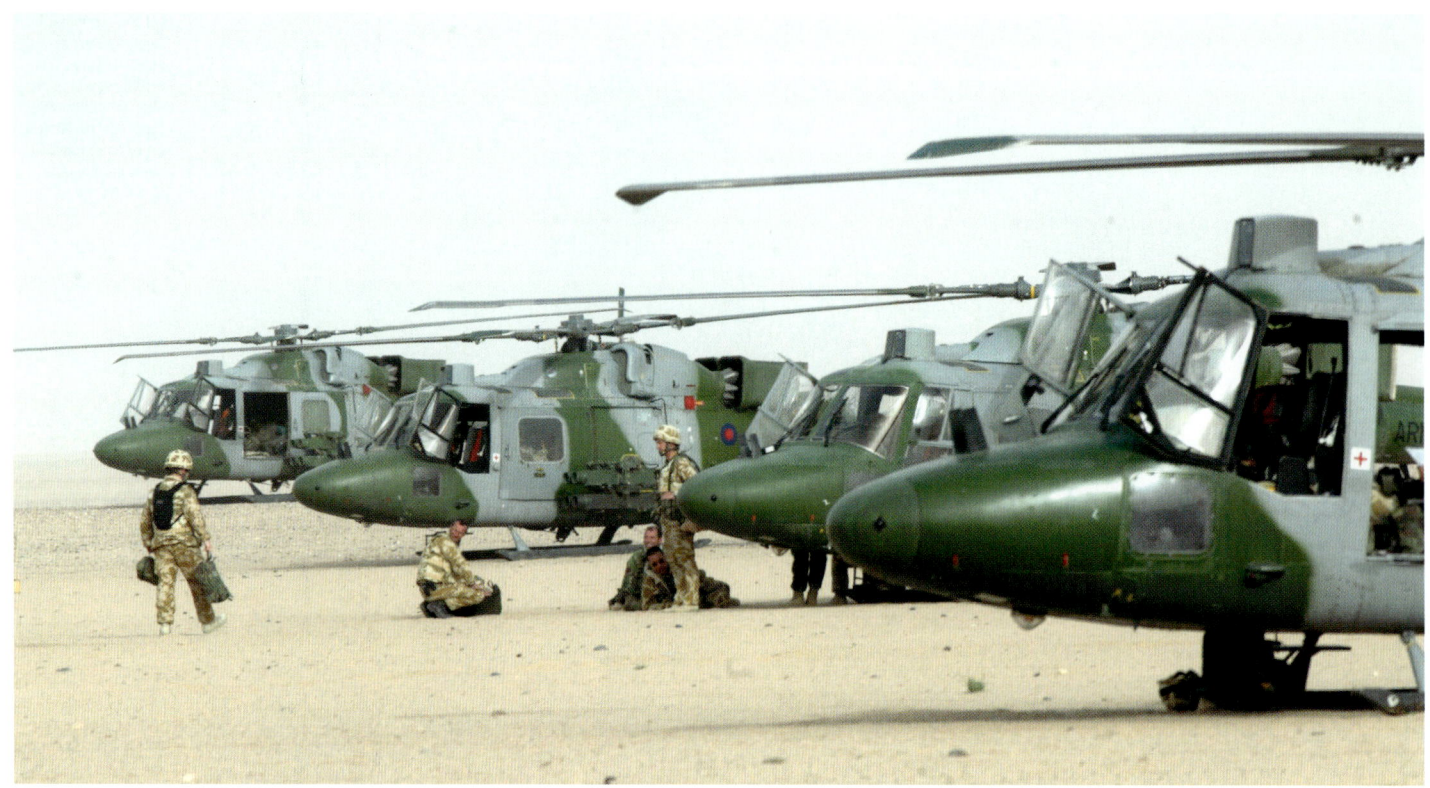

got too close to Iraqi infantry, volleys of rocket-propelled grenades could be expected.

In one typical incident during that period, Iraqi artillery and tank shells were exploding amidst the Scimitar-armoured vehicles of the Household Cavalry Regiment (HCR). An ARP of Lynx and Gazelle helicopters from 3 Regiment, led by Captain Richard Cathill, arrived overhead to give fire support. With visibility obscured

by sand thrown up by the Iraqi fire, Cathill manoeuvred his Lynx behind the Scimitars so he could line up and fire along the path of the 30mm tracer rounds fired by the HCR vehicles. He spotted the muzzle flash of an Iraqi self-propelled artillery piece and guided a TOW missile onto its target. This required him to fly his helicopter straight and level as shells exploded around it and his bravery won him the Distinguished Flying Cross.

In the first week of April, American troops were closing in on Baghdad and General Brims was getting ready to make his assault on Basra. Simultaneously, 16 Brigade was ordered to prepare to assault the 6th Division's positions at Ad Dayr and Al Qurnah to seize key bridges over the Euphrates.

Resistance in Basra appeared to be faltering and that was the cue for 3 Regiment to ramp up its support

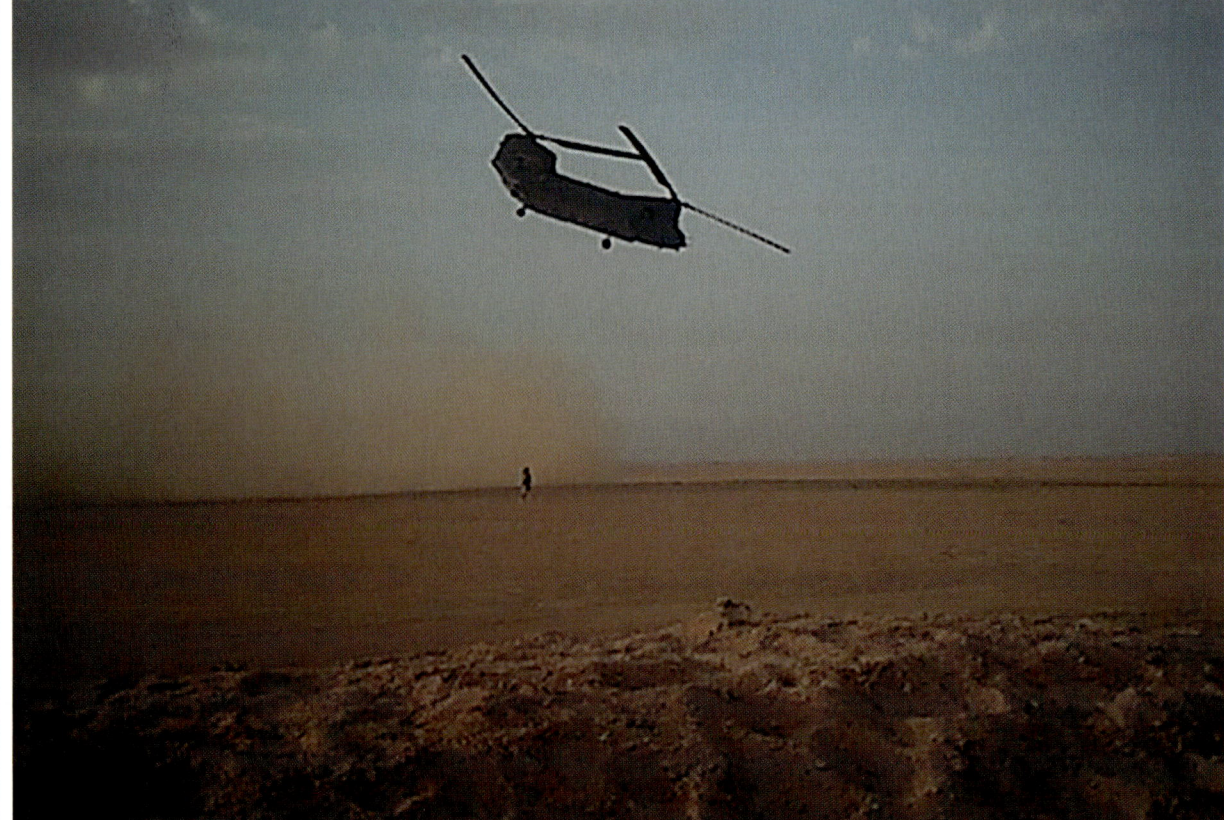

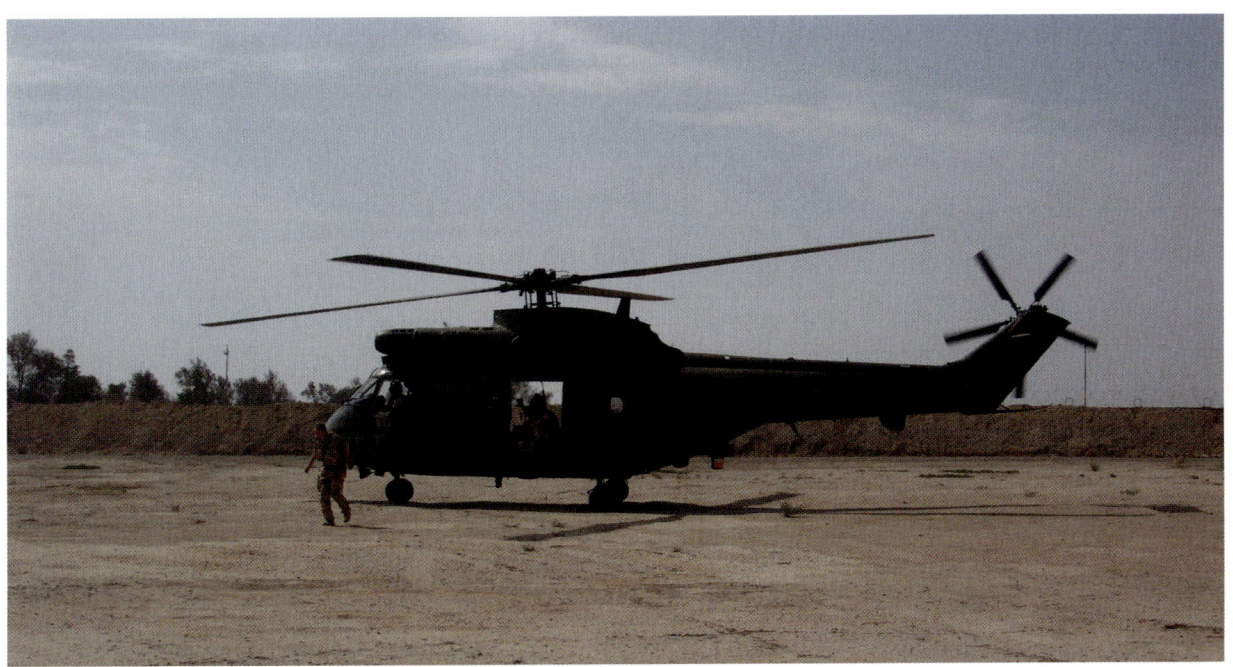

Westland Lynx AH7	
Powerplant:	2 × Gem 41-1 turboshafts
Length:	13.3m (43ft 9in)
Rotor Diameter:	12.8m (42 ft)
Height:	3.67m (12ft 0.5in)
Maximum take-off weight:	4,874kg (10,747lbs)
Speed:	296km/h (184mph)
Range:	596km (322nm)
Crew:	2-3
Capacity:	8 troopers

Armament

8 x TOW anti-tank guided missiles, 2 x 7.62mm General Purpose Machine Guns or .50cal Heavy Machine Gun

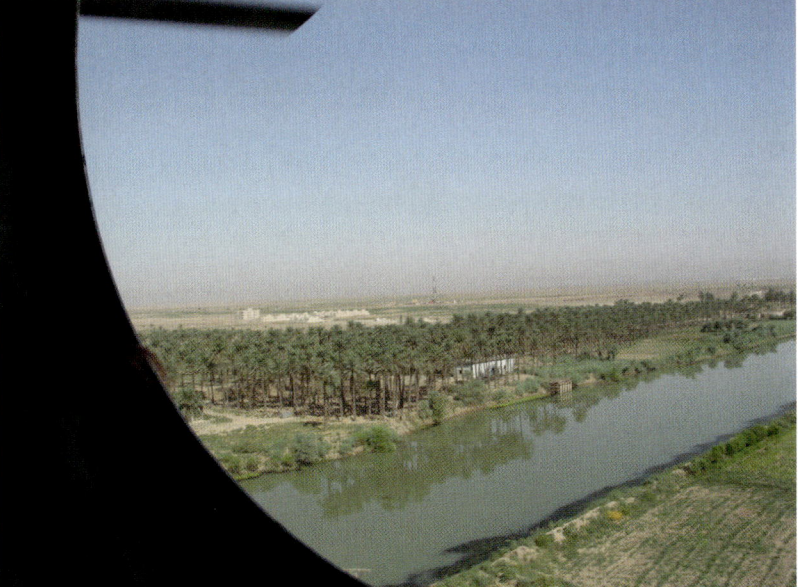

for 7 Brigade, with a regular rotation of ARPs organised to overfly the outskirts of Basra. One 622 Squadron ARP was engaged by an Iraqi surface-to-air missile on April 3, indicating that there was still some fight left in Iraqi defenders concealed in and around the city.

On April 6, US troops entered Baghdad. This was the moment General Brims had been waiting for and he ordered 7 Brigade to sweep into the city. The advance began on the morning of April 7, with 662 Squadron flying top cover, but it proved to be an anti-climax with cheering crowds of locals filling the streets to welcome the British troops.

This brought 3 Regiment's war to an end. It had played a key part in 16 Brigade's blitzkrieg advance through Iraq, and it gave crucial air support to 7 Brigade's drive on Basra. At the end of the war, 16 Brigade claimed the destruction of 86 Iraqi tanks, as well as hundreds of other vehicles and weapons. Out of these, 3 Regiment claimed four T-55s, two 2S1 self-propelled artillery pieces, a D30 howitzer, a BMP armoured vehicle and two 'technical' vehicles.

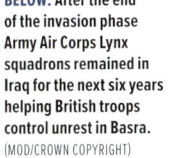

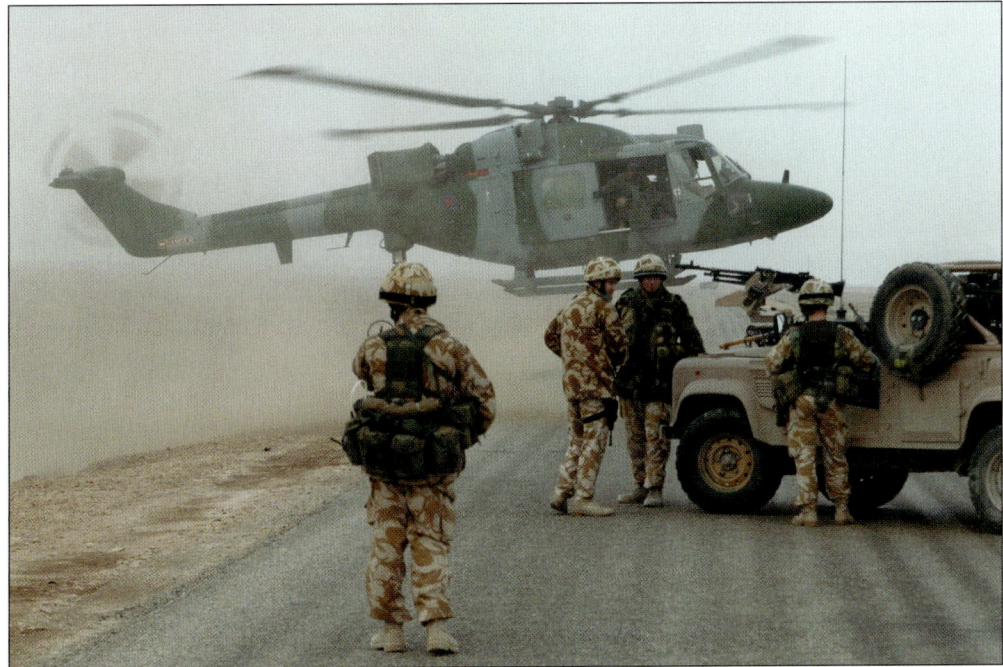

Britain's Apache over Helmand

Operation Herrick 2006 to 2007

RIGHT: The dramatic rescue mission into Jugroom Fort in 2007 saw AAC helicopter crews awarded decorations for valour.
(KANDAHAR MEDIA POOL)

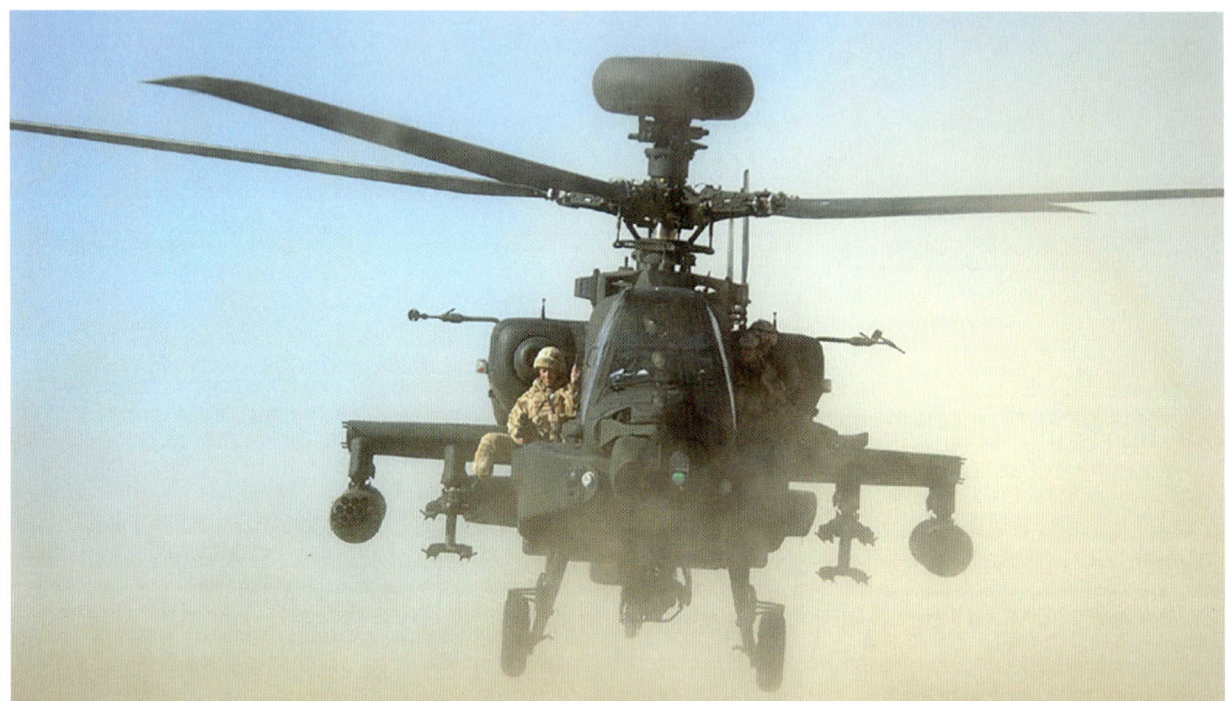

When the news emerged in January 2007 that three British Royal Marines and a Royal Engineer had strapped themselves onto the outside of two AgustaWestland Apache AH1 attack helicopters and been flown into the Taliban's Jugroom Fort, near the town of Garmsir in Afghanistan's southern Helmand province, to rescue a missing Royal Marine, it was greeted with incredulity. This was bravery of the highest order and left many people wondering why none of the participants received the country's highest decoration, the Victoria Cross for their part in the rescue.

The two Apache pilots, including Captain Tom O'Malley, received the Distinguished Flying Cross. The three Royal Marines did not receive decorations.

Warrant Officer Class 1 Ed Macy and Staff Sergeant Keith Armatage, both of 656 Squadron Army Air Corps, along with Captain David Rigg of the Royal Engineers, all received the British armed forces'

RIGHT: The rescuers seen riding on one of the Apache AH1's stub wings through the night vision system of the other rescue helicopter.
(MOD/CROWN COPYRIGHT)

third highest decoration for gallantry, the Military Cross for their part in the rescue of the body of Lance Corporal Mathew Ford. The medal citations needed little embellishment: "On 15 January 2007, Macy and Armatage were the Apache pilots supporting

a raid into a Taliban stronghold. Despite a heavy preparatory air and artillery bombardment, the ground assault had resulted in five British casualties around the walls of the fort. Following the confusion of the withdrawal one of the casualties,

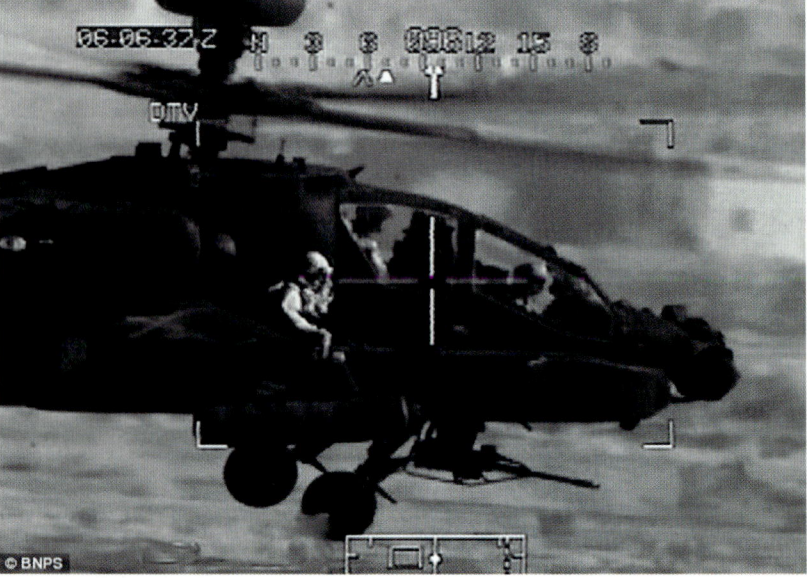

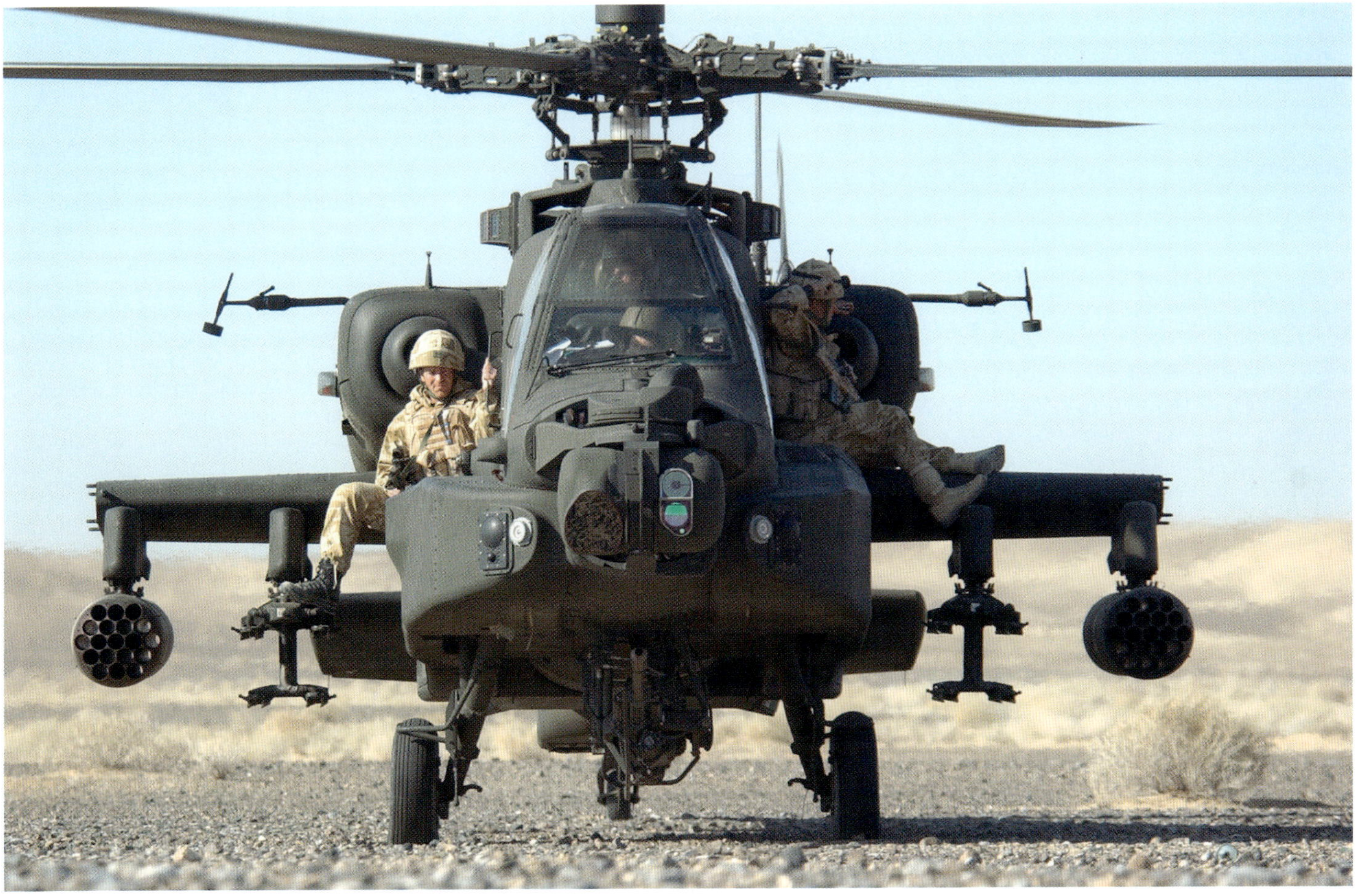

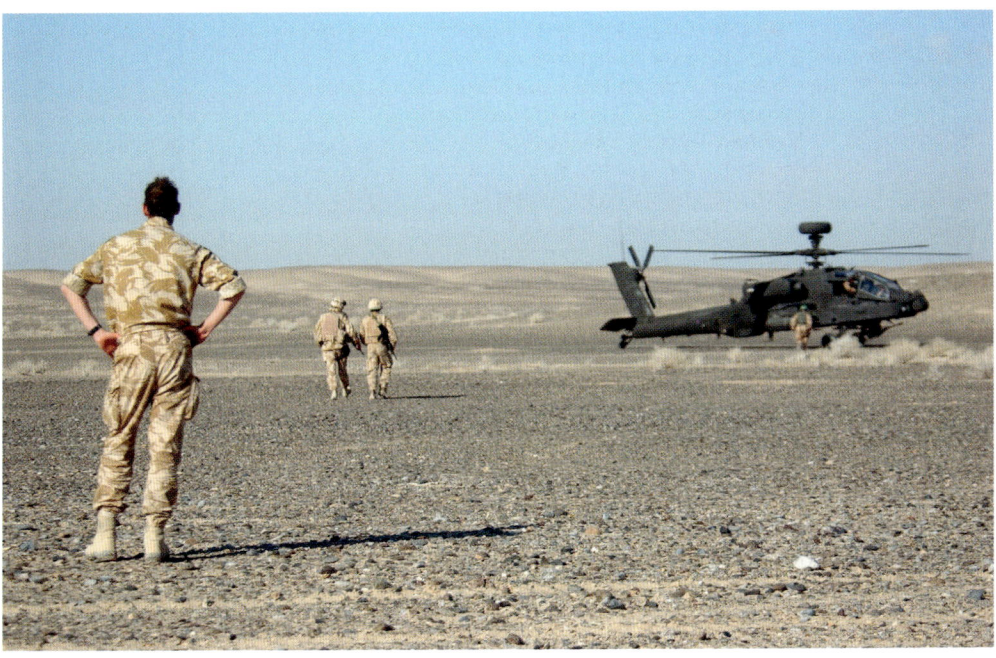

Lance Corporal Ford, was reported missing in action. A plan to rescue him was made.

"Macy demonstrated selfless gallantry and leadership as he helped inspire a hastily drawn together team to recover Ford. Macy's courage, quick thinking, and determination to find and recover Ford, with complete disregard for his own safety, was an outstanding act of valour and leadership.

"During the mission to recover Ford's body, Armatage was unable to land [his helicopter] where planned. The rescuers were disorientated and, seeing this, Armatage, armed only with a pistol, got out of his aircraft to lead them to the casualty. Almost immediately they came under enemy small arms fire. Throughout this audacious mission, Armatage's flying was impressively courageous and skilful. However, the fact that he evacuated his Apache armed only with a pistol to bring coherence to Ford's recovery was truly extraordinary."

"Rigg, despite thinking he was about to be thrown into a deliberate enemy ambush, volunteered immediately to take part in the rescue of Ford [strapping himself to the outside of an Apache]. He knew that he would be returning to face an aggressive, determined, and lethal enemy, who were already alert to the company's presence and were very likely to anticipate their return to find Ford. In the ensuing action Rigg displayed outstanding valour, clarity of thought and purpose to recover Ford and return him to his comrades, in the face of a lethal and determined enemy, with deliberate disregard for his own safety."

Over the summer of 2006 and into 2007, the Apache AH1 crews of 9 Regiment AAC were in action daily helping to protect isolated detachments of British Paratroopers and Royal Marines in Helmand province. Those battles have entered military folklore as, time after time, the arrival of pairs of Apaches would save the day by driving off hundreds of Taliban fighters besieging the British bases.

The Joint Helicopter Force (Afghanistan) (JHF(A)) had its headquarters at Kandahar Airfield and provided helicopters to work under the tactical command of the 3rd Battalion, The Parachute ➤➤

ABOVE: There was no shortage of volunteers to join the mission to rescue Corporal Ford from Jugroom Fort.
(MOD/CROWN COPYRIGHT)

BELOW: The rescue mission was launched from a remote site several miles from the Jugroom Fort, out in the Helmand desert.
(MOD/CROWN COPYRIGHT)

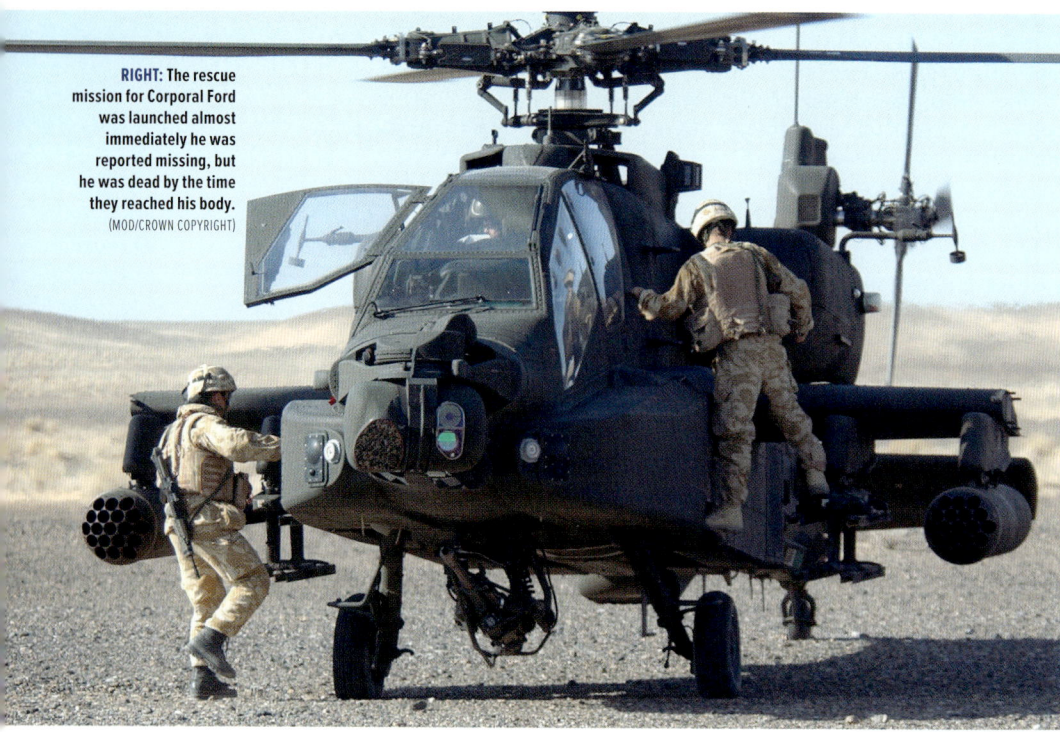

RIGHT: The rescue mission for Corporal Ford was launched almost immediately he was reported missing, but he was dead by the time they reached his body. (MOD/CROWN COPYRIGHT)

BELOW: The summer of 2006 saw troops of the Parachute Regiment cut off in isolated Platoon Houses across Helmand and they were dependent on helicopter support for survival. (MOD/CROWN COPYRIGHT)

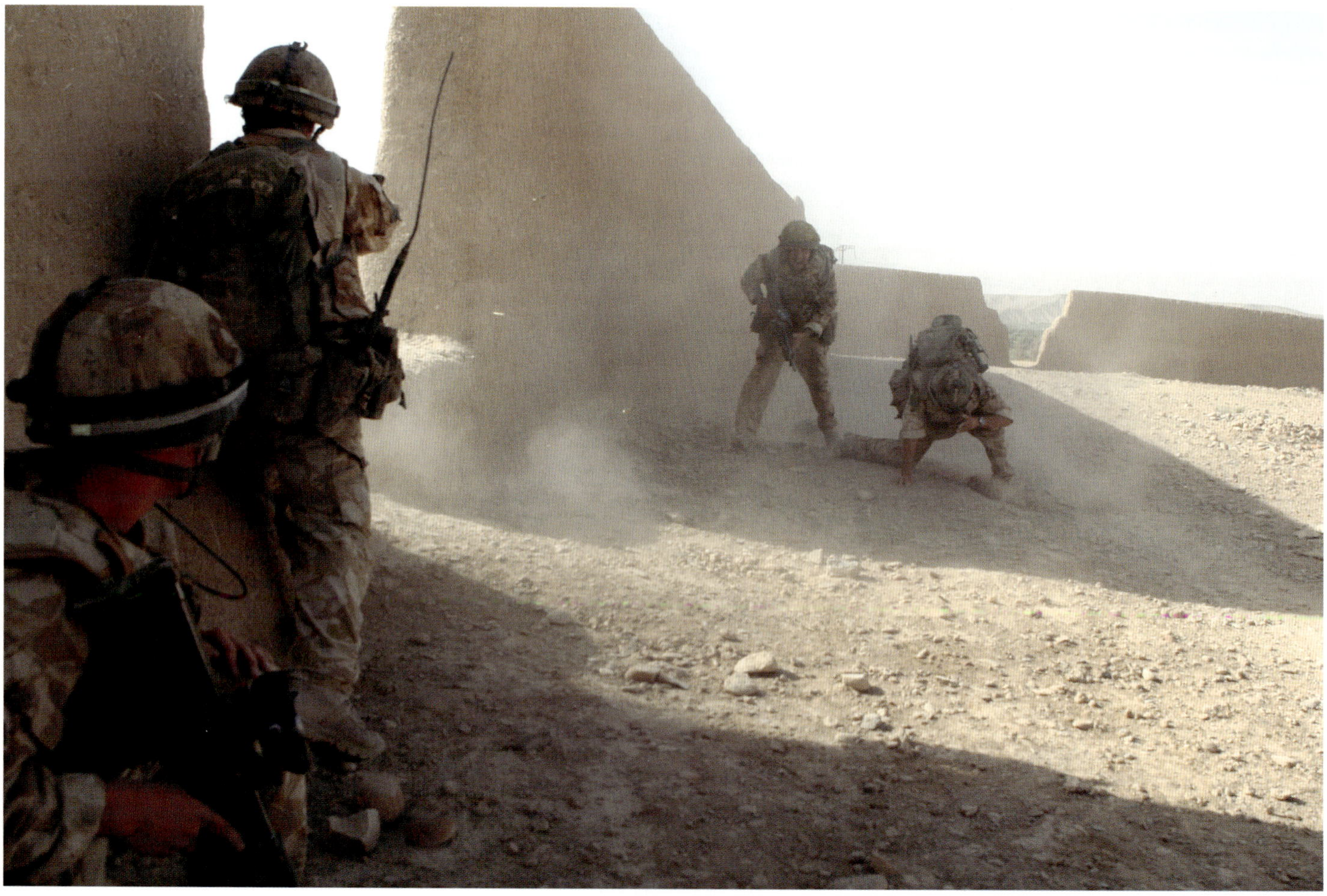

Regiment (3 PARA) at Camp Bastion. On each day during the summer of 2006, JHC(A) had to provide basic casualty evacuation and medical coverage for the British force and a reserve or reaction force element to respond to unforeseen events such as a helicopter crash. Any extra capacity was made available for deliberate or pre-planned British operations. Other NATO nations and the Afghans could also request British helicopter support when needed.

A flavour of the fighting in the summer of 2006 was provided by an RAF Flight Lieutenant who flew Boeing Chinook HC2s in Helmand during this period. "On a typical day, two Apaches and two Chinooks were deployed with the Immediate Reaction [medical] Team (IRT) and the [platoon-sized] Helmand Reaction Force (HRT) on standby at Bastion, 24/7," he said. "IRT/HRF were our priority and had to be sustained. They brought out wounded troops and responded to crises."

"We used Kandahar as our maintenance area and the remainder of our force was based [at Bastion]," recalled an AAC Apache AH1 pilot who served in Afghanistan in 2006. "Of our eight aircraft, four were up at Bastion at any one time. The Apache main effort was forward [at Bastion].

"The threat determined that we had to work as a team. The Chinook was the army's lifeline but because of the threat and the fact that the Apache provided fire support and eyes on target with its sensors, we did joint planning and preparation. You couldn't do it separately. To have any effect we worked closely as a team."

The Chinook pilot reinforced that point: "Working with Apaches was routine. There was no RAF/Army divide there. We just had different types of aircraft. We planned and briefed together."

The bulk of the HTF's combat troops was committed in the district centre and they were fighting for their

lives. With the summer heat pushing above 50°C, food, and water scarce and the troops fighting around the clock, senior officers wondered how long their men could keep fighting. Without the Chinooks and Apaches bringing in supplies and protecting road convoys, the troops would not have been able to hold on.

Brigadier Ed Butler, commander of 16 Air Assault Brigade, said 3 PARA could not have held out without the efforts of the RAF Chinook crews.

"They carried the most risk of anyone here – they can have 40 to 50 guys on board their helicopters," he recalled. "I must praise them for keeping going back, it was pretty close at times. They have done some awesome flying." By moving his troops by air the Brigadier said the Chinooks "saved many lives".

When the UK's helicopters were concentrated for a deliberate operation, considerable planning, and preparation was involved over a

48-hour period. "There was massive co-ordination of the many moving parts, not just aviation," said an AAC Captain who served in Helmand in the summer of 2006. "We used fast jets in support because we were the Airborne Forward Air Controllers in the fight. During deliberate operations we would talk in fast jets, monitoring the territory as the Chinook landed."

"We were busy, but it ebbed and flowed," said one Apache pilot. »

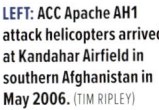

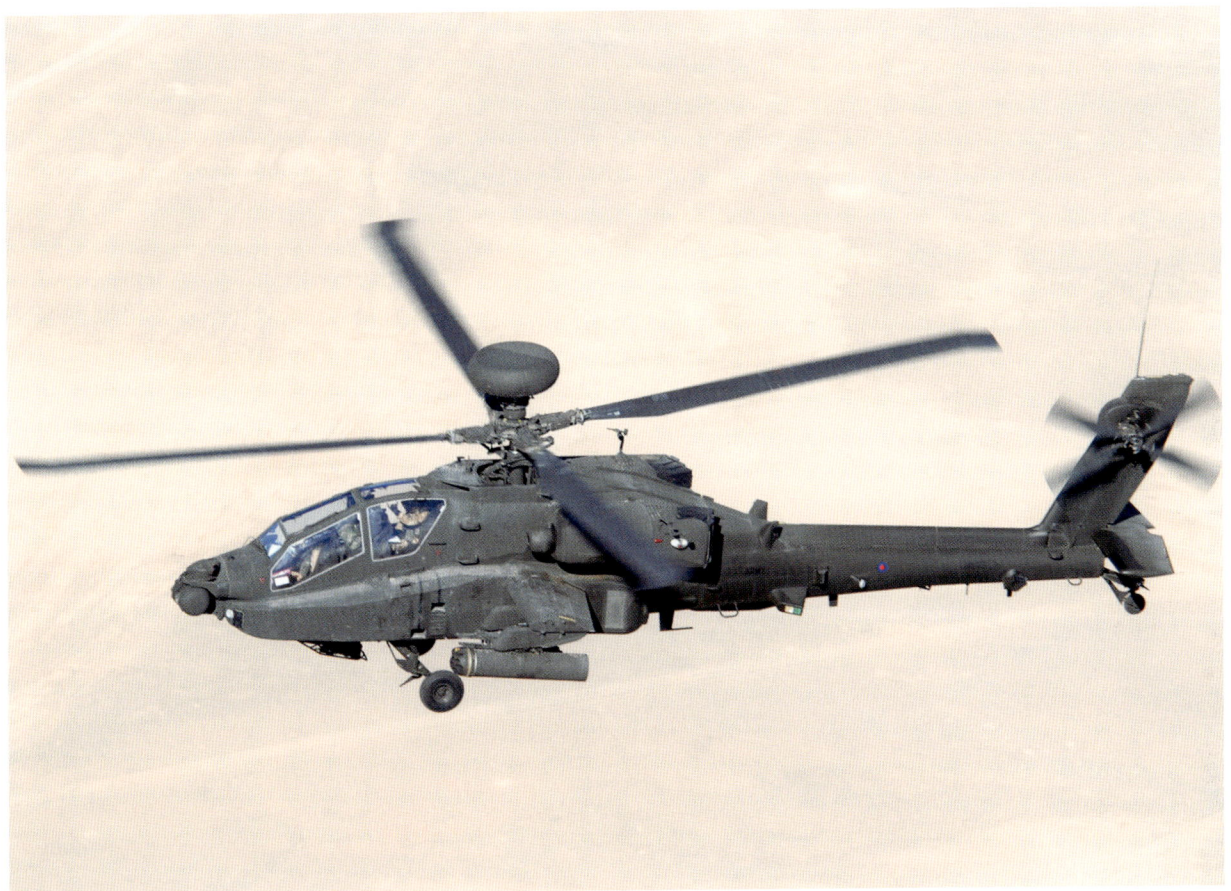

LEFT: ACC Apache AH1 attack helicopters arrived at Kandahar Airfield in southern Afghanistan in May 2006. (TIM RIPLEY)

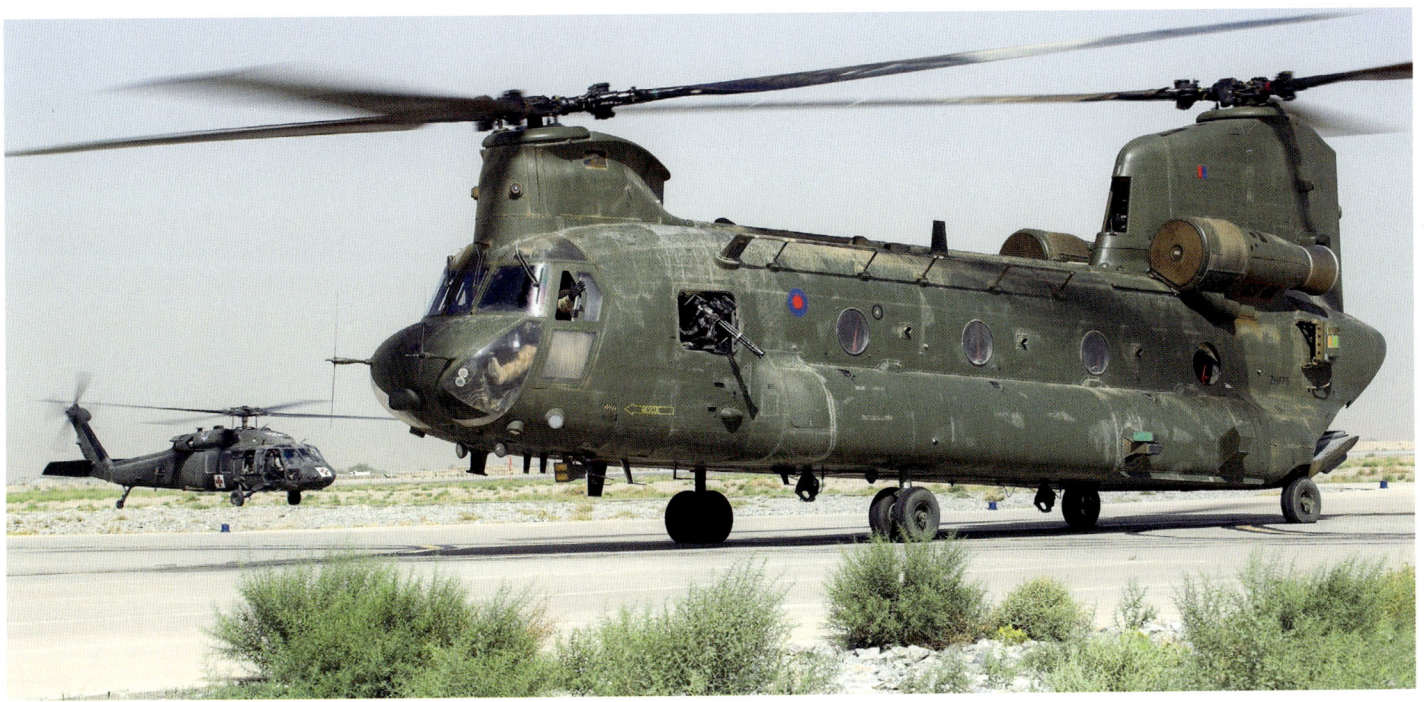

BELOW: Joint operations with RAF Chinook HC2 support helicopters to deliver assault troops deep into enemy territory soon became a regular feature of AAC Apache AH1 operations in Afghanistan. (CANADIAN MINISTRY OF NATIONAL DEFENCE)

Operation Herrick AAC Attack Helicopter Squadron deployments to Afghanistan 2006-2014	
Tour Dates	**Unit**
May to Aug 06	656 Squadron
Sept to Dec 06	664 Squadron
Jan to Apr 07	656 Squadron
May to Nov 07	662 Squadron
Dec 07 to Apr 08	663 Squadron
May to Aug 08	664 Squadron
Sept to Dec 08	654 Squadron
Jan to Apr 09	656 Squadron
May to Aug 09	662 Squadron
Sept to Dec 09	663 Squadron
Jan to Apr 10	653 Squadron
May to Aug 10	664 Squadron
Sept to Dec 10	654 Squadron
Jan to Apr 11	662 Squadron
May to Apr 11	663 Squadron
Sept to Dec 11	653 Squadron
Jan to Apr 12	654 Squadron
May to Aug 12	664 Squadron
Sept to Dec 12	662 Squadron
Jan to Apr 13	663 Squadron
May to Aug 13	653 Squadron
Sep 13 to Jan 14	654 Squadron
Feb to Jun 14	664 Squadron
Jul to Nov 14	662 Squadron

BELOW: A forward detachment of Apache AH1s operated from Camp Bastion during 2006 to provide a very high readiness alert capability. (AGUSTAWESTLAND)

"In general, our tactics were very different from the Chinooks. They had to go to lower levels but there was still the RPG threat and terrain [problems]. The enemy usually knew we were coming so we were always evolving our tactics. Ideas were always coming from the ground troops on better ways to flush out the enemy. Finding them in the first place was the most the difficult thing. This was very small-scale stuff but highly dangerous.

"Things were constantly changing. What you expected would not happen," said the Chinook pilot. "Big multi-ship operations were hairy. The locals expected us and so you had to do it fast. There was a real risk. You needed speed. We had a few hits when we had to go in and land. The Apaches stayed in the overhead, but we had to descend into the threat area."

"In district compounds they had Joint Terminal Attack Controllers (JTACs, formerly Forward Air Controllers) and they would call us in," said the AAC Captain. "We used close-in fire support (CIFS) procedures in one operation. The Paras were moving through an area,

flushing the [bad] guys out, when they came up on [radio] net asking us to engage the enemy in the wood line. It did work. The enemy ran when we appeared. If they did not, and were seen, they went to pieces – literally. The gun was our weapon of choice. It can be engaged quickly and accurately. You just kept your eyes on target. You only got a 10- to 15-second glimpse of the bad guys. If you chased them into a building, then you put in a Hellfire and if they were hiding in a field, you would use rockets."

The intensity of operations by the Apache force can be gauged by the fact that 664 Squadron flew 2,147 hours on its August to November 2006 tour, firing 9,100 30mm cannon rounds, 65 CRV-7 rockets and 28 AGM-114 Hellfire missiles.

Praise for the high level of integration between land forces and helicopters was repeated by Brigadier Ed Butler, who said: "3 PARA would not go anywhere without attack helicopters because of the effect they had on the enemy. There is an unprecedented bond between 3 PARA and the helicopter crews."

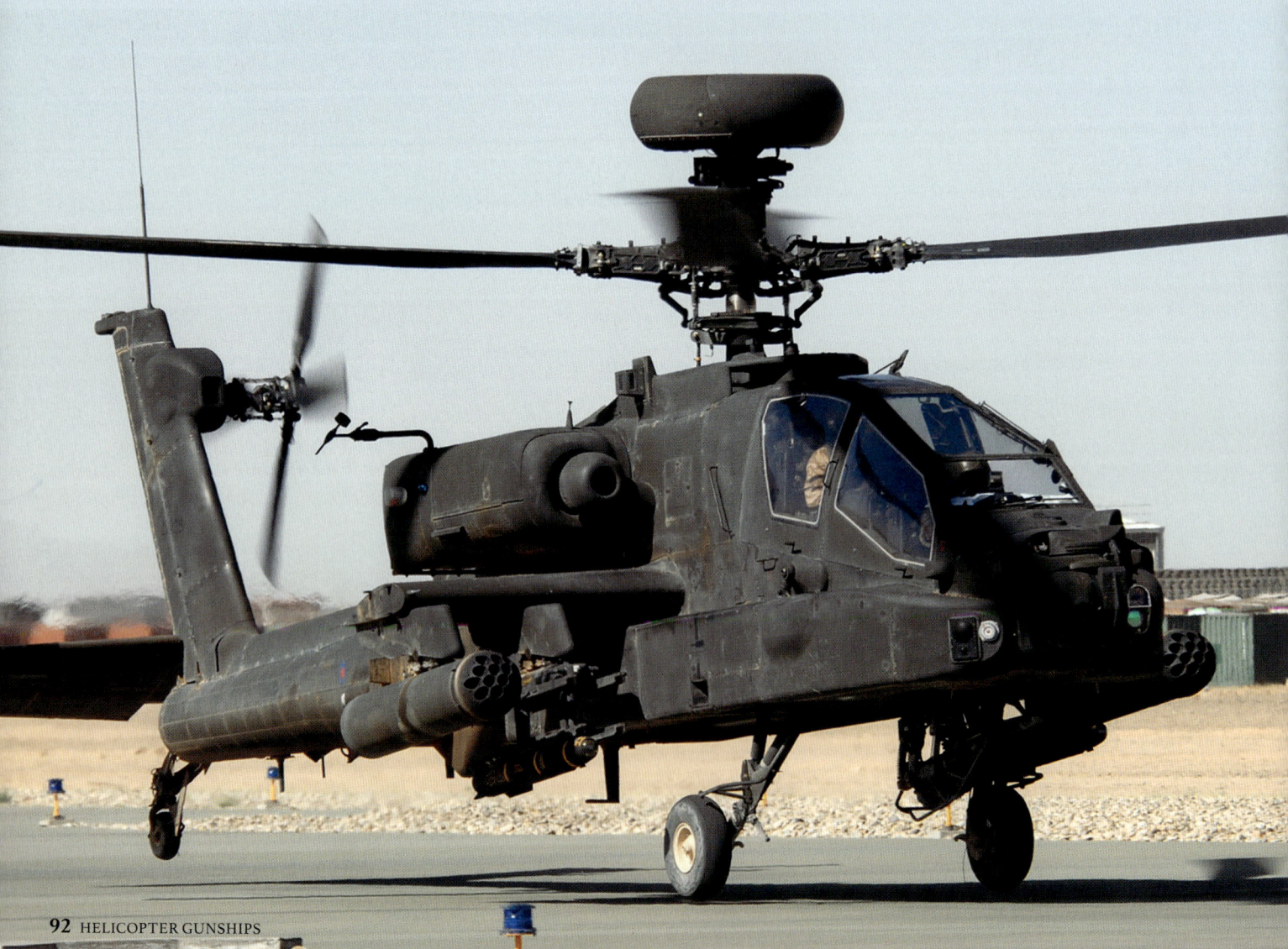

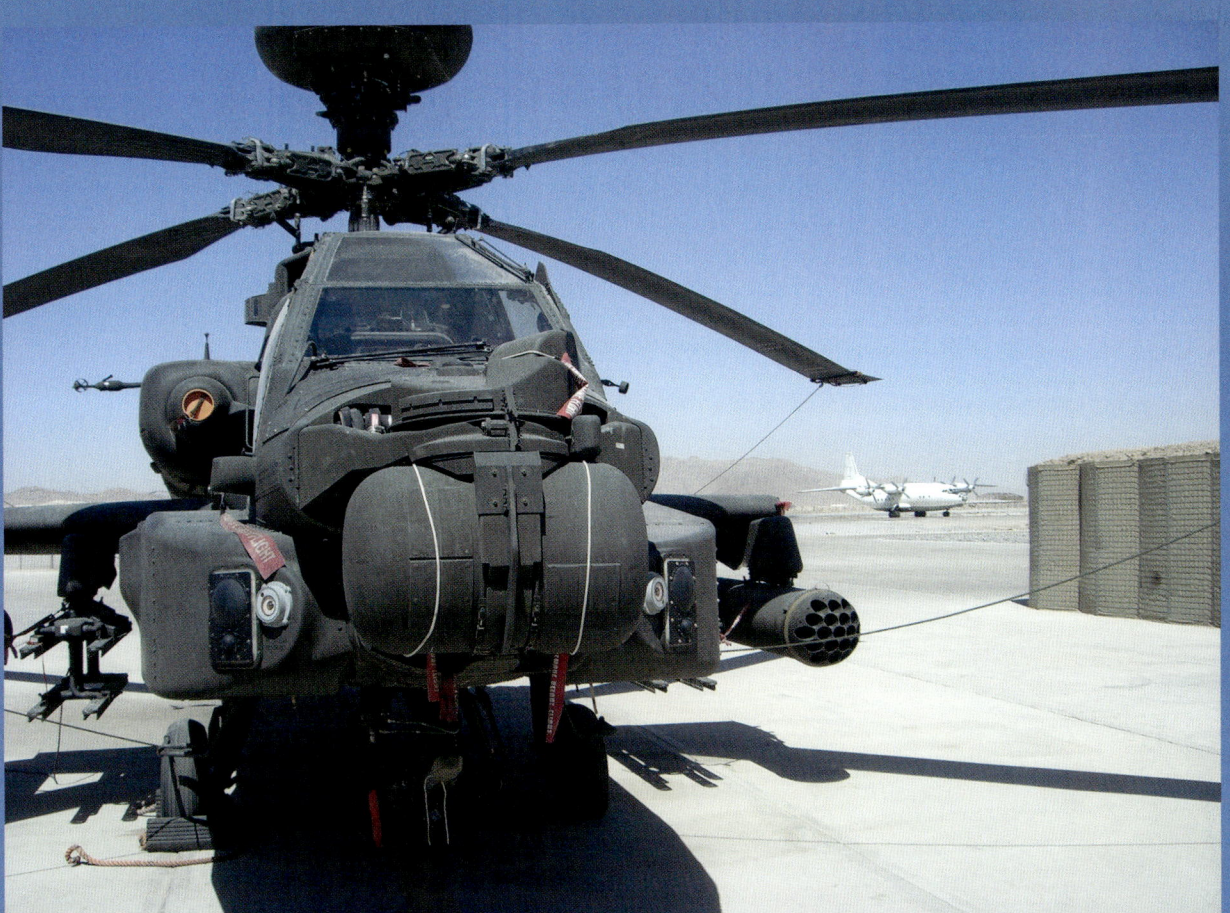

BELOW: The AAC's Apache force was in action around the clock during the summer of 2006 as British troops found themselves besieged in Platoon Houses.
(TIM RIPLEY)

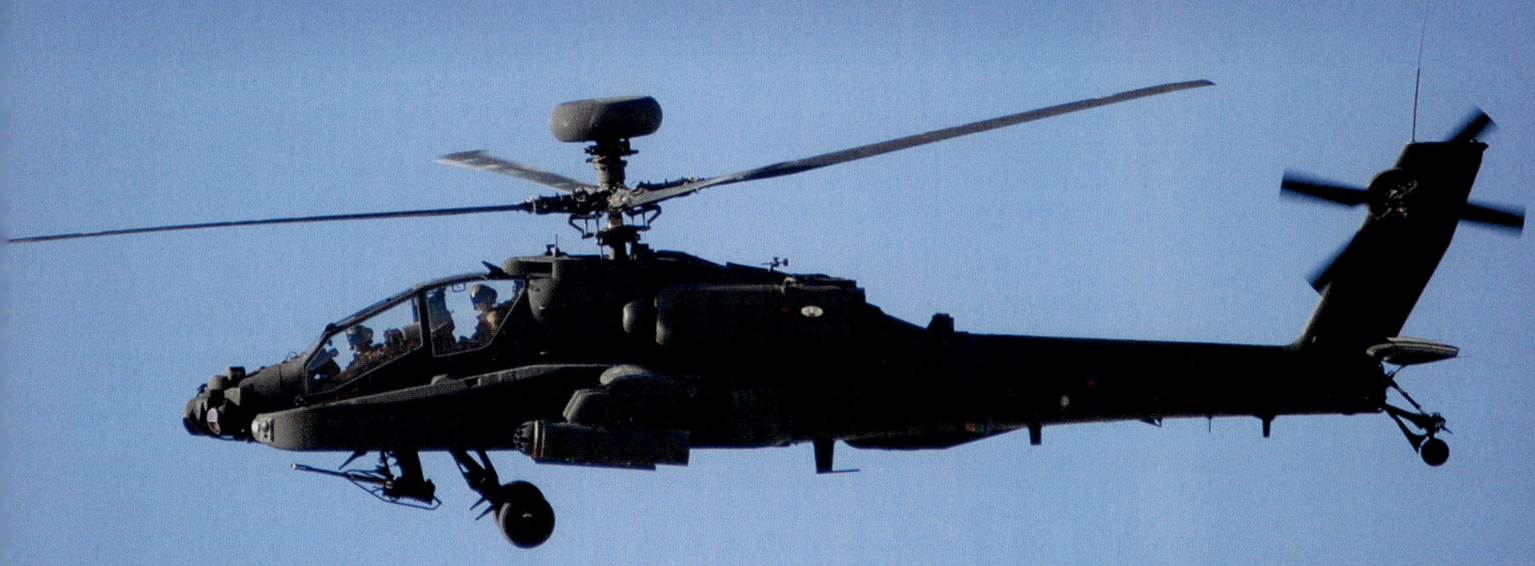

Operation Panther's Claw

British Army takes the Offensive in Afghanistan

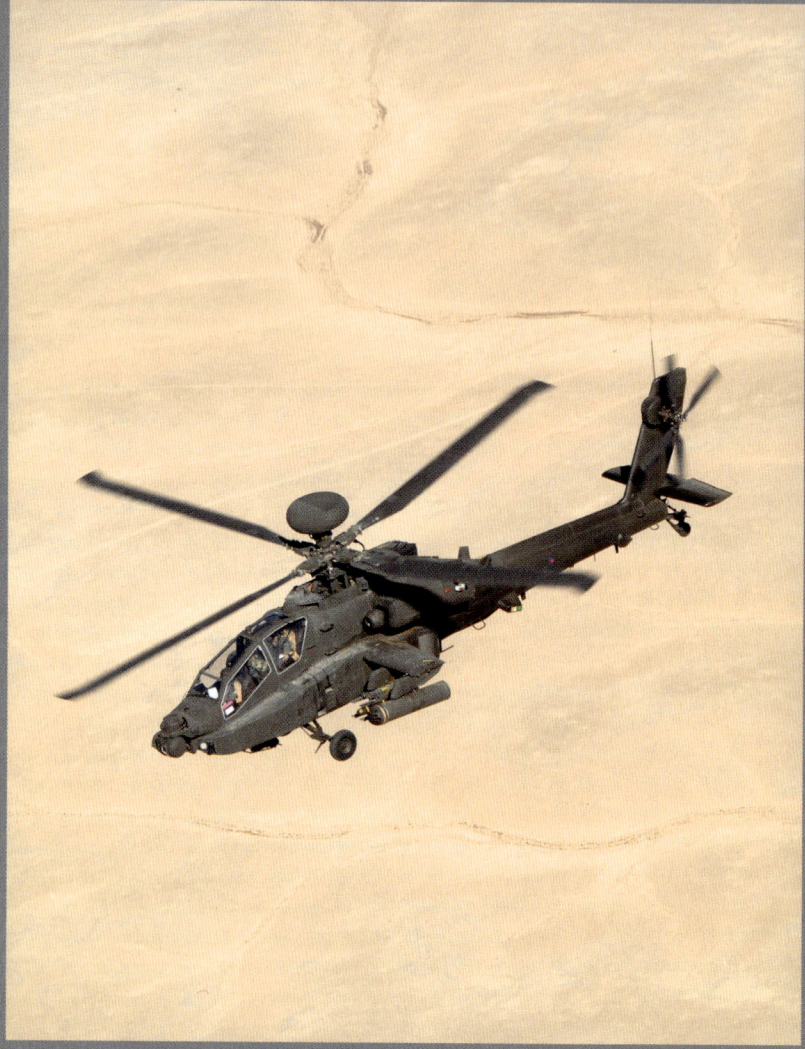

RIGHT: AAC Apache AH1 attack helicopters proved their worth time and time again in combat in Afghanistan. (AGUSTAWESTLAND)

operation, locating and then striking at insurgent bases and fighting positions.

Operation Panther's Claw was the largest British military operation since the 2003 invasion of Iraq, involving some 5,000 British troops backed by hundreds of Danish and Afghan allies. The mission of 19 Light Brigade was to push into Taliban sanctuary around Babaji, between the large towns of Nad-e Ali and Gereshk, to capture all the district's main villages. Other troops were to make surprise moves across the desert to set up a cordon of positions around the district to trap any insurgents who might try to escape the clearance operation led by the 800 troopers of the Light Dragoon's Battlegroup.

While the initial moves were underway, at the main British base at Camp Bastion maintenance technicians and armourers of 662 Squadron AAC were working to prepare its eight Apaches for around-the-clock missions. Boxes of 30mm cannon ammunition, CRV-7 2.75in rockets and AGM-114 Hellfire missiles were being stacked next to the landing pads and the squadron's pilots were resting to dramatically increase their flying, or ops, tempo during the assault. Two flights, each with a pair of helicopters, were scheduled to be in the air as the first troops of the Light Dragoons crossed their start line – the

During a hot Afghan night, thousands of British, Danish and Afghan troops had driven across miles of desert to their assembly points. Within hours Operation Panther's Claw would start with the aim of surrounding and then clearing hundreds of heavily armed and determined Taliban insurgents from the villages and woods around the run down town of Babaji. Overhead, British Army attack helicopters and unmanned aerial vehicles (UAVs) were flying top cover for the approaching columns of armoured vehicles and scouting ahead to gather intelligence on enemy positions and movements. As the month-long battle unfolded, Army Air Corps (AAC) AgustaWestland Apache AH1 attack helicopters and Royal Artillery UAVs would play decisive roles in the

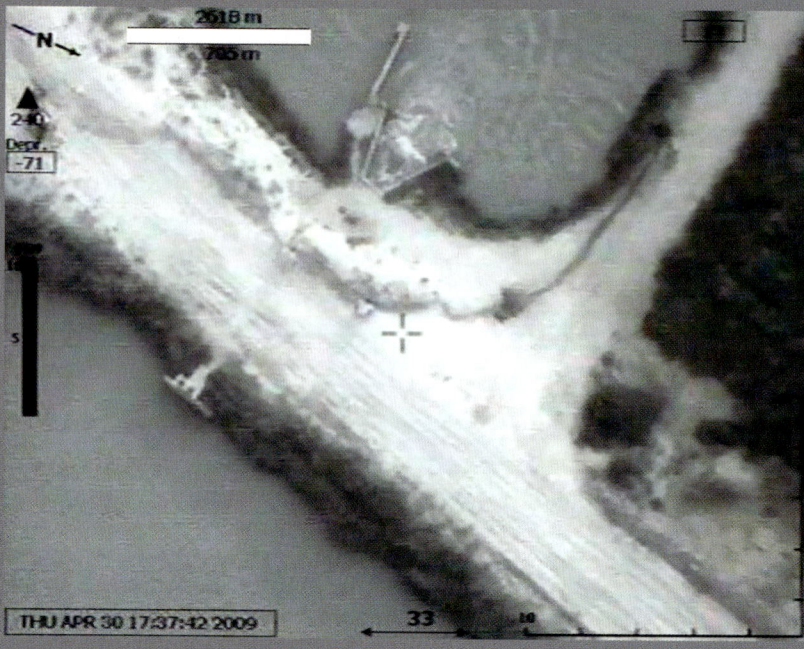

RIGHT: Video imagery of Taliban insurgents recorded by Hermes 450s gave British commanders early warning of insurgent attacks. (THALES)

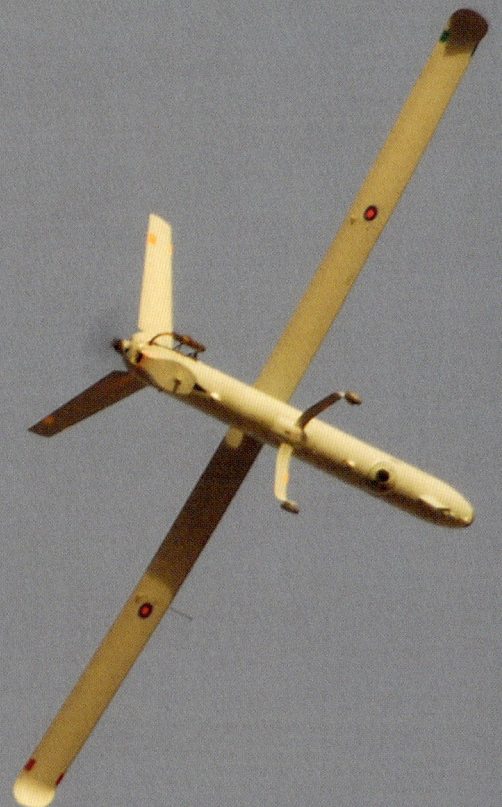

point at which Taliban resistance was expected to be heaviest. Two more Apaches were held back at very high readiness (VHR) on Camp Bastion's heli-pad, prepared to lift at a few minutes' notice to react to emergencies. These were most likely to be the close escort of Royal Air Force Boeing Chinook HC2 heavy-lift helicopters containing medics of the immediate reaction team (IRT) to pluck casualties from landing zones close to insurgent positions.

On the other side of Camp Bastion, in a non-descript group of air-conditioned pre-fabricated buildings, Royal Artillery imagery analysts were peering at large computer screens showing live video of the battlefield, beamed from Hermes 450 UAVs orbiting high over Babaji. The analysts were not just looking for signs of enemy movement or insurgents planting deadly Improvised Explosive Devices (IEDs) along the Light Dragoons' intended line of advance, they were also watching for signs of unusual behaviour amongst the local population. This so-called 'pattern of life analysis' would tell them if the British had lost the element of surprise and the degree to which the population was helping the Taliban. »

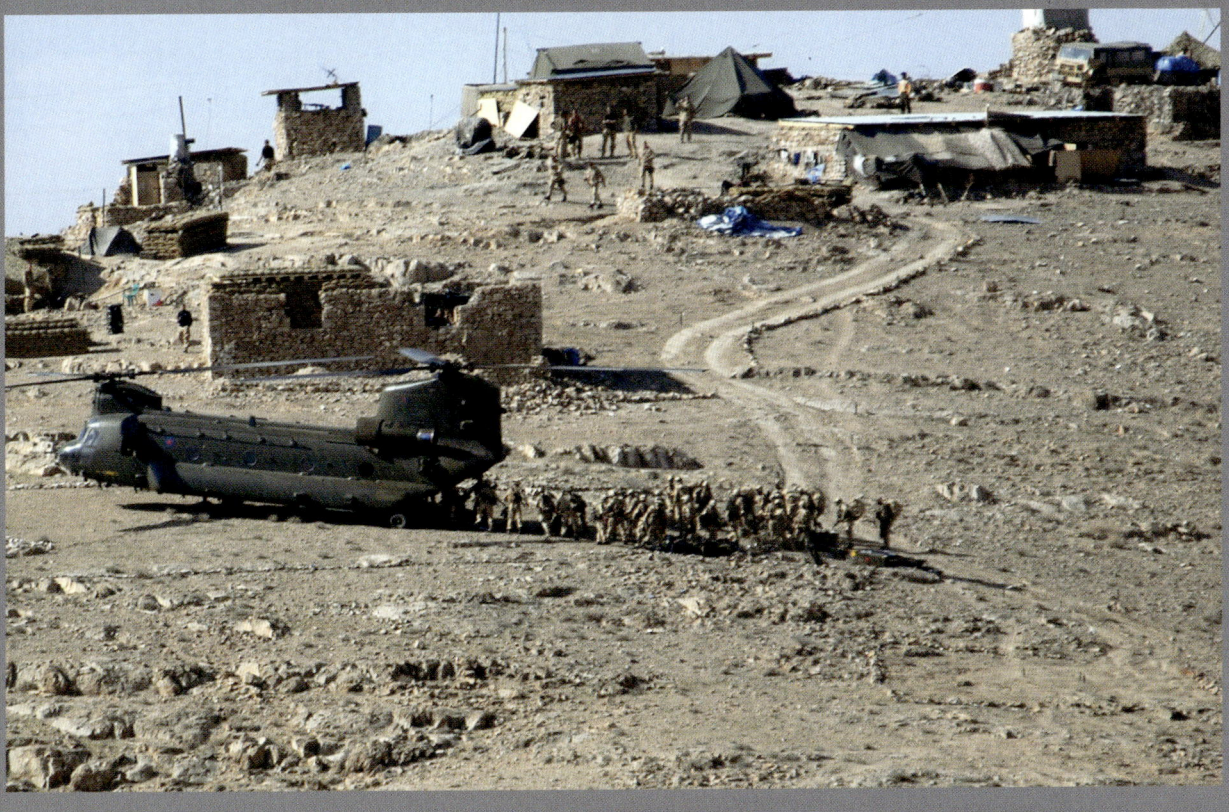

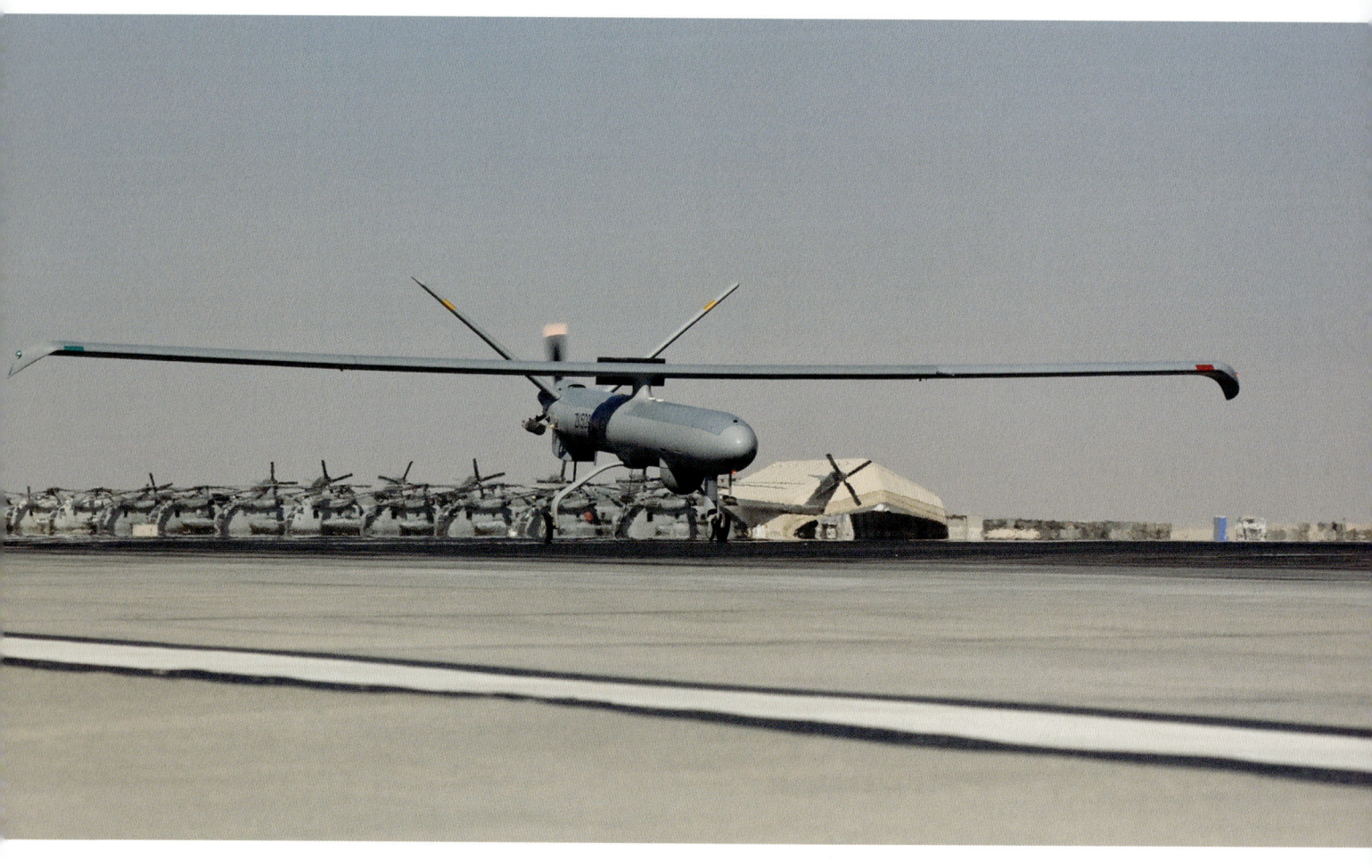

ABOVE: Royal Artillery Hermes 450 unmanned aerial vehicles were airborne around the clock over Helmand province to protect British troops from insurgent attack. (THALES)

For the gunners of 22 Battery Royal Artillery, this was no remote control video game. Several of their comrades were there with the advance guard of the Light Dragoons, sweating under the weight of heavy body armour, water containers and hundreds of rounds of SA-80 rifle ammunition. Crucially, they had receivers that allowed the senior officers of the Light Dragoons to watch the same video feed as the analysis team at Camp Bastion. Other gunners with the Light Dragoons assault troops were standing by, ready to launch Lockheed Martin Desert Hawk III mini-UAVs to provide close surveillance over the battlefield. To the troops of the Light Dragoons, the Royal Artillery UAVs were known as 'Greeneyes' and for the next month they would be constantly overhead, giving them unprecedented view of the action. Unlike some bigger UAVs operated by the Royal Air Force and allied air forces, that were controlled from the coalition air headquarters in the Gulf state of Qatar, Greeneyes were owned and operated by 19 Light Brigade and they could be tasked immediately to the meet the needs of British troops, 24/7. Operation Panther's Claw would see all the British Army's air assets in Afghanistan used to maximum effect.

The operation kicked off on July 3, 2009, and within minutes of the British troops advancing they had called in Apaches to neutralise enemy positions. Over the first week the intensity of AAC attack helicopter operations can be gauged by the fact that 662 Squadron flew 191 hours and fired 3,000 rounds of 30mm cannon ammunition, 10 Hellfires, and 24 rockets.

On the ground, the Light Dragoons had to fight for every building in every village as they pushed forward. Babaji district had been heavily seeded with IEDs to such a degree that British Army combat engineers described it as the "biggest minefield in the world". The officer commanding 662 Squadron, Major Phil Cook, and his flight of two Apaches were engaging two compounds containing six Taliban fighters resisting the Light Dragoons' advance on July 6 when a British Scimitar light tank was hit by a rocket-propelled grenade. As British troops tried to free the vehicle's wounded crew, they set off two IEDs and three more soldiers were wounded, including the forward air controller or Joint Terminal Attack Controller (JTAC) with the assault wave. The IRT Chinook was scrambled from Camp Bastion and Major Cook's two Apaches were diverted to provide top cover for the extraction mission.

The heavy casualties meant the Chinook had to make three landings to lift off all the wounded men, but the landing zone was being swept by Taliban fire. So each time the Chinook approached, Major Cook and his wingman flew ahead and put down 30mm cannon suppressive fire into the Taliban trenches. Over a 20-minute period they fired some 600 rounds to allow the Chinook to pull out all the casualties safely.

The break-in phase of Operation Panther's Claw lasted just over a week, with heavy fighting. Gradually the enemy began to realise the precarious nature of their position, with British troops squeezing them from four sides and their fighters started to make their escape. The British, Danish and Afghan battlegroups had set up blocking positions along the series of drainage canals that bounded Babaji district. These canals provided ideal patrol lines for the Hermes 450s and their operators started to spot an increasing number of suspicious individuals attempting to cross them during the hours of darkness. Ground troops were dispatched to intercept them or, if they were openly carrying weapons, Apaches and fast jets were cleared by the UAV operators to engage the targets.

Likely locations for the positioning of IEDs were also kept under surveillance by the Greeneyes in the build-up and for the duration of the

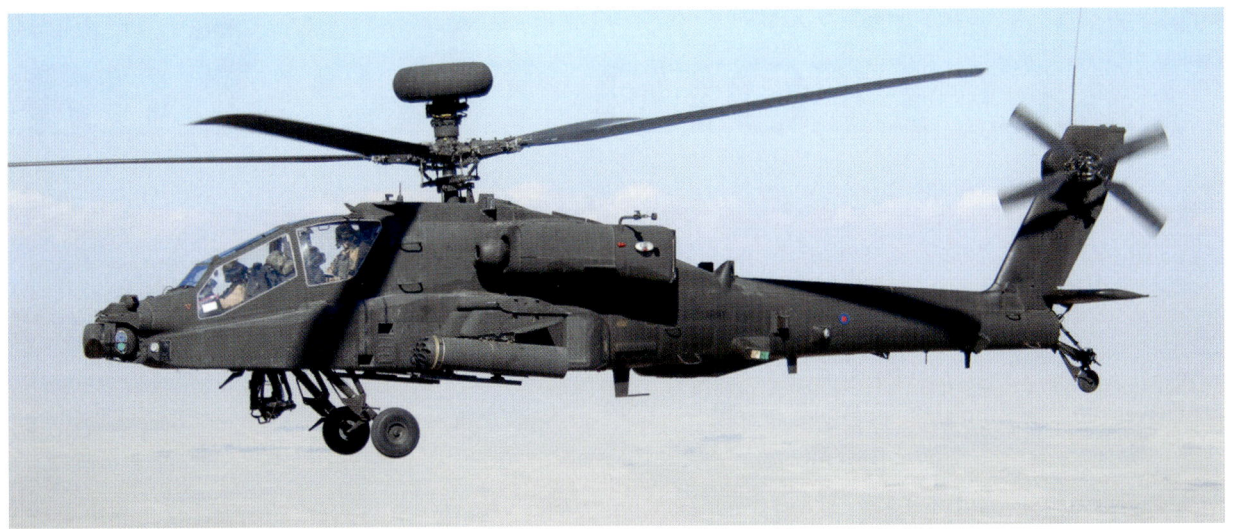

operation, leading to several Apache strikes on Taliban IED teams. During one incident a pair of Apaches were directed to a location where a Hermes 450 had detected several men acting suspiciously. They located the men and watched them for several minutes through the Apaches' night vision sensors at 3km range until the Taliban gave themselves away as bomb makers. Within minutes they had been successfully engaged and killed, which caused a major boost to morale among the assault troops which had already taken dozens of casualties from the hated IEDs.

The finale of Operation Panther's Claw got under way on July 25, as reserve troops from the 3rd Battalion, The Royal Regiment of Scotland (3 SCOTS) battlegroup were helicoptered forward to occupy and secure several villages in the district that had yet to be cleared by the Light Dragoons. This was the battalion's fourth major air assault mission of Panther's Claw. Royal Artillery UAVs generated intelligence briefing packs full of detailed pictures of target areas to allow the assault troops to make comprehensive plans for their mission. At first light on July 25 two Apaches led six Chinooks into action to land nearly 200 troops. The operation caught the Taliban by surprise and within a few hours the Adera Cemetery area had been secured.

Operation Panther's Claw was a major success for British integration of air assets – fixed wing, helicopters, and UAVs – flying above a complex battlefield. The operation would be repeated on an even larger scale in January and February of 2010 during Operation Moshtarak in central Helmand province.

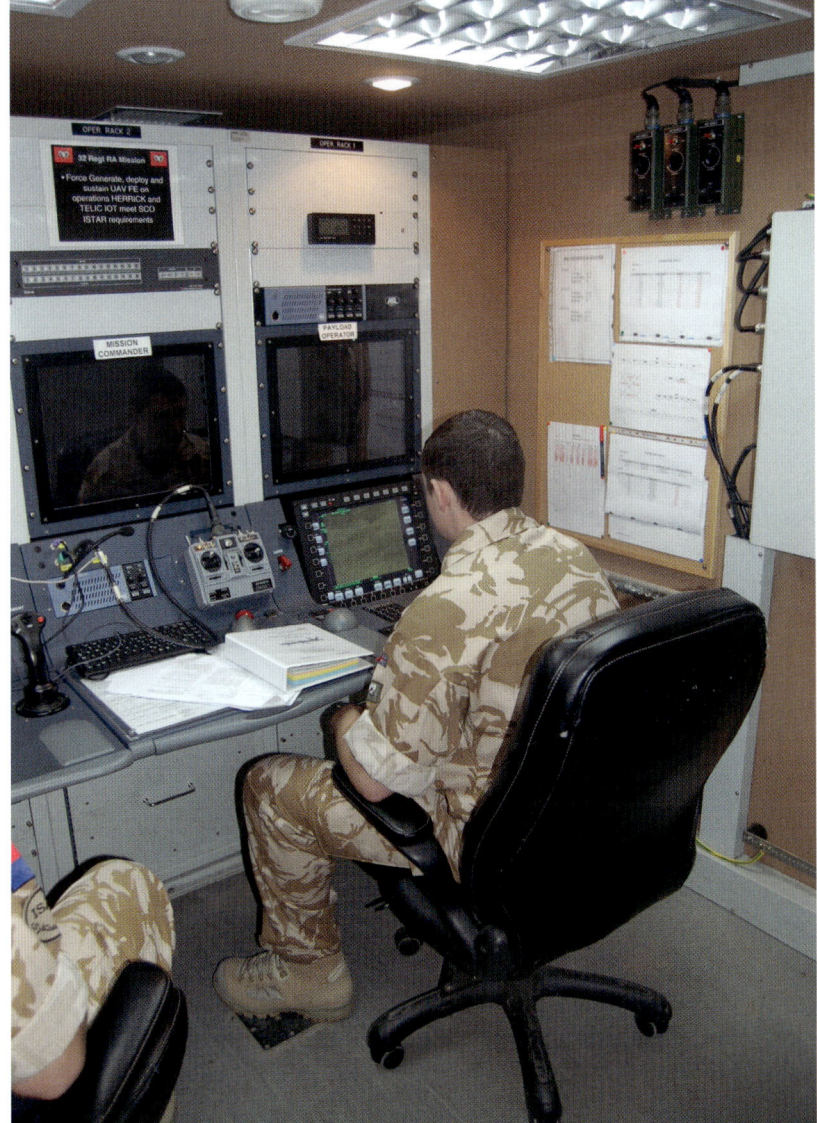

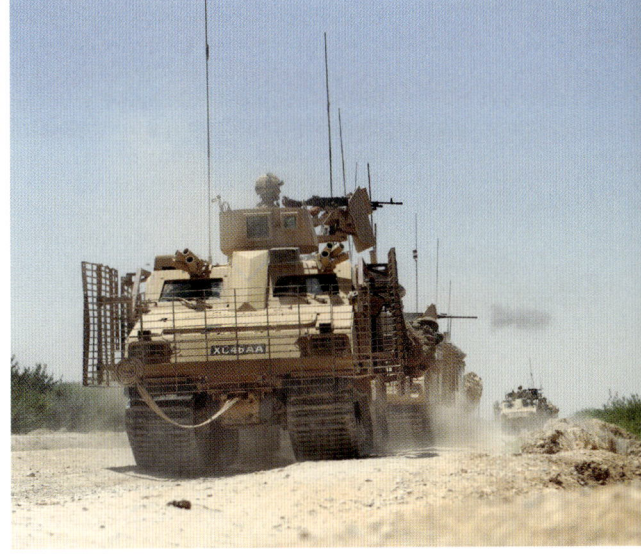

Strike from the Sea

Attack Helicopters Hit Libya

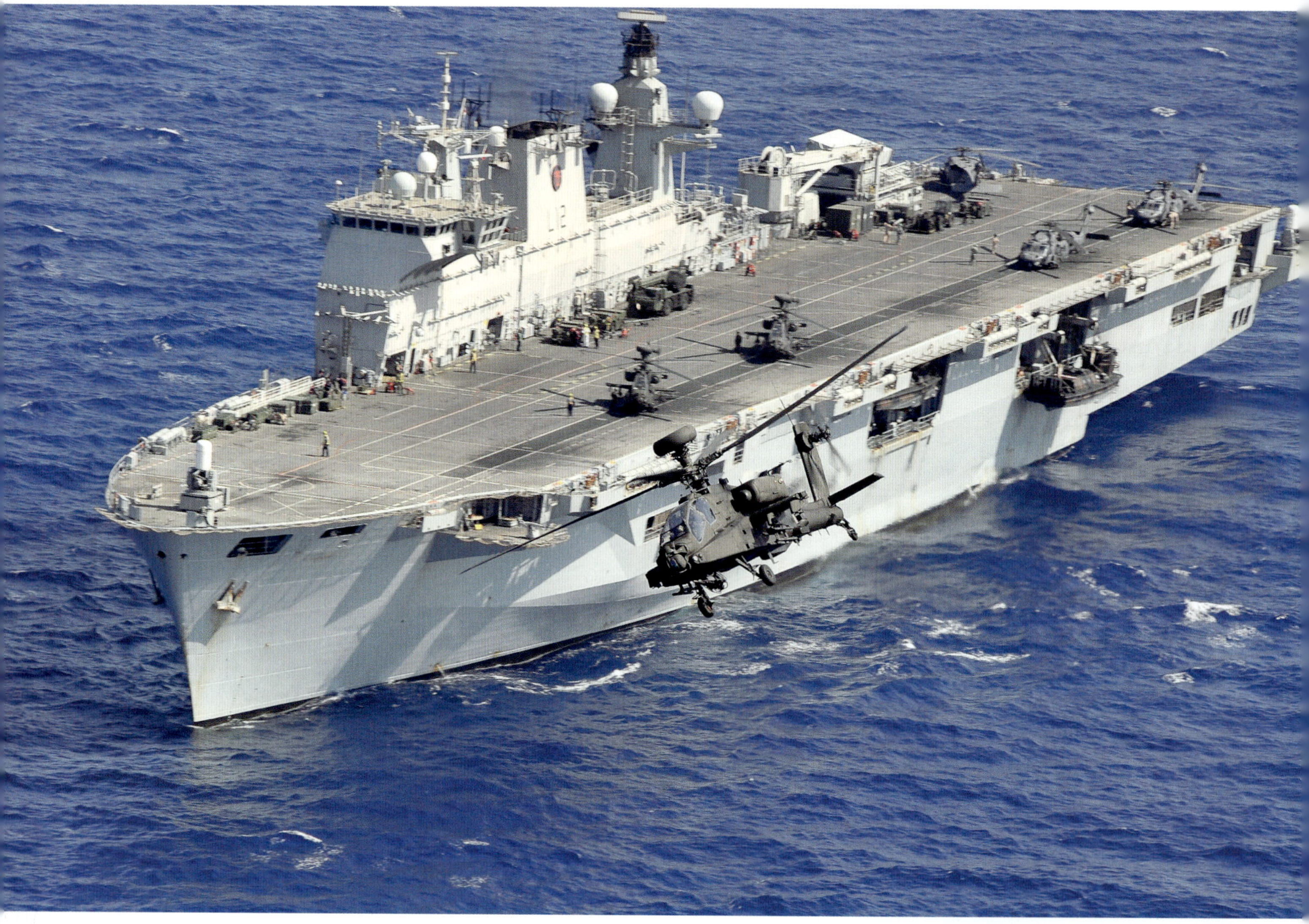

ABOVE: AAC Apache AH1 carried out the first-ever maritime strike operations by AH-64s from HMS *Ocean* during the 2011 Libyan war.
(MOD/CROWN COPYRIGHT)

Pooled Media News Report from HMS *Ocean*:

"1.04am on Saturday June 4, the pilot of an Apache helicopter gunship, hidden in the inky black sky, pressed the trigger of the 30mm cannon, bringing down concentrated fire on a pick-up truck and ripping it open. Ammunition stored inside set off secondary explosions, spreading the swirling flames. Three men who had been trying to open fire with the vehicle's anti-aircraft gun mounted at the back of the truck, were now terrified, scrambling to get away."

The first-ever offensive operation by UK Army Air Corps AgustaWestland Apache AH1 attack helicopters

RIGHT: RAF Tornado GR4 strike jets co-ordinated their missions closely with the AAC Apache AH1s for maximum effect.
(MOD/CROWN COPYRIGHT)

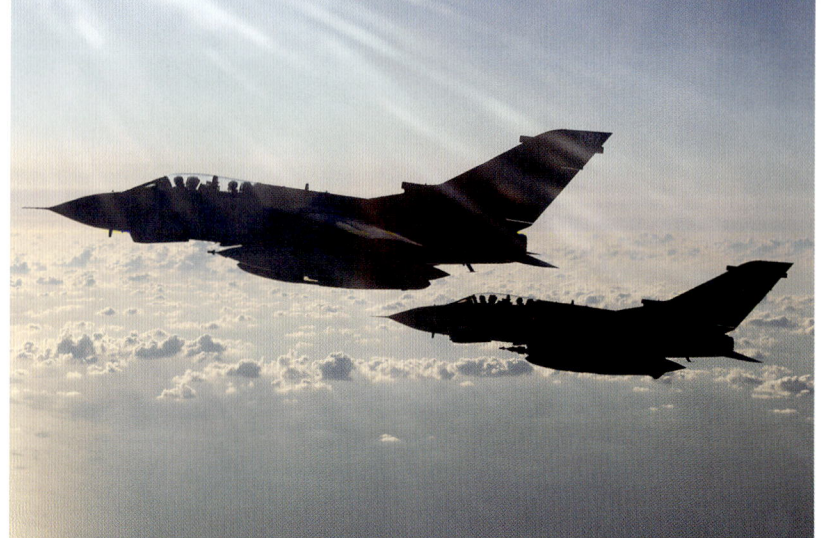

embarked on the warship in the early hours of June 4, 2011, was the culmination of joint Royal Navy and British Army efforts to bring rotary wing combat power within range of Libya. This attack had come three months after UK and NATO forces had been committed to action in the North African country following an insurrection against the 40-year rule of Colonel Muammar Gaddafi.

Under the code name Operation Cougar, the Royal Navy's Response Force Task Group (RFTG), commanded by Commodore John Kingwell, set sail for the Mediterranean Sea from a number of UK ports during April 2011. It eventually boasted 15 helicopters and more than 2,000 personnel embarking on eight Royal Navy warships and Royal Fleet Auxiliary (RFA) support ships.

The first elements of the RFTG, led by the amphibious ship HMS *Albion*, the Type 23 frigate HMS *Sutherland,* and the landing ship RFA *Cardigan Bay*, sailed on April 6. The second wave of the RFTG sailed at the end of April led by the helicopter carrier HMS *Ocean*, with five Apache attack helicopters of 656 Squadron AAC, more HC4 helicopters of 845 Naval Air Squadron and a pair of Westland Sea King ASaC7 airborne command and control helicopters of 857 Naval Air Squadron.

As HMS *Ocean* entered the Mediterranean, her Apaches carried out the first-ever live firing of Hellfire

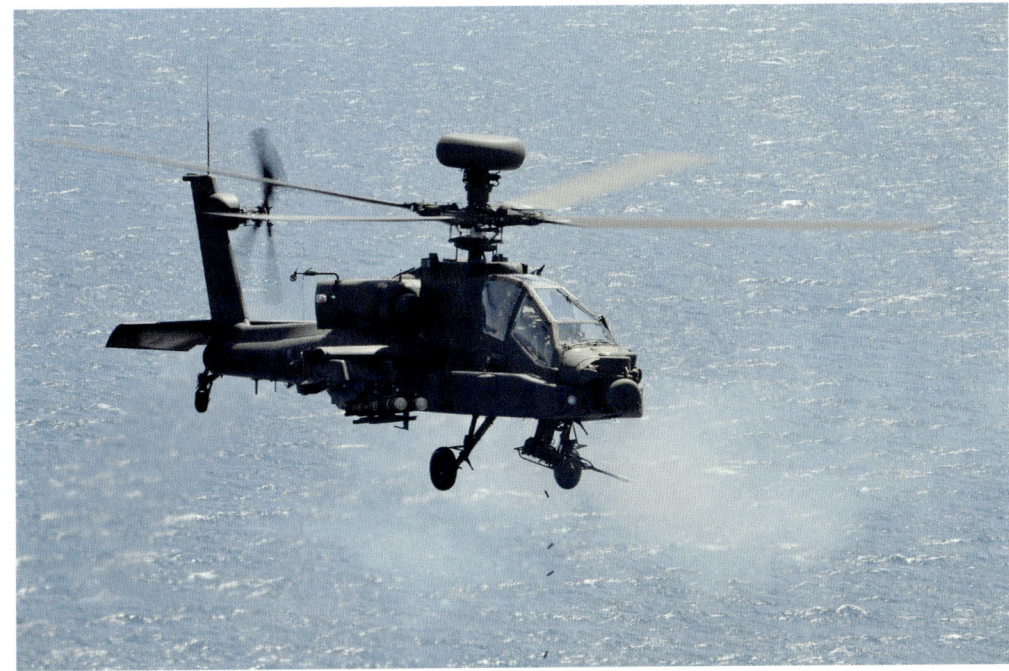

missiles from attack helicopters embarked on a Royal Navy warship, as well as test firing their 30mm cannons and CRV-7 rockets.

The helicopters on HMS *Ocean* and HMS *Albion* had, by then, been combined into a Tailored Air Group (TAG) led by a command team provided by the UK's Joint Helicopter Command (JHC). The team had been working up options for using the TAG in the Libyan campaign, in conjunction with NATO fixed-wing strike aircraft and French helicopter assets embarked

on the assault ship FNS *Tonnerre*, which had set sail from Toulon for the central Mediterranean on May 20.

On May 27, UK Prime Minister David Cameron agreed to proposals from Britain's Chief of Defence Staff, General Sir David Richards, to commit the TAG to NATO's Operation Unified Protector. Preparation now began in earnest for the British and French helicopters to join the action in Libya. Planning teams were dispatched from the helicopter units to the NATO Combined Air Operations Centre ➤➤

ABOVE: En route to Libya, the Apache crews of 656 Squadron AAC carried out the first maritime live firing of their weapons. (MOD/CROWN COPYRIGHT)

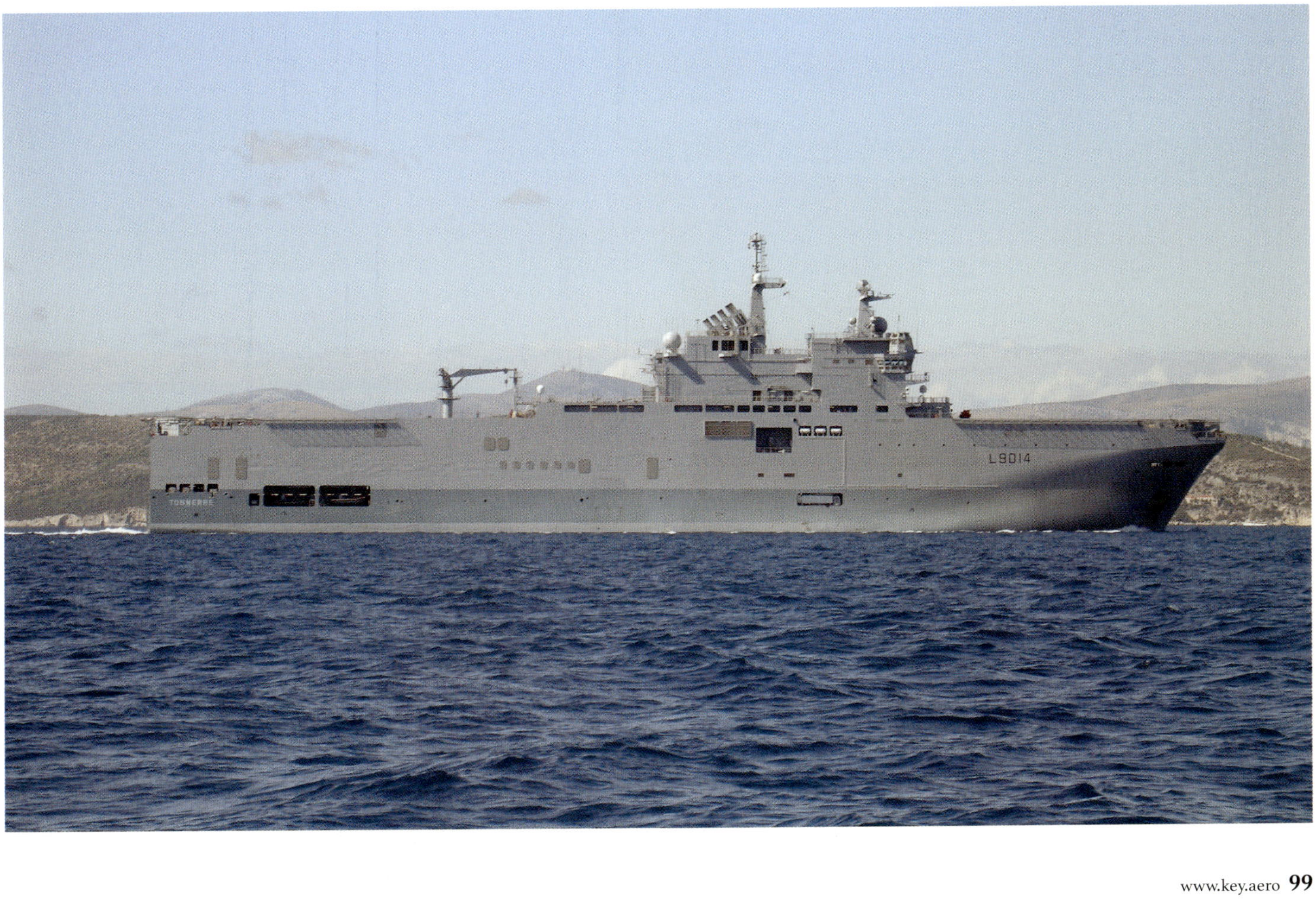

BELOW: The French landing ship FNS *Tonnerre* proved a useful base for ALAT Tiger, Gazelle and Puma helicopters during the joint French-UK operation off the Libyan coast. (FRENCH MOD)

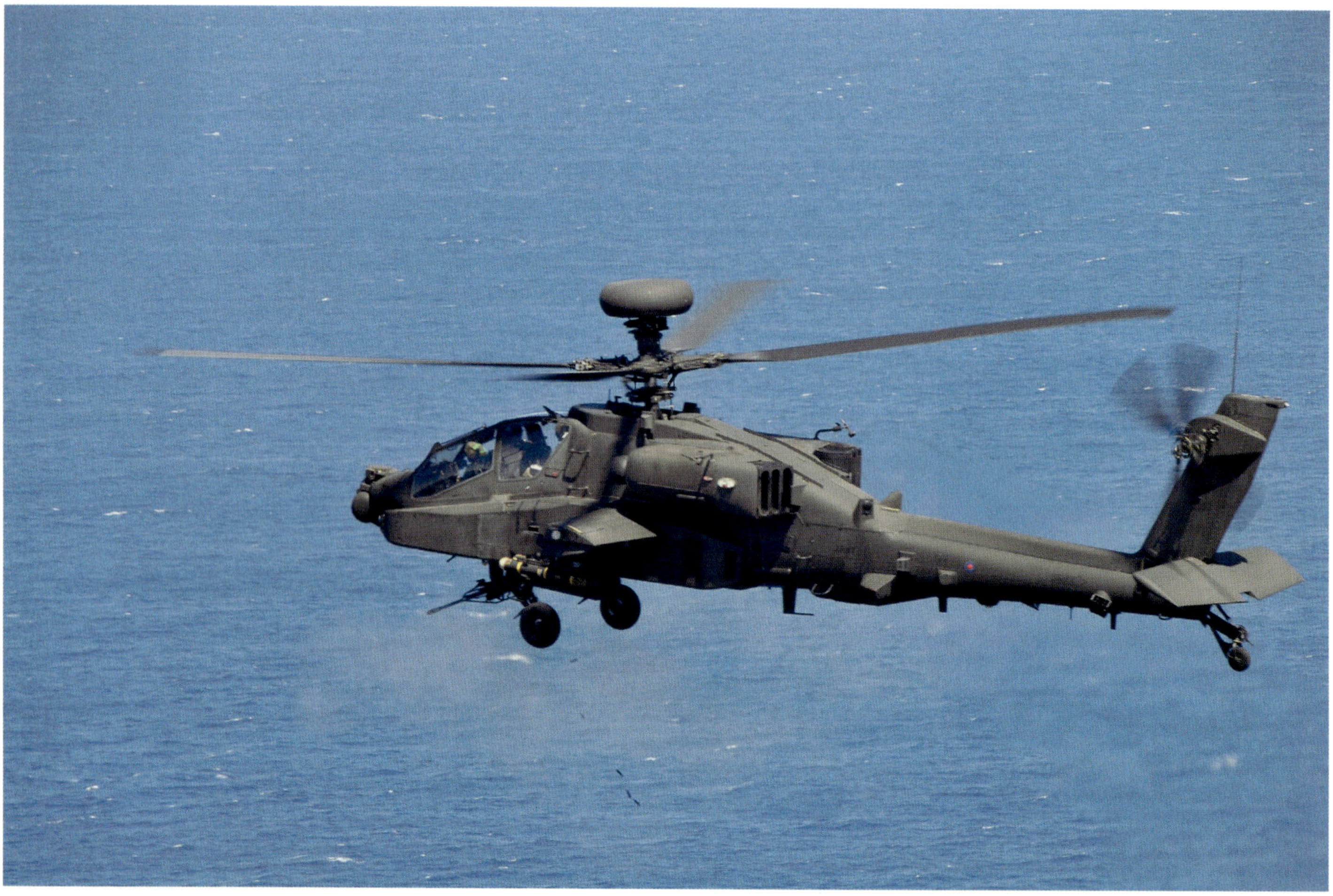

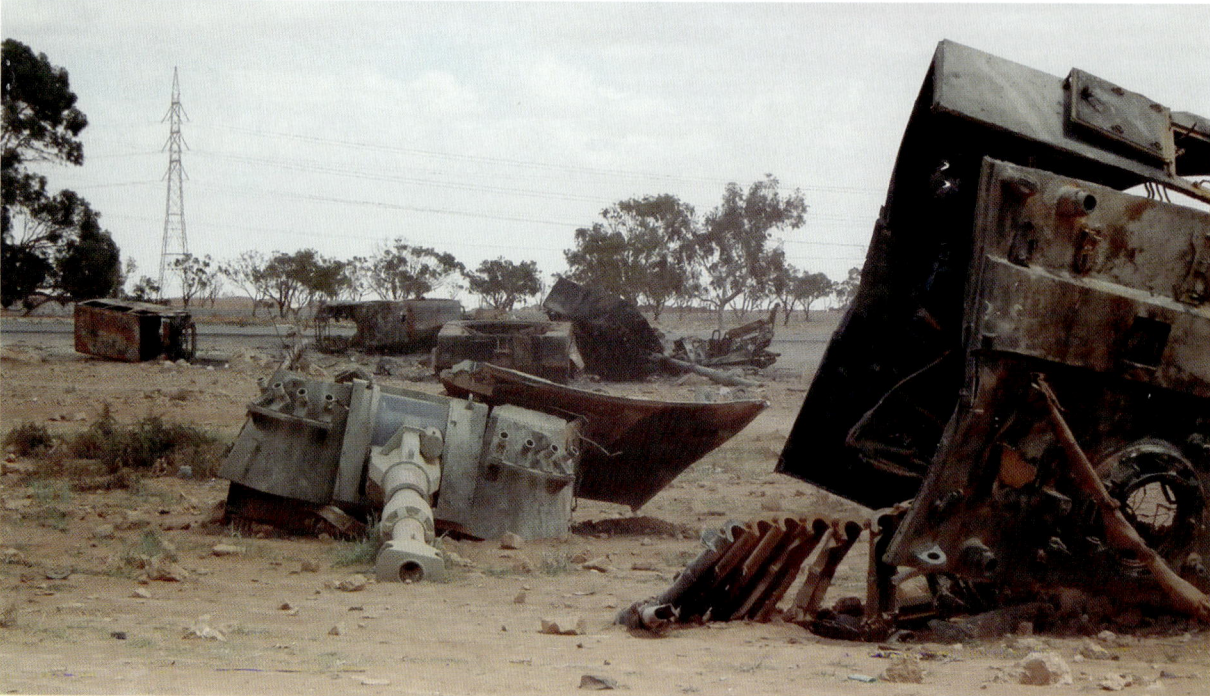

ABOVE: 656 Squadron AAC was the first British Apache unit to take the helicopter into action in Afghanistan in 2006 and it was the first AH-64 unit to operate in the maritime strike role. (MOD/CROWN COPYRIGHT)

RIGHT: Libyan tanks and armoured vehicles were devastated in the British and French attack helicopter strikes. (MOD/CROWN COPYRIGHT)

(CAOC) at Poggio Renatico in central Italy, to co-ordinate their efforts with Alliance fixed-wing air units that would support them over Libya.

An intelligence, surveillance, targeting and reconnaissance (ISTAR) plan was developed to put the first tranche of intended targets of the British and French attack helicopters under around-the-clock surveillance from NATO reconnaissance aircraft – led by RAF Raytheon Sentinel R1 airborne stand-off radar aircraft – to build a picture of Libyan forces deployed around them. This was to try to reduce the number of surprises the attack helicopters might encounter on their first mission.

The first UK attack helicopter operation involved precision strikes on June 4 against a Gaddafi-regime radar installation and a military checkpoint, both located around Brega. The UK Ministry of Defence reported that both targets were destroyed, and the helicopters had returned safely to HMS *Ocean*.

French Army Light Aviation (ALAT) Eurocopter EC625 Tiger HAP and Aerospatiale SA342 Gazelle attack helicopters went into action at almost the same time and destroyed a command and control post and 15 military vehicles on the eastern edge of Brega.

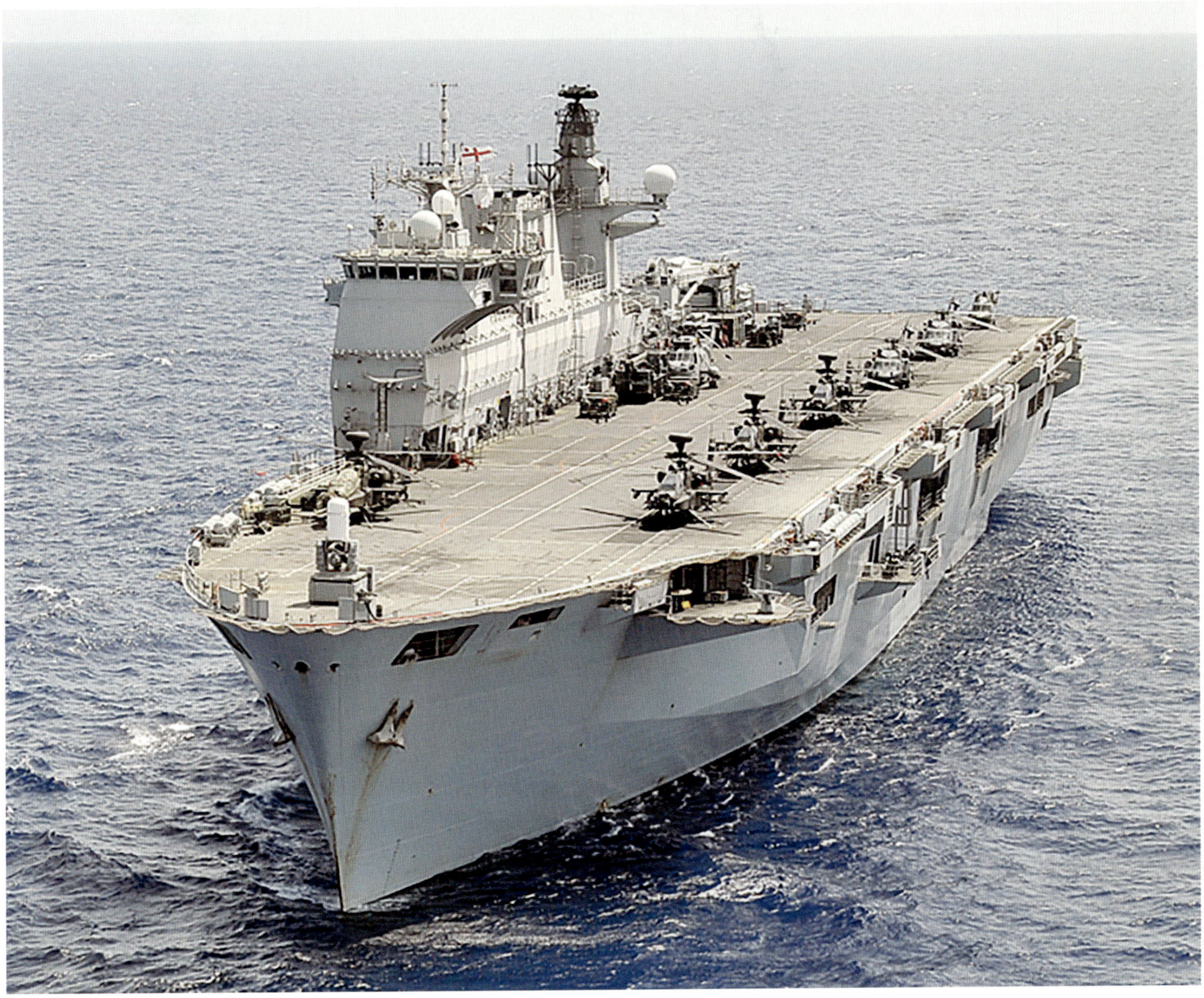

Supporting the helicopter strikes were a fixed-wing package of Royal Air Force ground attack aircraft, which destroyed another military installation in eastern Libya, and a separate RAF mission that attacked two ammunition bunkers at the large Waddan depot in central Libya.

Throughout these operations, a Sea King ASaC7 of 857 Squadron was airborne providing command and control co-ordination for both the helicopters and fixed wing jets, as well as monitoring Libya vehicle movements with its Searchwater radar in ground moving target indicator mode.

The British Apache helicopters reportedly received fire from Libyan troops armed with AK-47s, but none hit the Apaches. After a period of maintenance back on HMS Ocean, there was a further strike in the Brega area in the early hours of

June 5 by two Apaches, with a Sea King ASaC7 helicopter providing intelligence. This destroyed a multi-barrelled rocket launcher mounted on a truck and placed in an abandoned building.

For the leaders of the rebel resistance to Colonel Gaddafi, the first wave of British and French attack helicopter strikes took place in what they considered to be the wrong place. The focus of rebel efforts was to punch through the lines of Libyan

government troops defending the strategic town of Zliten, to the west of the rebel stronghold of Misrata. According to the rebels, if Zliten could be taken then the road to Gaddafi's capital, Tripoli, would be open.

During June 9, the rebel's requests were met when HMS Ocean moved up the coast to Misrata and launched Apache helicopters to attack the regime's military communications installation and multiple rocket launchers near the city. »

ABOVE: Five Apache AH1s eventually operated from HMS Ocean at the peak of the Libyan conflict. (MOD/CROWN COPYRIGHT)

BELOW: French EC625 Tiger attack helicopters joined the maritime strike operation. (FRENCH MOD)

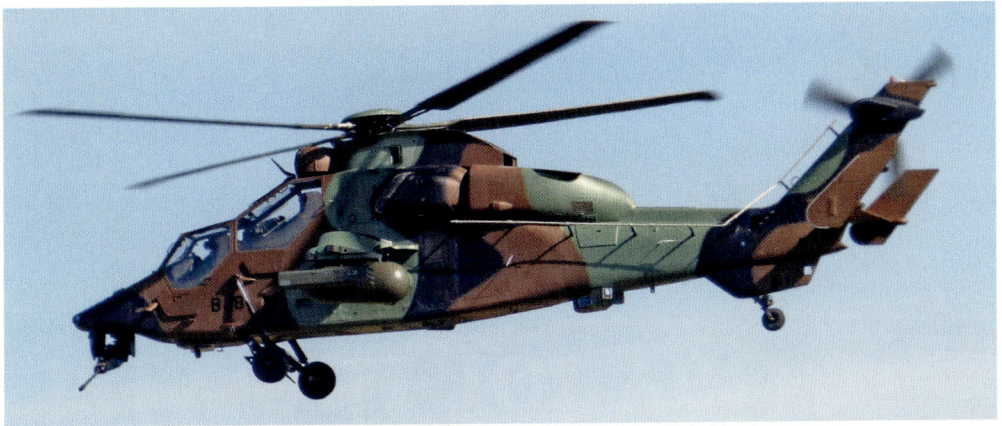

UK and French attack helicopters then embarked on a concerted raiding strategy along the length of Libya's coastline to keep regime forces off balance and uncertain where the next attack would come, according to AAC commanders involved in the mission to the North African country.

"AH attacks were a visible demonstration of NATO resolve," Lieutenant Colonel Phil Cook, head of the Joint Helicopter Command (JHC) Air Manoeuvre Planning Team (AMPT) recalled. "We operated from Brega [on the eastern edge of regime-controlled territory] to Zuwara [between Tripoli and the Tunisian border]. This increased the risk and sense of uncertainty among regime forces and provided a vital psychological effect."

"In a 24-hour period, HMS *Ocean* and FNS *Tonnerre* could appear anywhere on the Libyan coast and then the regime would not know where we would strike next," said an AAC officer who served on HMS *Ocean* off Libya. "Over the first 30 days of the operations either our or French helicopters were in action for 20 to 25 nights somewhere in Libya."

Cook described a typical attack helicopter mission off the besieged Libyan city of Misrata in June. "Our Apaches were on deck alert on HMS *Ocean* off Misrata before a planned mission," he said. "Royal Navy Westland Sea King ASaC7s detected regime special forces patrol boats and cued the attack helicopters to engage them. The Apaches then continued on their pre-planned mission against two vehicle check points. While this was happening, a UAV located a ZSU-23-4 self-propelled anti-aircraft system. Then they hit another check point and destroyed a technical vehicle."

During and after Apache missions, a pair of 857 Naval Air Squadron Sea King ASaC7s monitored the local area with their Thales Searchwater radars looking for emerging land and maritime threats. In the first months of operations the Sea King detachment on HMS *Ocean* flew some 200 hours.

By the end of August 2011, Gaddafi's regime had fallen and rebel forces had occupied the capital, Tripoli. Between June and August 2011, 656 Squadron

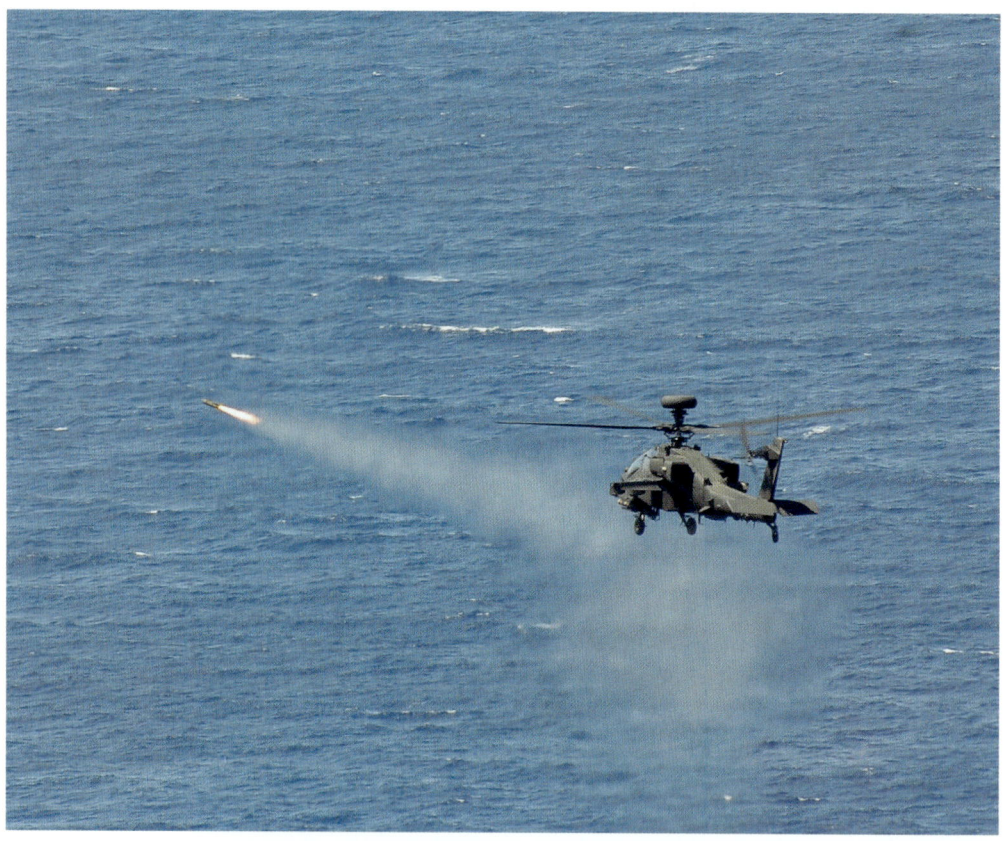

ABOVE: Maritime operations are now routine for British Apache AH1 units, as a result of the success of the Libyan mission. (MOD/CROWN COPYRIGHT)

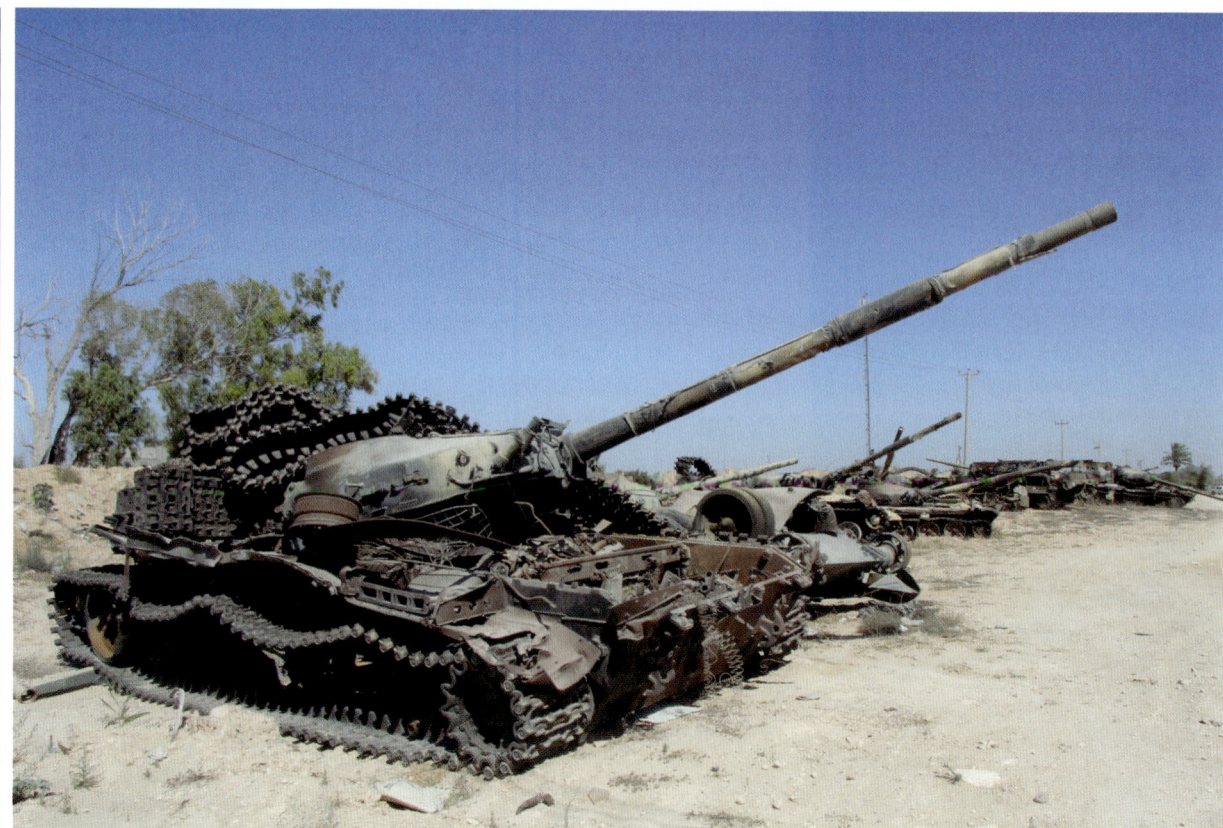

RIGHT: Libyan defences outside the city of Misrata were broken by the British and French missile attacks, opening the way for the rebel advance on Tripoli. (MOD/CROWN COPYRIGHT)

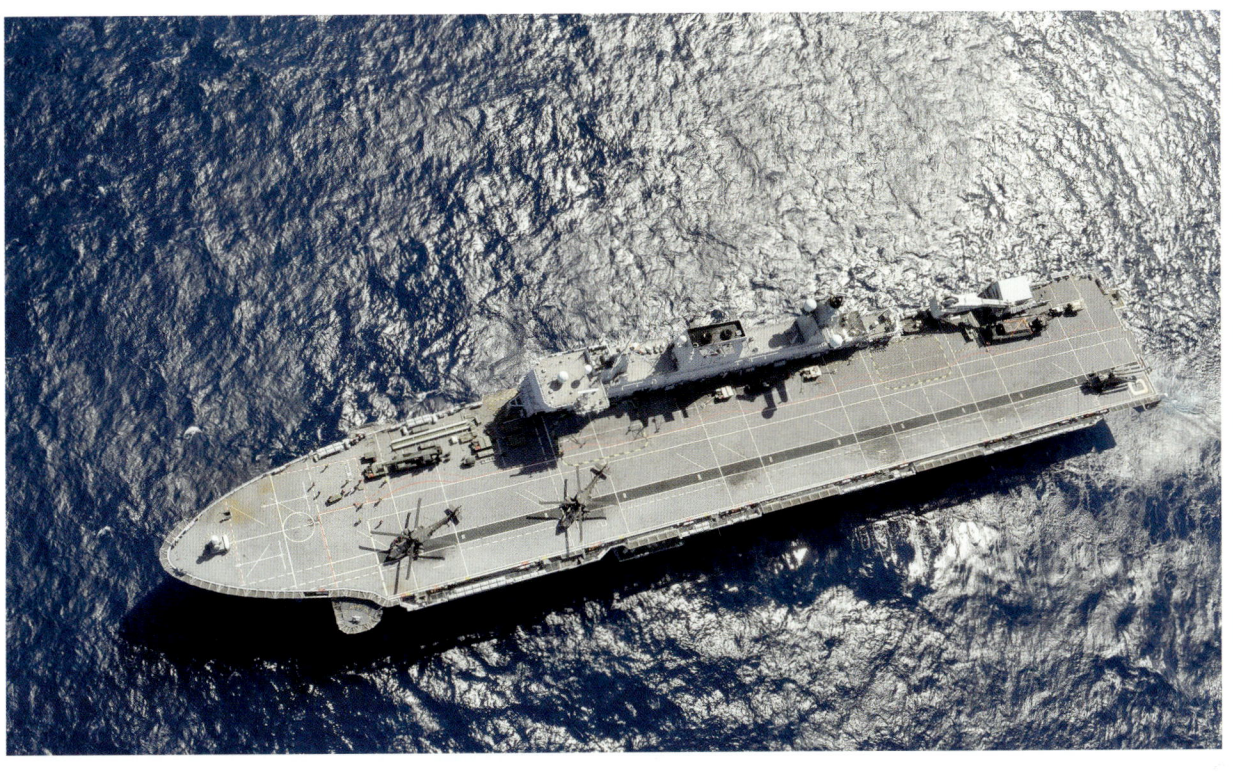

LEFT: Apache operations against Libya from HMS *Ocean* opened a new chapter in the history of the Army Air Corps. (AGUSTAWESTLAND)

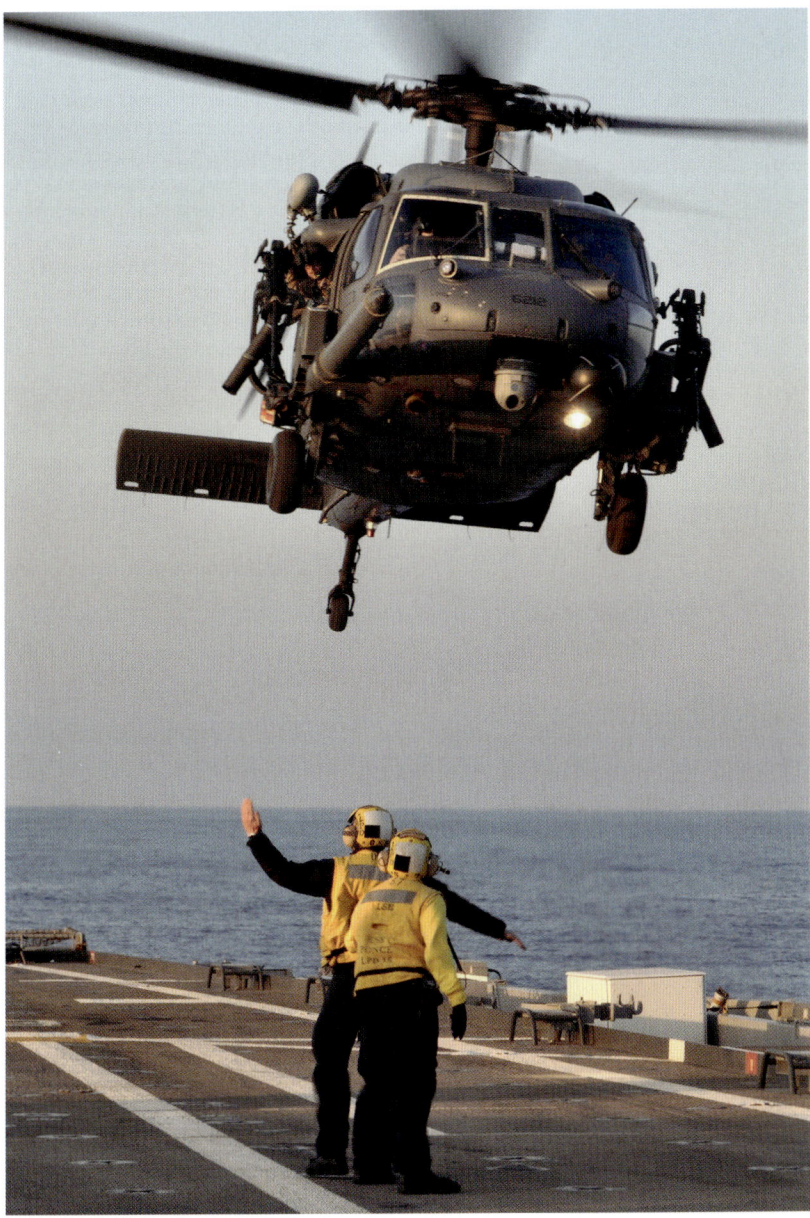

spent 155 days at sea. It flew 48 combat sorties, firing 99 Hellfire missiles and 3,000 rounds of 30mm cannon and striking 116 targets.

"Some commentators said it couldn't be done," commented 656 Squadron's commander, "that it was too risky: that we would be shot down, and that it could not contribute to the campaign. To us, no problem is insurmountable, and we knew we would succeed in Libya. Attack helicopters are menacing, they manoeuvre in and out of sight and sound at any time of day and in almost all weather. They create uncertainty and deep unease in the mind of the enemy and they are precise with their weapons. With the additional element of surprise by launching from a floating platform capable of moving hundreds of miles a day, the new player in the air campaign was potent and presented a very difficult problem to the adversary. This was the message we wished to transmit to the pro-Gaddafi military.

"I shall never forget the anticipation of launch [on our first mission], the low-level flight across the sea and the subsequent Hellfire strikes. Everything that happened that night was a new operational experience for us. We repeated it with growing complexity throughout June, July and into August a further 21 times, flying deliberate strike missions across the full breadth of Libya. However, we succeeded on every mission. Every target was struck, often in the face of significant ground fire, every pilot came home safely, and no aircraft were damaged."

LEFT: USAF HH-60H Rescue Hawks of the 56th Rescue Squadron embarked on HMS *Ocean* to provide combat search and rescue cover for the British and French attack helicopters. (USAF)

Apache Gunships Against ISIS

US Army Aviation in Operation Inherent Resolve

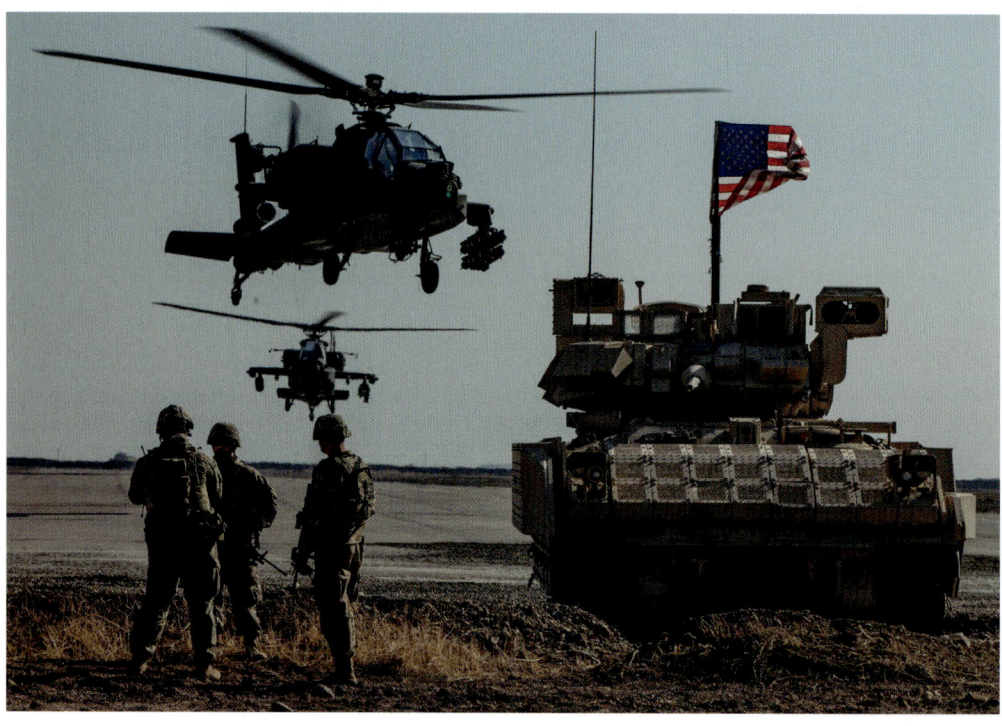

ABOVE: US Army Apaches provided much of the aerial fire power that turned the tide against ISIS fighters in Iraq and Syria. (US DOD/COMBAT CAMERA)

US and British warplanes had already been bombing the advancing ISIS columns, but US commanders now thought it was time to ramp up the air support available to hard-pressed Iraqi troops trying to establish a defence line to the west of Baghdad.

At Baghdad airport, the US Army's 3rd Battalion, 159th Aviation Regiment was winding up its US Army McDonnell Douglas AH-64D Apaches to join the fight. They had arrived earlier in the summer from Camp Buehring in Kuwait to protect the US base at the airport. The heavily armed helicopters had originally been limited to perimeter patrols around the airport and escorting US transport helicopters flying visiting generals and diplomats around Baghdad.

Now the 3rd/159th Aviation would take the fight to the enemy. US and British Special Forces were operating with Iraqi troops on the ground near the frontlines, identifying where the ISIS fighters were massing to attack.

Once cleared for action, the first Apaches struck on October 5, 2014, hitting fighters in Fallujah, in Iraq's Anbar province west of Baghdad, where battles were raging. A US military spokesman reported that the

O ver the autumn of 2014, fanatical fighters from the so-called Islamic State (ISIS) surged across Iraq capturing town after town. By early October the Jihadi army was approaching the outskirts of the Iraqi capital, Baghdad. US soldiers inside the large coalition base in the city could hear the sound of mortar and artillery fire a few kilometres to the west.

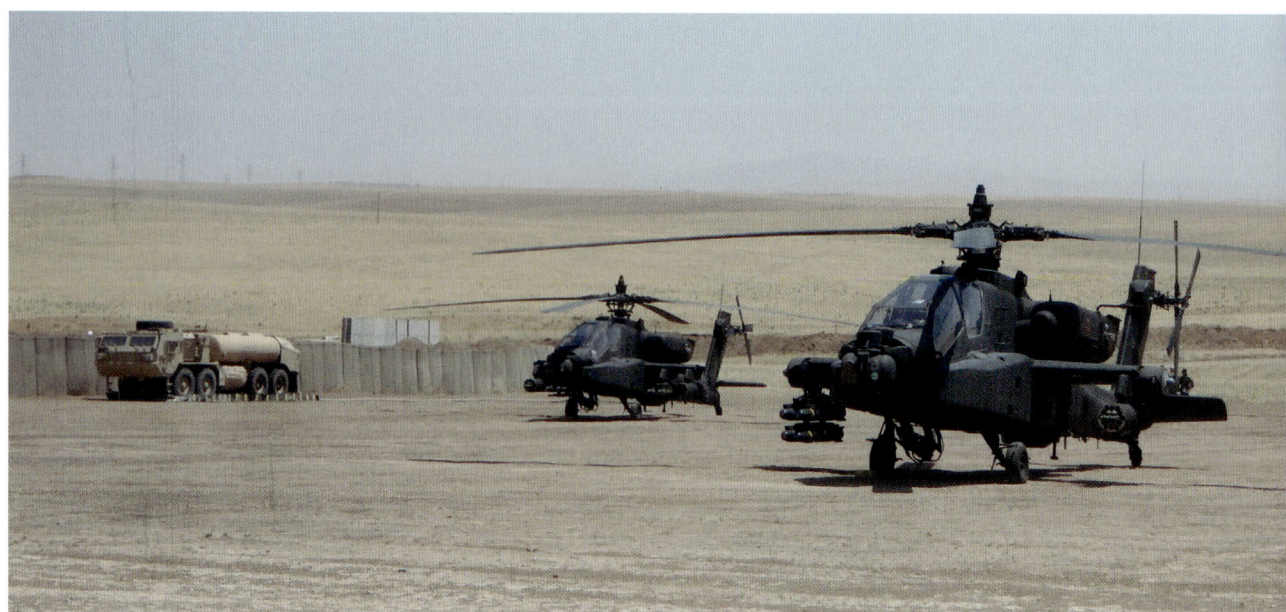

RIGHT: The US Army deployed its Apaches to forward operating bases across Syria and Iraq to increase their operational effectiveness. (US DOD/COMBAT CAMERA)

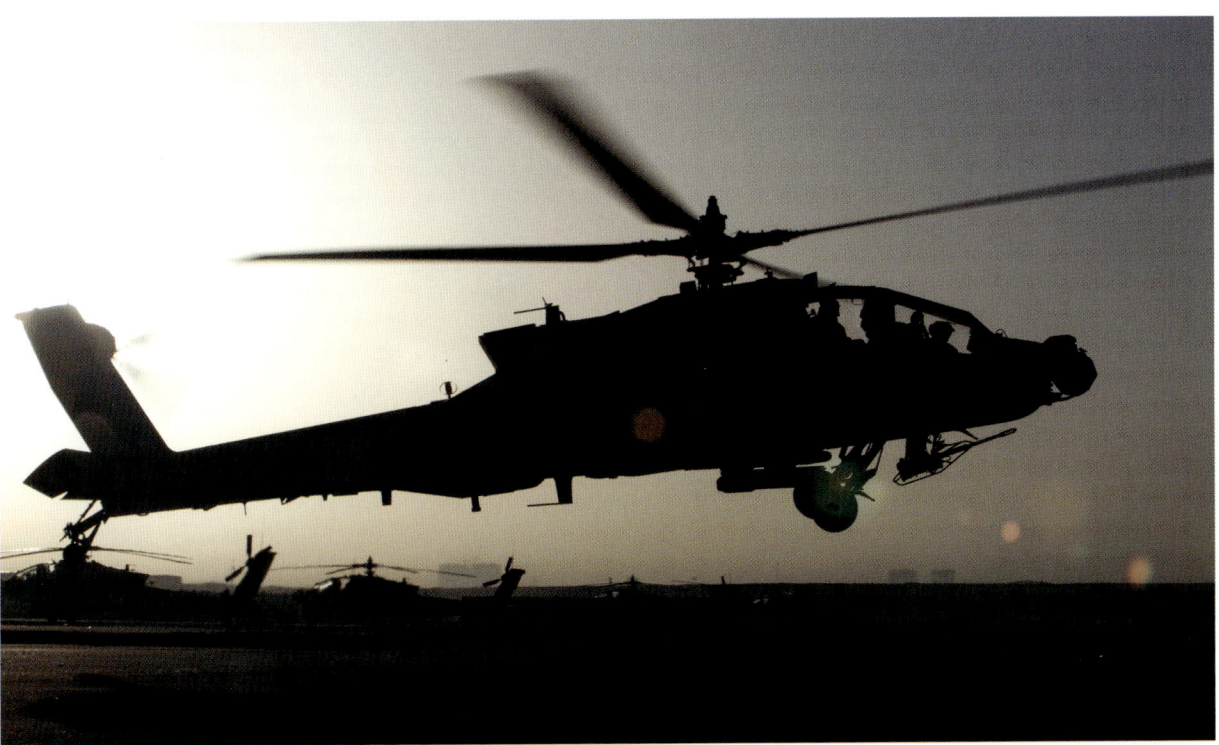

AH-64Ds hit ISIS mortar positions, fighting units and a bunker.

US President Barack Obama was determined that there would be no US ground combat troops on the ground in the Middle East to support the Iraqi army and anti-ISIS militia forces in Syria. The US would rely on airpower – fixed-wing and attack helicopter, artillery, advisers, and special forces raiding teams – to provide war-winning capabilities to local forces. This was not a recipe for a quick victory and the US military began rotating units into Iraq and Syria to support the campaign. US commanders made sure that they had at least one battalion with 24 Apache helicopters in Iraq and Syria throughout the war to protect coalition forces and take the offensive deep into ISIS territory. »

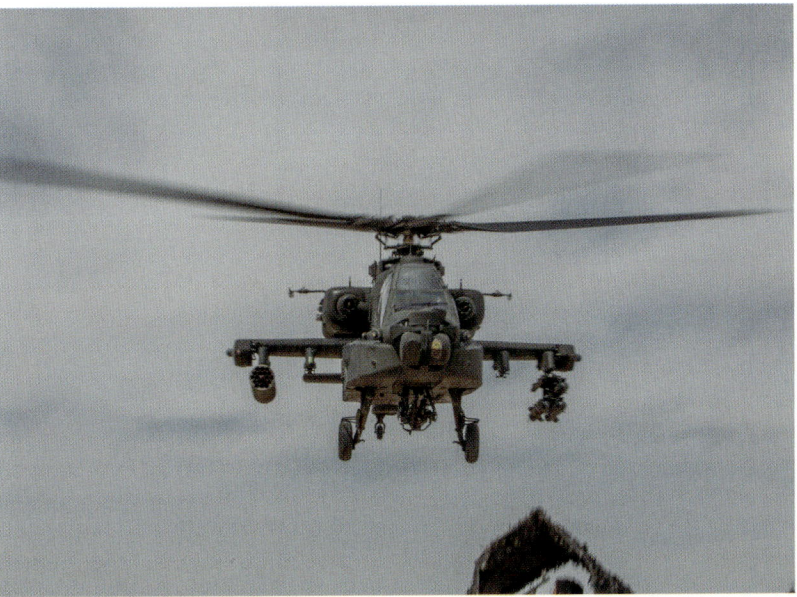

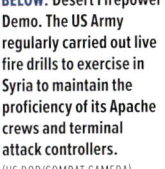

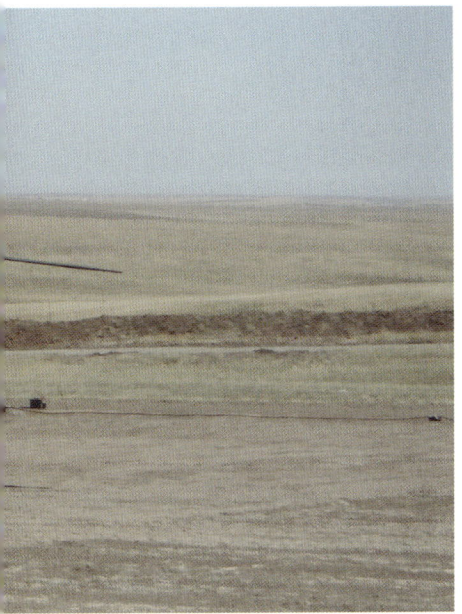

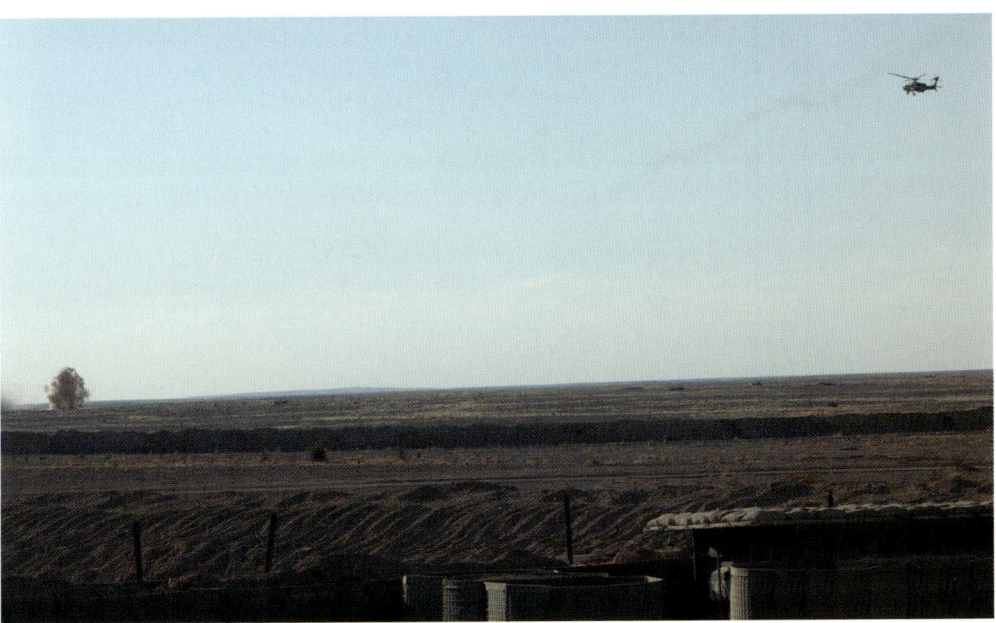

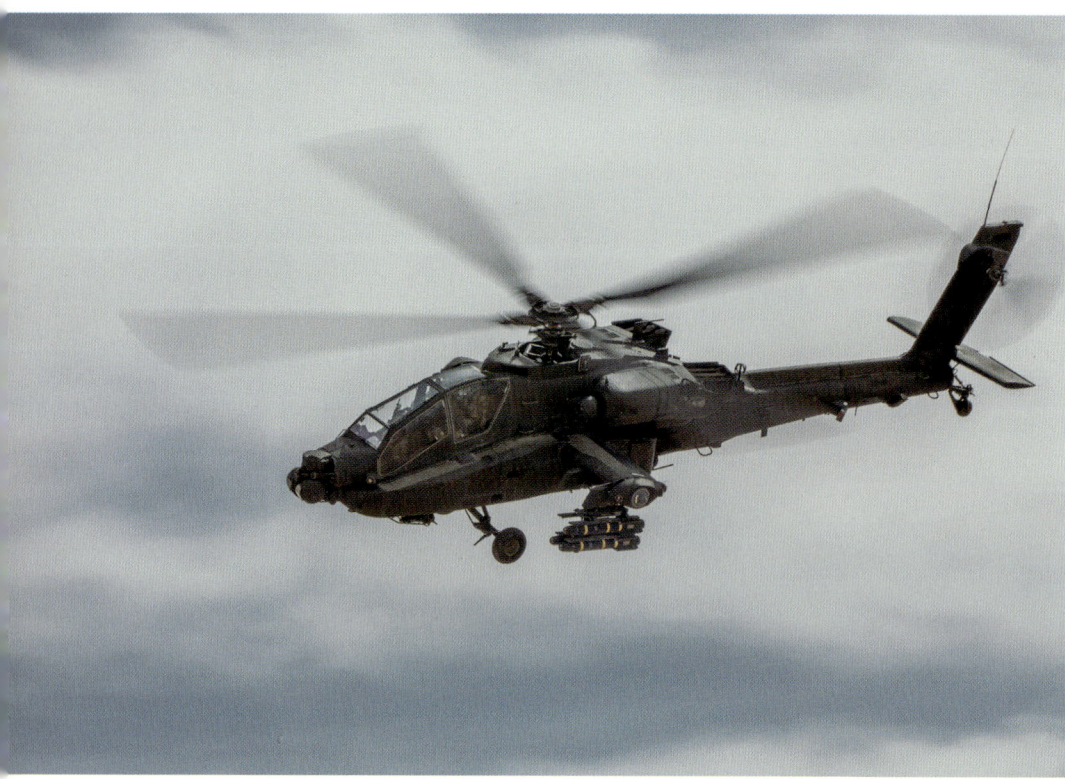

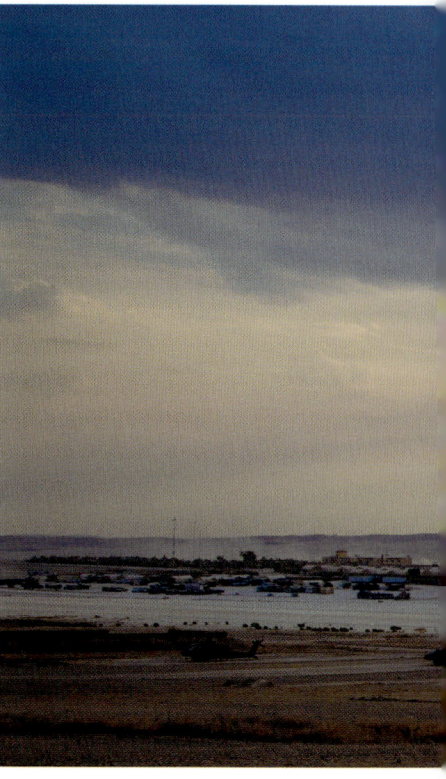

The US Army always kept a combat aviation brigade in the war zone, and it usually comprised an attack helicopter battalion, an air assault battalion with Sikorsky UH-60 Black Hawks and a heavy lift battalion of Boeing CH-47 Chinooks. The deployment of the brigade's helicopters reflected the ebb and flow of the battle. So, in 2014 and 2015, as the fight was focussed on Baghdad and in Anbar province, US helicopters flew most of their missions around the Iraqi capital.

In the summer and autumn of 2016, Iraqi troops were on the offensive and they set their sights of capturing the northern city of Mosul from ISIS. Tens of thousands of Iraqi troops were massed around Mosul with an unprecedented amount of coalition airpower, including US Apaches operating from a forward operating base at Qayyarah Airfield West, to the south of the city.

As Iraqi troops were battling around Mosul, the US military was also ramping up support for Kurdish fighters of the Syrian Democratic Forces (SDF). Small US Special Forces advisory teams were on the ground in Syria with the SDF, helping them to plan an offensive to capture the ISIS capital, Raqqa, and call down coalition air strikes. To supply its Special Forces operatives, US military engineers headed into Syria to build a series of airstrips and forward operating bases (FOB).

The biggest American airstrip, dubbed the Kobani Landing Zone (KLZ), was built to the northwest of

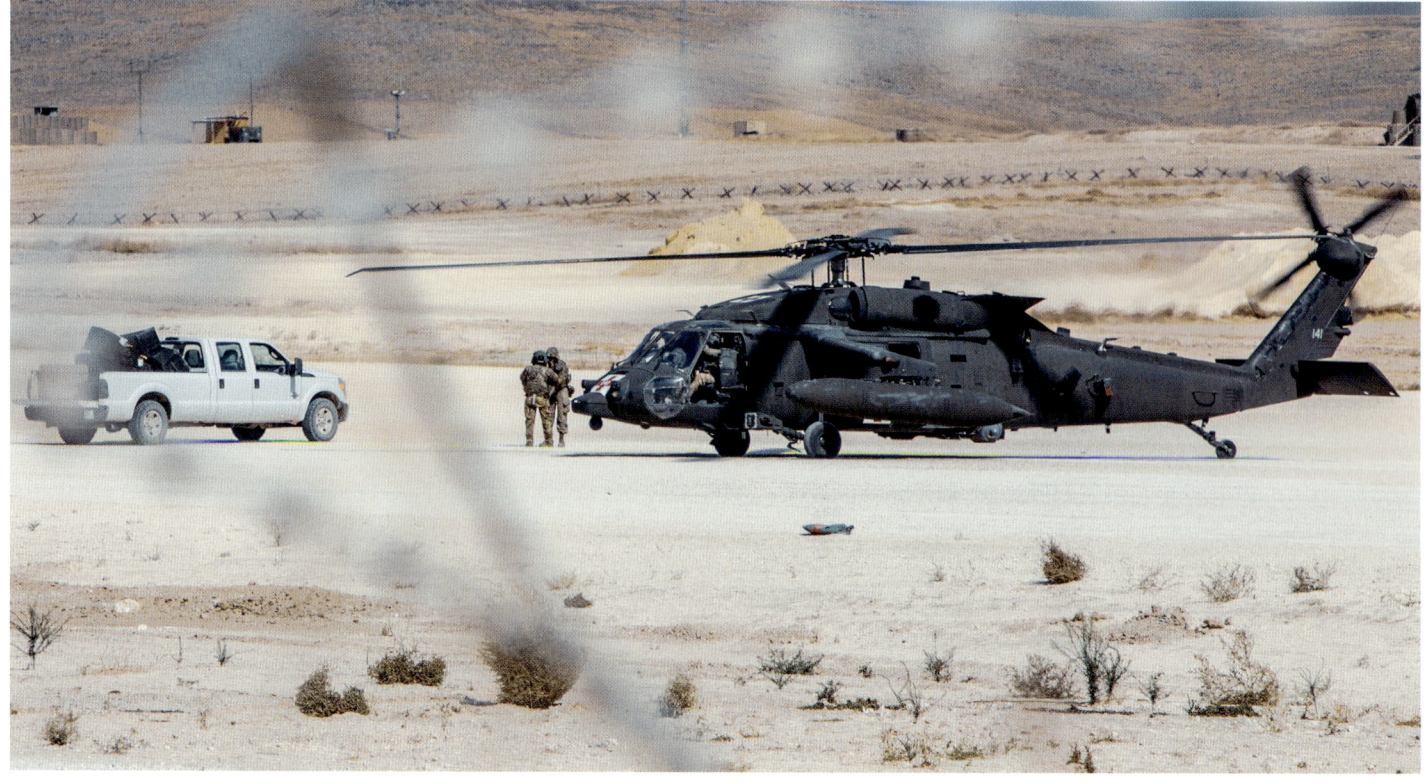

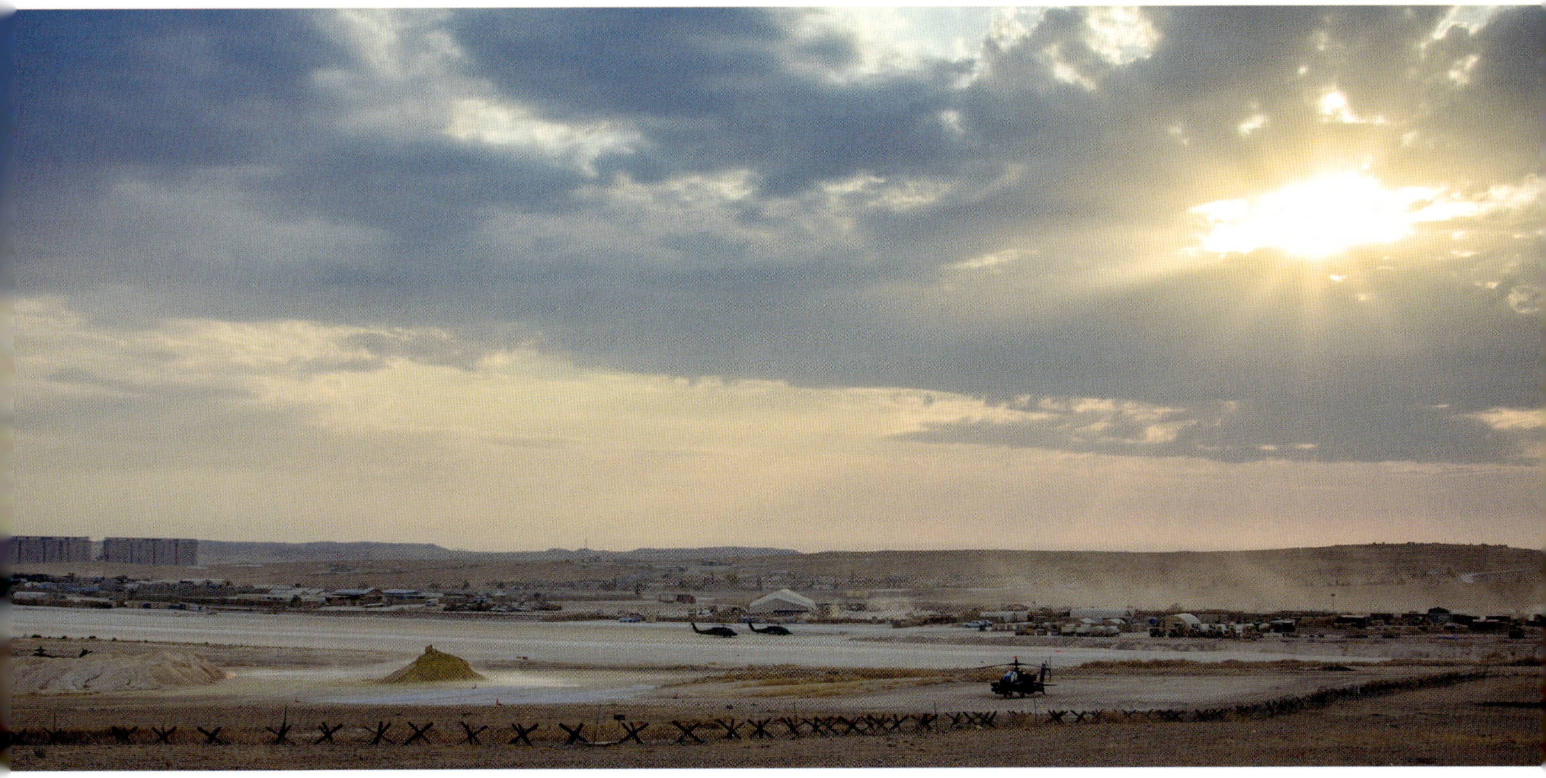

ABOVE: Kobani Landing Zone in northwest Syria was the main US helicopter base during the battle to take Raqqa from ISIS in 2017. (US DOD/COMBAT CAMERA)

Raqqa. It opened the way for giant cargo aircraft to land the heavy arms needed by the SDF. By the end of 2016, US Air Force Boeing C-17 Globemasters and Lockheed Martin C-130J Hercules were flying into these improvised airstrips on a daily basis. The massive base included helicopter landing pads, fuel dumps, ammunition bunkers and prefabricated accommodation for several hundred troops.

In the first months of 2017, the SDF was advancing towards Raqqa, and to boost the offensive US Army Apaches were sent to a FOB to the north of the city. On March 22, 2017, hundreds of SDF fighters and a contingent of US Special Forces troops operating as their advisers, launched a large-scale helicopter-borne assault on ISIS around the area of the Tabqa Dam, to the south west of Raqqa, in a bid to encircle the city and trap its fighters inside.

The assault force was inserted on the southern bank of the Euphrates river by US Army Chinooks, escorted by AH-64Es, and this took the Jihadi fighters by surprise. The following day an ISIS force counter-attacked, prompting the US advisors to call up flights of Apaches to bring down gun, rocket, and missile fire on the enemy.

Over the next four months the fighting intensified as the SDF closed up to the edge of Raqqa's suburbs and then pushed into the city in the face of fanatical resistance. At any point in time eight AH-64Es and a similar number of UH-60s were operating from KLZ, ready to answer calls from help from the SDF. »

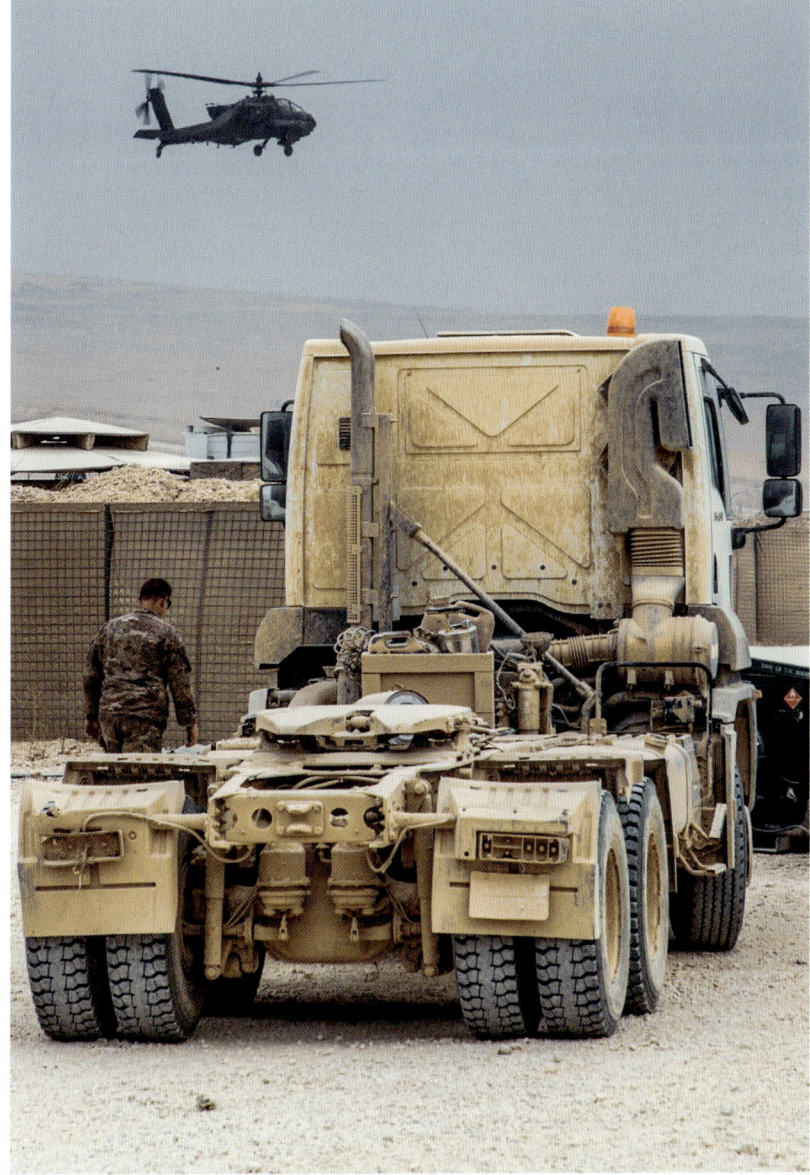

LEFT: Road convoys bringing supplies to US Special Forces contingents in Syria often received Apache escorts. (US DOD/COMBAT CAMERA)

The Battle for Raqqa turned into a brutal street fight, with the SDF and ISIS battling over every building. US and British air controllers were always close by and when an enemy strong point needed to destroyed, an AH-64E would be called up to blast it with pinpoint accuracy.

In October 2019, US President Donald Trump struck a deal with Turkey to allow it to attack Kurdish units of the SDF inside Syria. He ordered US troops to step aside and let the Turks attack the local militia, who only days before had been their allies in the war against ISIS.

As the withdrawal operation gathered momentum, the US, British and French special forces started pulling out of a string of small forward bases across northwestern Syria and falling back to the US airstrip 25km south of Kobani. The US base at KLZ was in a precarious position. Russian, Syrian, Turkish and SDF troops were all within 10 miles of it and the political situation was evolving by the hour in a very unpredictable way. An added layer of protection was provided by the presence of four AH-64Es from the 1st Attack Reconnaissance Battalion,

RIGHT: Senior US commanders regularly visited the US aviation forces inside Syria. (US DOD/COMBAT CAMERA)

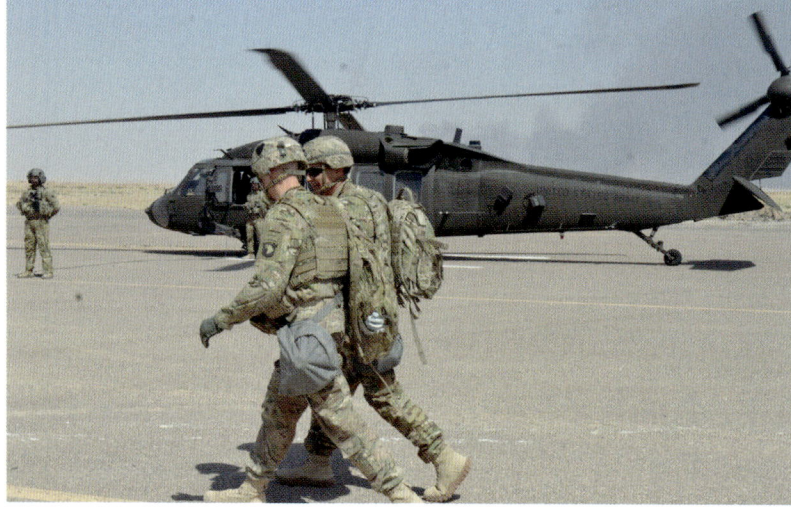

BELOW: In October 2019, US Apaches supported a Special Forces raid in north western Syria that led to the death of the ISIS founder, Abū Bakr al Baghdadi. (US DOD/COMBAT CAMERA)

Syria: Reported ISIS-Leader Al-Baghdadi Compound

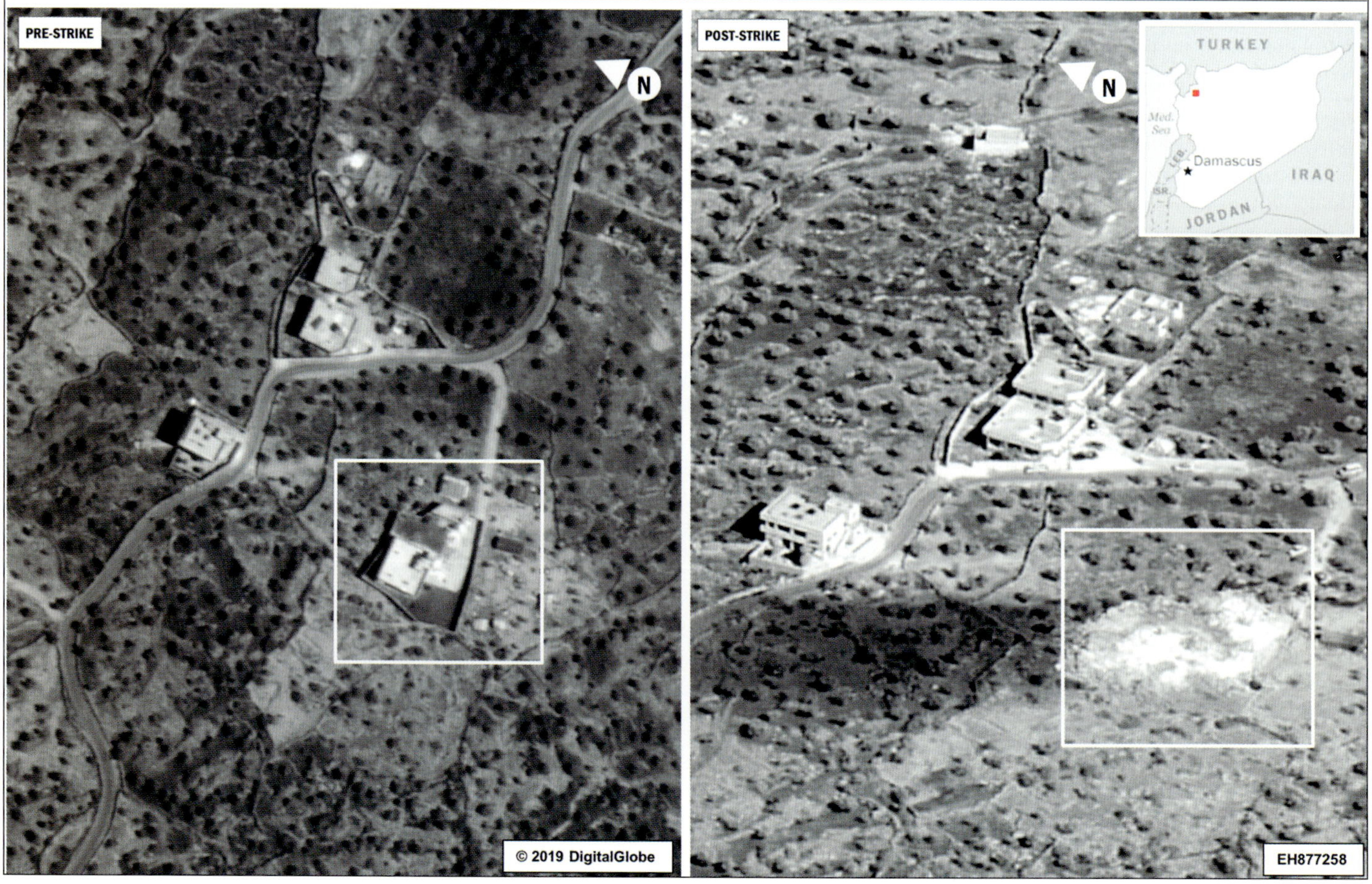

PRE-STRIKE

N

© 2019 DigitalGlobe

POST-STRIKE

N

TURKEY

Med. Sea

Damascus

IRAQ

JORDAN

EH877258

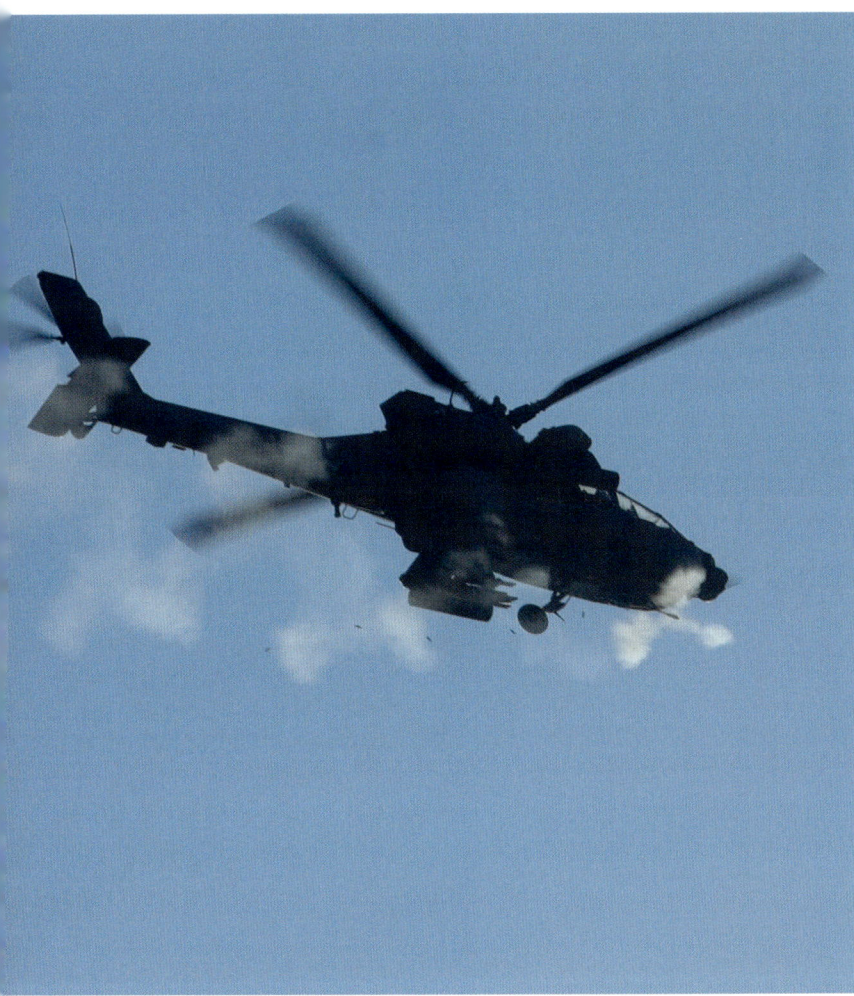

US Army Attack Reconnaissance Battalions Deployed for Operation Inherent Resolve 2014-2022	
Major Unit	**Deployment Date**
34th Combat Aviation Brigade	August 2014
3rd Battalion, 159th Aviation Regiment (AH-64D)	March 2014
4th Battalion, 501st Aviation Regiment (AH-64D)	December 14
185th Theater Aviation Brigade	April 2015
3rd Squadron, 6th Cavalry Regiment (AH-64D)	August 2015
40th Combat Aviation Brigade	December 2015
1st Battalion, 10th Aviation Regiment (AH-64E)	April 2016
77th Combat Aviation Brigade	August 2016
4th Squadron, 6th Cavalry Regiment (AH-64E)	December 2016
29th Combat Aviation Brigade	April 2017
2nd Squadron, 17th Cavalry Regiment (AH-64E)	September 2017
449th Theatre Aviation Brigade	December 2017
7th Squadron, 17th Cavalry Regiment (AH-64E)	February 2018
35th Combat Aviation Brigade	August 2018
4th Battalion, 4th Aviation Regiment (AH-64E)	July 2018
244th Expeditionary Combat Aviation Brigade	May 2019
1st Battalion, 1st Aviation Regiment (AH-64E)	June 2019
34th Expeditionary Combat Aviation Brigade	January 2020
1st Battalion, 227th Aviation Regiment (AH-64E)	January 2020
28th Expeditionary Combat Aviation Brigade	October 2020
4th Battalion, 4th Aviation Regiment (AH-64E)	September 2020
40th Expeditionary Combat Aviation Brigade	May 2021
1st Battalion, 82nd Combat Aviation Brigade (AH-64E)	March 2021
11th Expeditionary Combat Aviation Brigade	January 2022
1st Battalion, 227th Aviation Regiment (AH-64E)	October 2021

1st Aviation Regiment, flying from KLZ.

The value of the Kobani Landing Zone was dramatically illustrated in October 2019 when it provided the launch pad for the raid that led to the death of the ISIS founder, Abū Bakr al Baghdadi. SDF and US intelligence had tracked the infamous Jihadi to a hideout in Idlib province, some 120km to the west of KLZ.

Troops from the secretive Joint Special Operations Command (JSOC) strike unit, the famous Delta Force, were given the job of leading the raid and they were carried to the target by Boeing MH-47G Chinooks from the 160th Special Operations Aviation Regiment. While most media reports claimed that the strike force launched from an air base near Irbil, subsequent briefings in the Pentagon said the raiders had staged through a forward base in Syria, close to Idlib. That base could only have been KLZ.

The raid was a dramatic success. Apaches from the detachment based at KLZ machine-gunned several insurgents who tried to fire on the assault force. This allowed the raiders to land from the Chinooks and then storm Baghdadi's hideout. The assault team in its MH-47Gs then successfully recovered to KLZ to refuel, en route to its home base at Harir in Iraq. The Apaches remained in Syria to cover the US withdrawal to the east of the country. President Trump then changed his mind and US troops maintained positions around Syria's eastern oil fields. US Army Apache helicopters remained on duty to provide them with air cover.

LEFT AND BELOW: The aerial fire power of the AH-64E repeatedly proved decisive during the war against ISIS. (US DOD/COMBAT CAMERA)

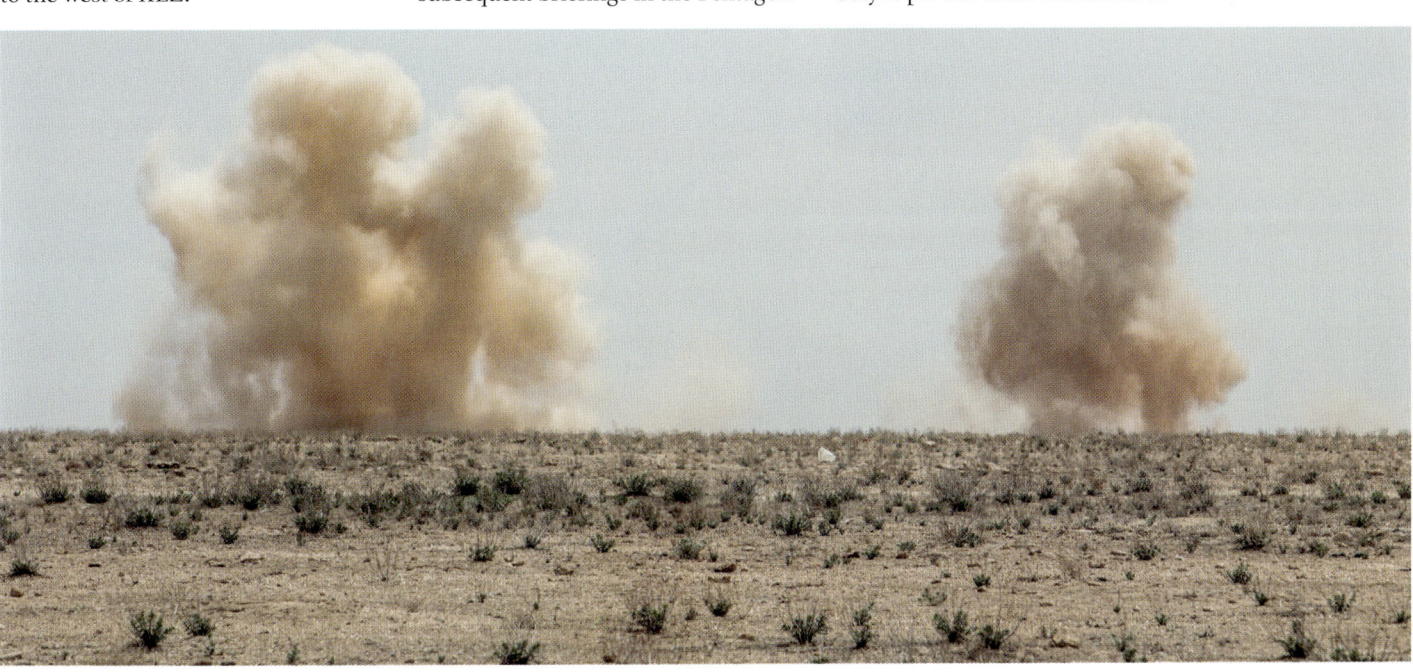

Seize Kiev

Russian Gunships over Ukraine

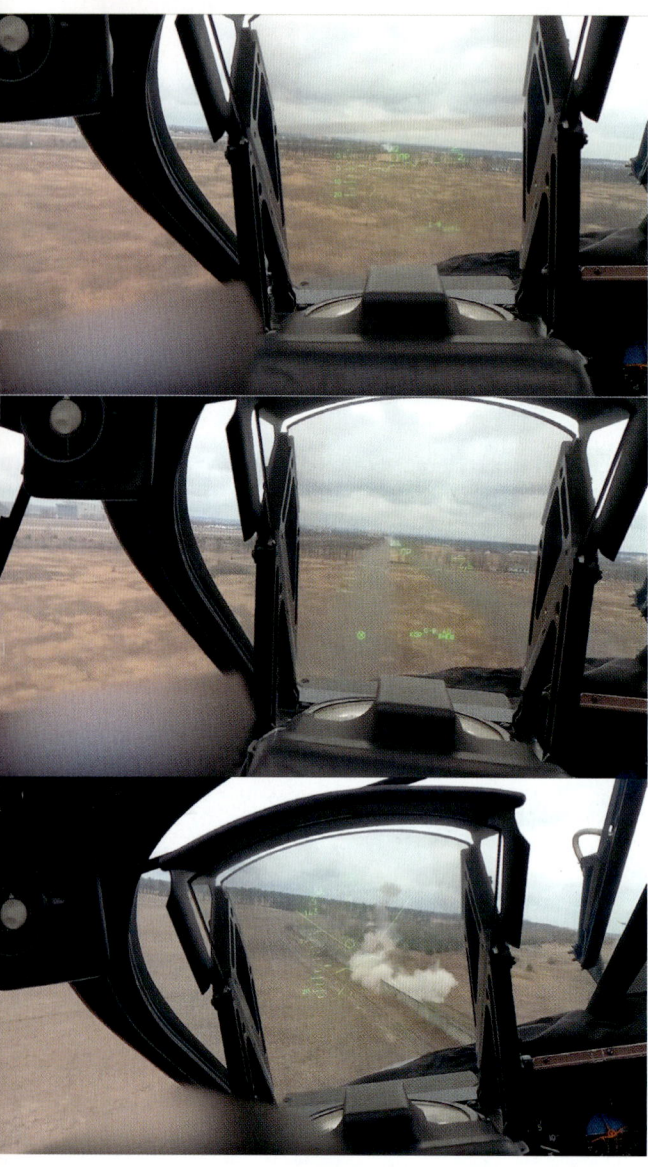

ABOVE: The attack on Hostomel airport outside Kiev as seen from the cockpit of Russian Aerospace Force Ka-52 attack helicopter. (RUAF)

RIGHT: Bolshoy Bokov airfield near Mazyr in southern Belarus became the hub for Russian helicopters operating around the Ukrainian capital, Kiev. (MAXAR TECHNOLOGIES/VIA TIM RIPLEY)

Early on the morning of February 24, 2022, a long line of helicopters could be seen flying down the Dnieper River toward the Ukrainian capital, Kiev. As they neared the city, the Kamov Ka-52 gunships and Mil Mi-8 assault helicopters turned westward. On the shore Ukrainian soldiers readied a salvo of Igla heat-seeking man-portable surface-to-air missiles to take aim at the Russian helicopters. One of the Ka-52s was hit and crashed into the river. The formation kept going and within minutes the Mi-8s were landing Russian paratroopers on the runway of the Antonov International Airport in the Kiev suburb of Hostomel.

The speed of the daring Russian raid caught the Ukrainian army by surprise. There were no Ukrainian troops defending the airport buildings and the Russian paratroopers were soon giving interviews to American television crews. This calm would not last long and by the end of the day the Russians troops were fighting off determined Ukrainian counter-attacks and diving for cover as artillery fire burst around them. The battle was recorded on camera phones by local people and was soon being posted online – they looked like scenes from the epic Vietnam war movie *Apocalypse Now.*

Once the helicopters had dropped off their paratroopers they lifted off and headed back to bases in Belarus, over 100km to the north. Ground support crews were waiting at two forward operating bases in fields near the town of Mazyr to refuel and re-arm the in-bound helicopters.

The Russian Aerospace Forces' (RuAF or VKS) deployment to Belarus began in January 2022 under the cover of Exercise Allied Resolve 2022, which saw the deployment of an all-arms combat group from the Eastern Military District to the country. A joint Russian-Belarus rapid reaction force was being tested during the exercise, according to Moscow's cover story.

The day before the invasion a large force of RuAF helicopters were photographed in a field-operating location in southeastern Belarus. Satellite images subsequently identified more than 30 assorted helicopters, including Ka-52s and Mi-18s, at a temporary base on a road south of Chojniki. The site had also been photographed by local people, who posted images of it online.

Another forward operating location for Russian helicopters was identified in social media images in another field near the town of Mayzr.

Other satellite imagery from that period showed that a large logistical operation was underway to convert a former airfield at Bolshoy Bokov, near Mayzr, into a major helicopter base. This site was not up and running when the war started but several days later the helicopters re-located from the temporary base to Bolshoy Bokov.

There was a steady flow of RuAF transport aircraft heading to Machulishchy airfield, near Minsk, from locations across Russia after the start of the Exercise Allied Resolve 2022. A detachment of Mil Mi-26 heavy lift helicopters also took up residence at the air base. The 11th Air and Air Defence Army set up its forward command post at Machulishchy to co-ordinate all Russian air operations in Belarus.

From its field locations the RuAF helicopters had been flying daily sorties around Kiev. The Russian helicopters had been repeatedly filmed flying in the vicinity of Kiev and shuttling back to their base in Belarus.

A video was posted online on February 25 showing a Russian Mi-24 making a daytime low-level attack on a convoy of Ukrainian Buk air defence missile systems on a motorway on

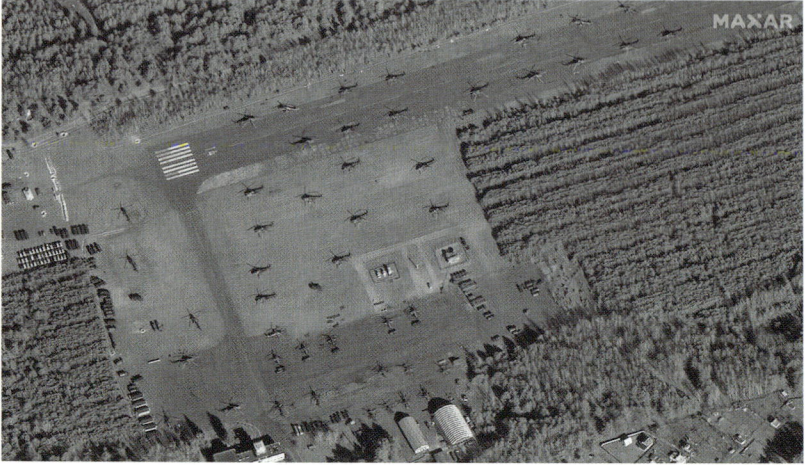

the eastern outskirts of Kiev, which left one launcher and several support vehicles burning.

As Russian troops become bogged down in fighting around the northern edge of Kiev, the RuAF's Mi-8s were required to fly casualty evacuations missions deep into the combat zone. One video clip from a Russian UAV showed an Mi-8 landing at Hostomel airfield, only a few hundred metres from the frontline, to pick up wounded soldiers on stretchers.

Intriguingly, up to mid-March the Russian high command had not committed the bulk of its 180 or so helicopters in Belarus into action. Satellite imagery dating from March 3 and March 6 indicated that only half had so far been deployed to forward operating sites near to the Ukrainian border. The remainder were positioned at Machulishchy air base, including more than 15 Mil Mi-26 heavy lift helicopters and more than 70 Mi-8 assault helicopters. These seemed to be overwhelmingly RuAF assets. The Belarus Air and Air Defence also operated helicopters from the base before the war, but usually had fewer than 10 helicopters there, according to satellite imagery.

In the first phase of the Ukraine invasion, the Russian military operated around 80 helicopters from three forward operating sites in southeast Ukraine, to bring them within operating range of Kiev. Satellite imagery indicated 16 Kamov Ka-52, 65 Mi-8s, four Mi-35s and five Mil Mi-28Ns were present at these bases between February 24 and March 1.

In early April, the Russian high command decided to call off the advance on Kiev and switch the focus of its offensive to the Donbas region in the southeast of Ukraine. Units that had previously been based in Belarus for the advance on Kiev were relocated to the region around Valuyki in Russia, including several helicopter detachments, to operate with the 4th Air and Air Defence Army. These Ka-52, Mi-28N, Mi-35 and Mi-8 helicopters were identifiable by their 'V' recognition markings, which indicated they were from the 15th Army Aviation Brigade, normally home-based at Ostrov.

There was already a strong Russian helicopter force operating in the Donbas, including Ka-52 and Mi-28N attack helicopters and Mil Mi-8 transport helicopters from the 16th Army Aviation Brigade. The helicopters had flown to forward operating bases in separatist-held territory around Donetsk to bring them closer to the front. Before they were re-deployed, the helicopters had

the infamous 'Z' recognition mark applied to prevent friendly troops opening fire on them.

Ka-52s, Mi-35s and Mi-28Ns were routinely filmed by local citizens in Donetsk and Luhansk cities, heading to the front. They were all flying at ultra-low level, even weaving between high rise buildings, signalling that their pilots were very aware of the

threat posed by Ukrainian surface-to-air missile batteries.

Russian forces lost several aircraft and helicopters along the Donbas front during April, including at least one Mi-28N shot down apparently by a British-supplied Starstreak man-portable surface-to-air missile. Two Ka-52s were also lost to other light anti-aircraft missiles.

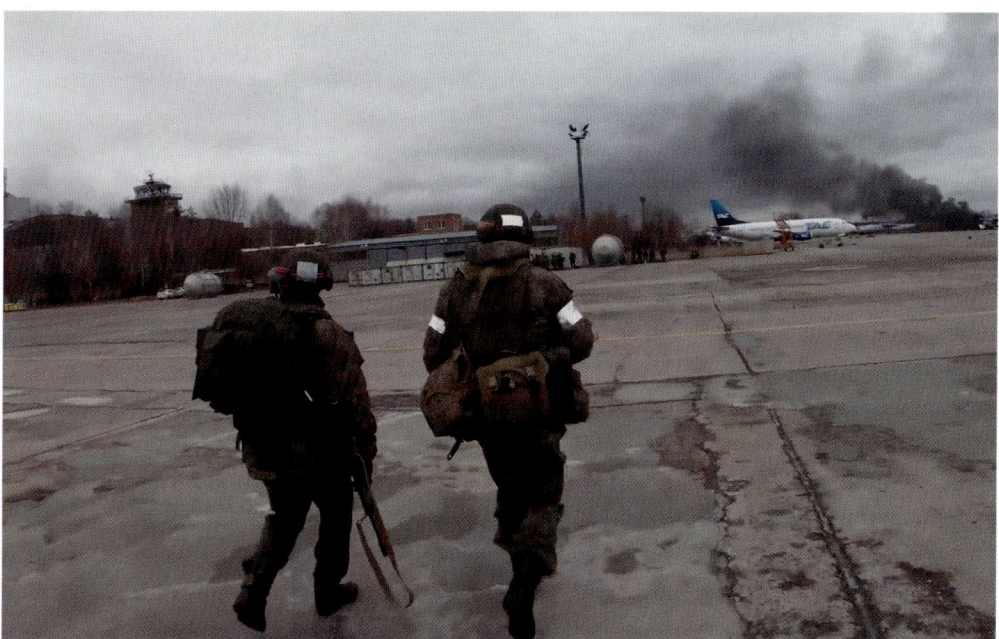

BELOW: Russian paratroopers advance across the tarmac of Hostomel airport outside Kiev after being landed by helicopter in the opening hours of the invasion. (RUAF)

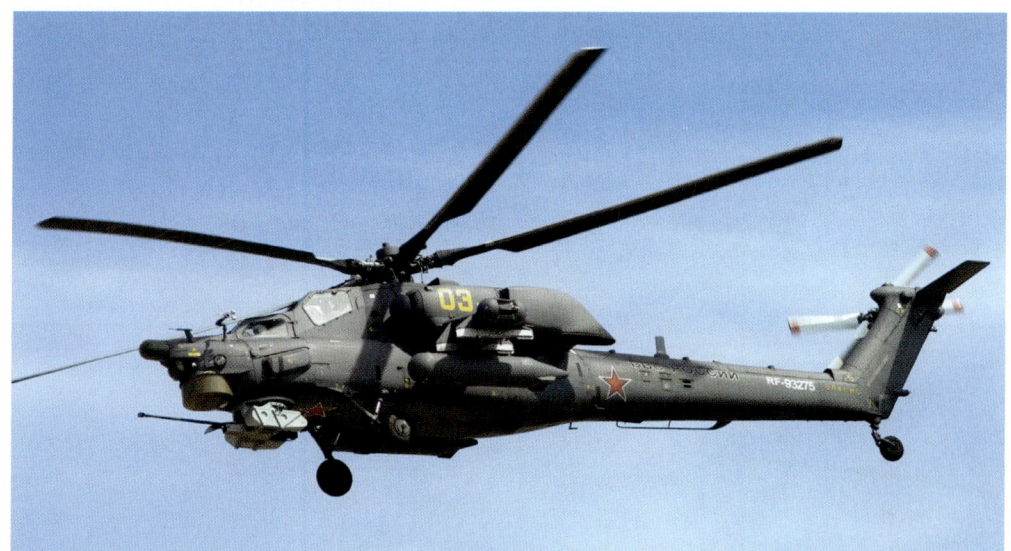

ABOVE: Russian Aerospace Forces' Mi-29Ns saw extensive service on all fronts during the Russian invasion of Ukraine. (RUAF)

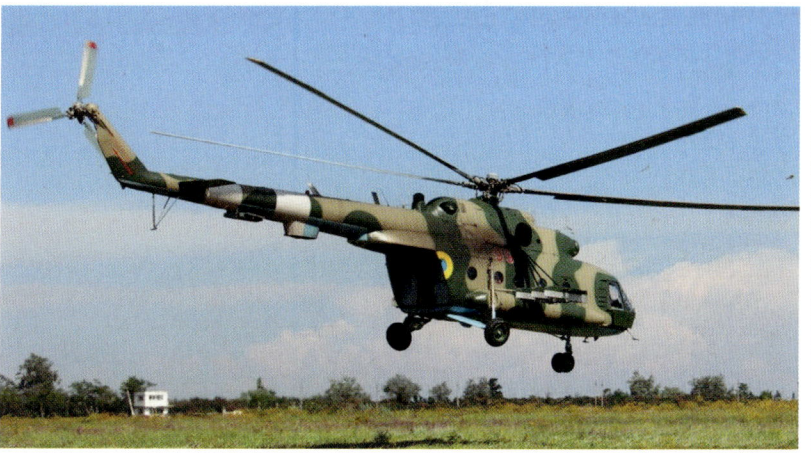

LEFT: Ukraine's Mi-8s played an import role delivering arms and other supplies to front line troops including the besieged garrison in Mariupol. (UKRAINIAN AIR FORCE)

Air Cav for the 21st Century

Future of Attack Helicopters

RIGHT: The Future Attack Reconnaissance Aircraft, or FARA, will be the US Army's next generation attack helicopter. (BELL)

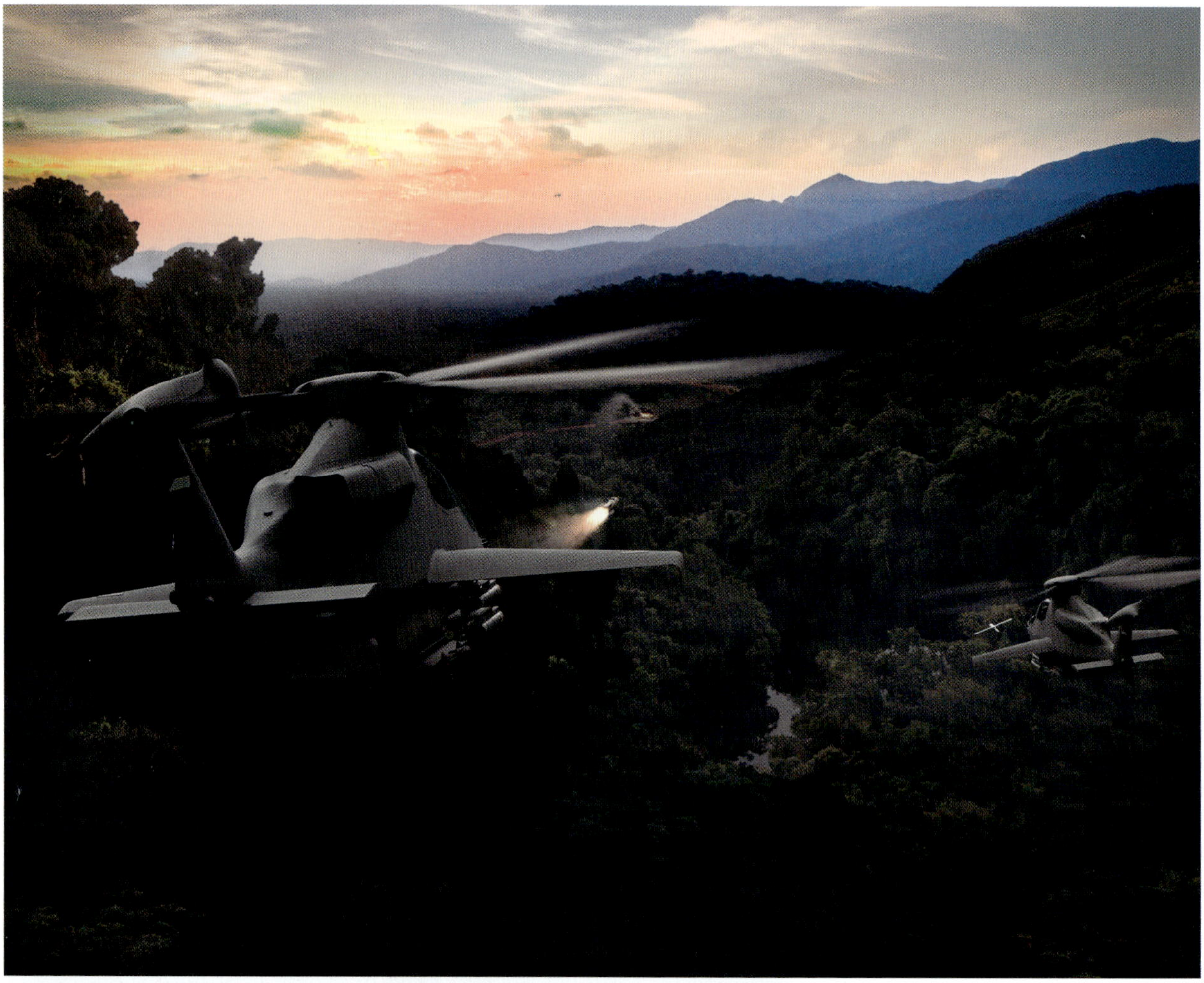

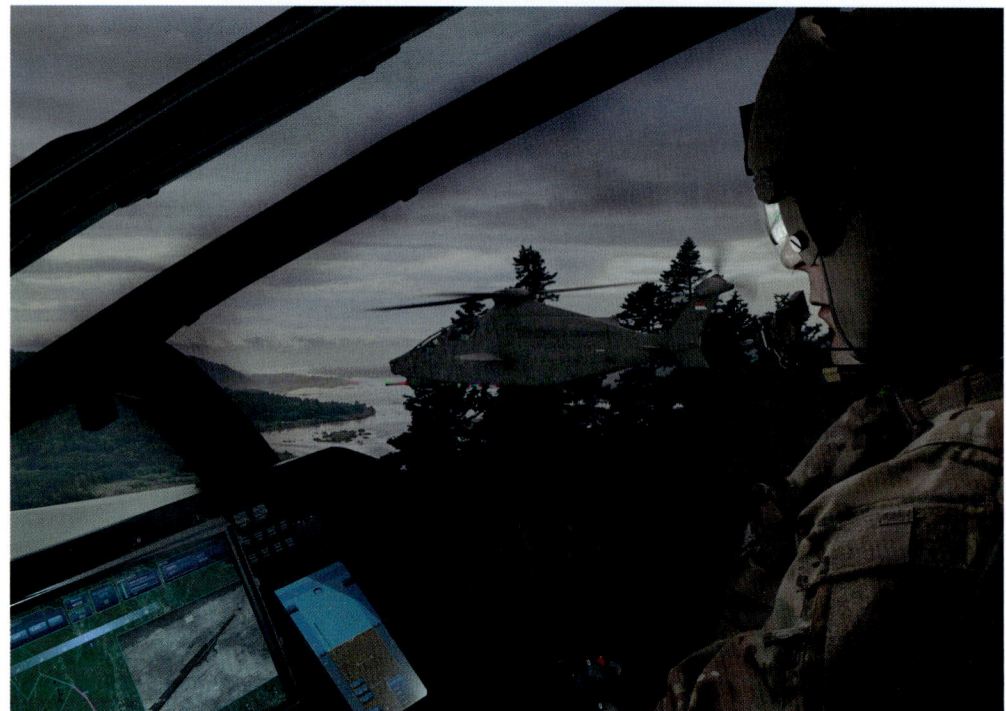

BELOW: Advanced cockpit avionics and interfaces are central to the FARA project. (BELL)

In the six decades since the "Air Cav went tear-assing around 'Nam" the attack helicopter has now been firmly established as a 'must have' weapon for any serious army.

The ability to delivery precision firepower close to friendly troops has proven to be decisive in almost every war that has involved attack helicopters. The psychological impact on the enemy of the sudden appearance of low-flying helicopter gunships over the battlefield cannot be underestimated, while the presence overhead of friendly attack helicopters repeatedly proves to be a major morale boost for ground troops.

Over the past two decades armed unmanned aerial vehicles, or drones, have made an appearance on battlefields around the world. At the top of the range, the US General Atomics Predator and Reaper armed drones have proved potent weapons to find and destroy high-value targets on

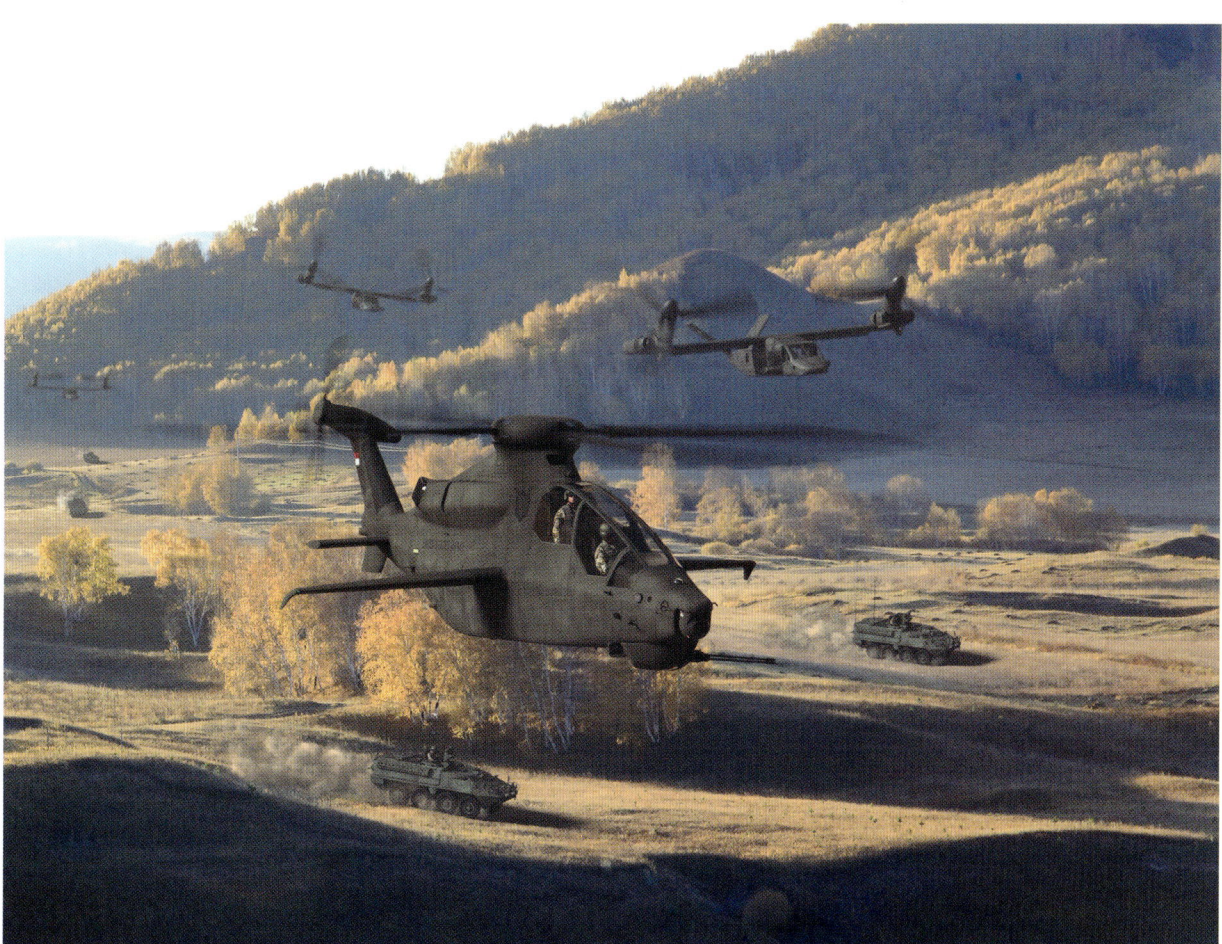

confusing battlefields. For armies, or even militia groups, that can't afford high-end drones such as the Predator, low cost hobby drones have been turned into attack systems by fitting them with rudimentary weapons. In some cases, this is as basic as strapping hand grenades or mortar bombs to the drone and flying it into the intended target. Extremely basic, but deadly.

Drone enthusiasts have claimed that their new weapons have revolutionised the battlefield and allowed air support to be delivered at a fraction of the cost of old-tech weapons such as attack helicopters. The US$60m price tag for a state-of-the-art Boeing AH-64E Apache is eye-watering and that is without all the weapons, training and logistical support needed to get one into action.

In stark cost terms, the gunship looks like its days are numbered, but few armies have been prepared to put all their eggs in the drone basket yet. Although attack helicopters are expensive, they do things that drones cannot, and they are not dependent on air-to-ground communications. If the enemy jams a drone's radio links it cannot operate. Thanks to having a pilot, an attack helicopter can press on to its target even if its communications have been disabled.

Drones also fly at very slow speeds and so can be easily spotted, tracked, and engaged by the enemy. Attack

helicopters can duck, dive and weave around the battlefield, all at very high speeds. This is a critical advantage that even the smartest drone cannot yet do. The ability to fly from field sites just behind the frontline is also a key advantage of attack helicopters that few other aircraft or drones can replicate.

So, the world's armies are not about to give up their attack helicopters any time soon. The US Army, as the largest operator of all types of helicopters, is continuing to invest in keeping its

current Apaches in fighting condition and eventually replacing them with more powerful helicopters.

It is expected that the US will keep funding the conversion of its D model Apache into AH-64E until all 800 are up to the same configuration. It is also funding the development of a new armed helicopter, dubbed the Future Attack Reconnaissance Aircraft (FARA), that is expected to enter service around 2030. It was originally conceived as a replacement for the old Bell OH-58D Kiowa »

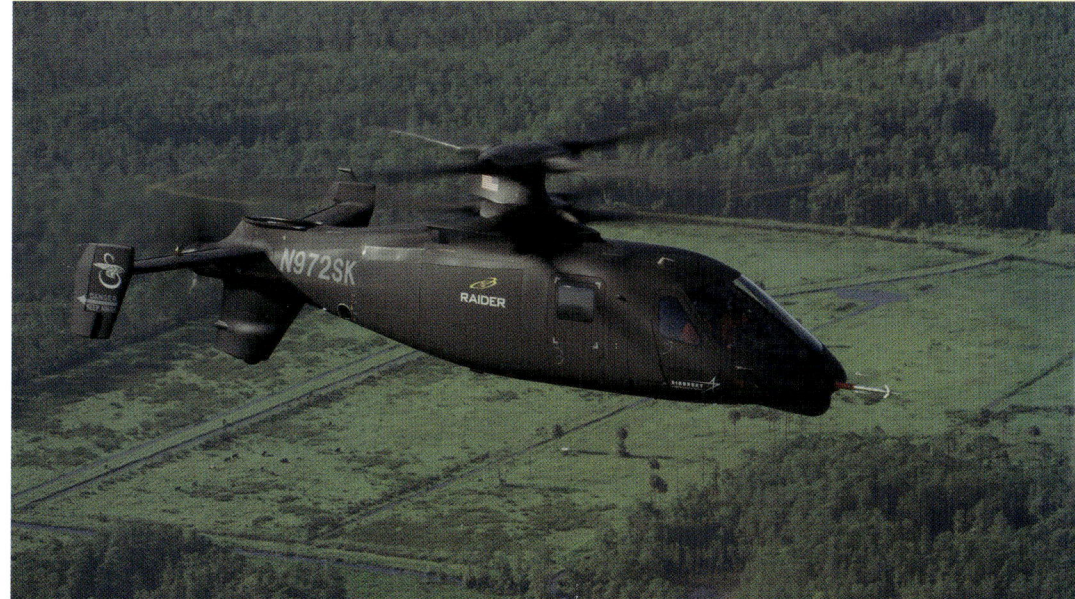

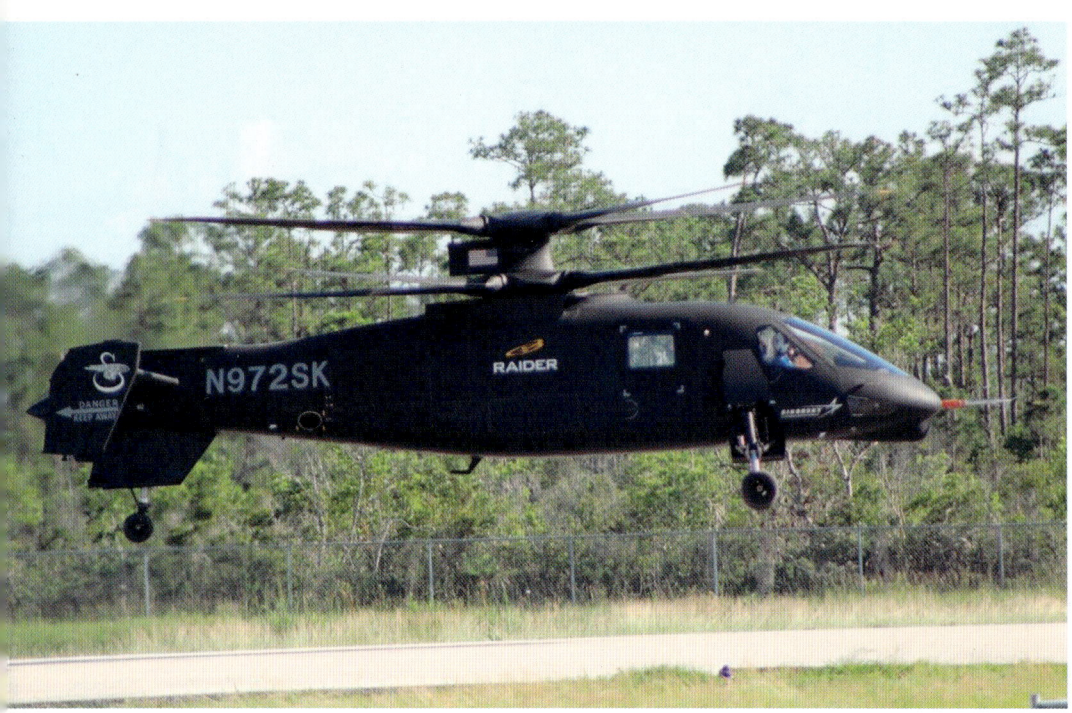

calls for a cruising speed in excess of 330kmph (180 knots).

Bell's design is called the 360 Invictus and it features a winged helicopter with a single rotor and ducted tail rotor. It has a two-seat tandem cockpit with sighting optics and/or a laser designator above a 20mm cannon gun turret at the chin position below the cockpit, mid-mounted stub wings below the shrouded rotor hub and four 40-foot (12m) diameter rotor blades, an active horizontal stabiliser and a tilted and shrouded tail rotor. Missiles are mounted on integrated launchers and unfold to fire. The stub wings are intended to provide lift equivalent to approximately 50% of the weight of the aircraft at moderate to high speed. Combat radius will be 250km (135nm) with at least 90 minutes time on station.

Sikorsky's Raider X incorporates compound coaxial rotors and a pusher propeller design that was originally used on its X2 and S-97 Raider helicopters. It uses a single General Electric T901 engine. The cockpit has side-by-side seats instead of the tandem seating typical of American attack helicopters, and internal weapons and sensors are mounted using a modular system in accordance with FARA specifications and to anticipate future upgrades and obsolescence.

Whichever design wins the FARA contest will likely be in US Army service until the second half of the century, and it is likely to attract significant export orders. Few armies are ready to park up their attack helicopters just yet.

Warrior armed scout helicopter which was retired without a replacement in 2014, but the Apache and armed MQ-1 Grey Eagle drones have taken over the armed scout role, so there is much speculation that the FARA will end up replacing the US Army's Apache.

The FARA is part of a major drive to re-capitalise all the US Army's transport, attack, reconnaissance, and utility helicopters over the next 20 years. The FARA is called the 'knife-fighter' of future Army Aviation capabilities, providing maximum performance in a small package.

FARA candidates will use the engine selected under the Improved Turbine Engine Program (ITEP).

The US Army launched a competition for the development of the FARA and five companies – AVX/L3, Bell, Boeing, Karem/Northrop/Grumman/Raytheon and Sikorsky – all threw their hats in the ring. In 2020, the US Army down-selected Bell and Sikorsky and now aims to choose the winner in 2023, to allow a prototype to be built by 2025. Both designs are required to use the General Electric T901-900 turboshaft engine that won the ITEP competition in February 2019. The US Army also

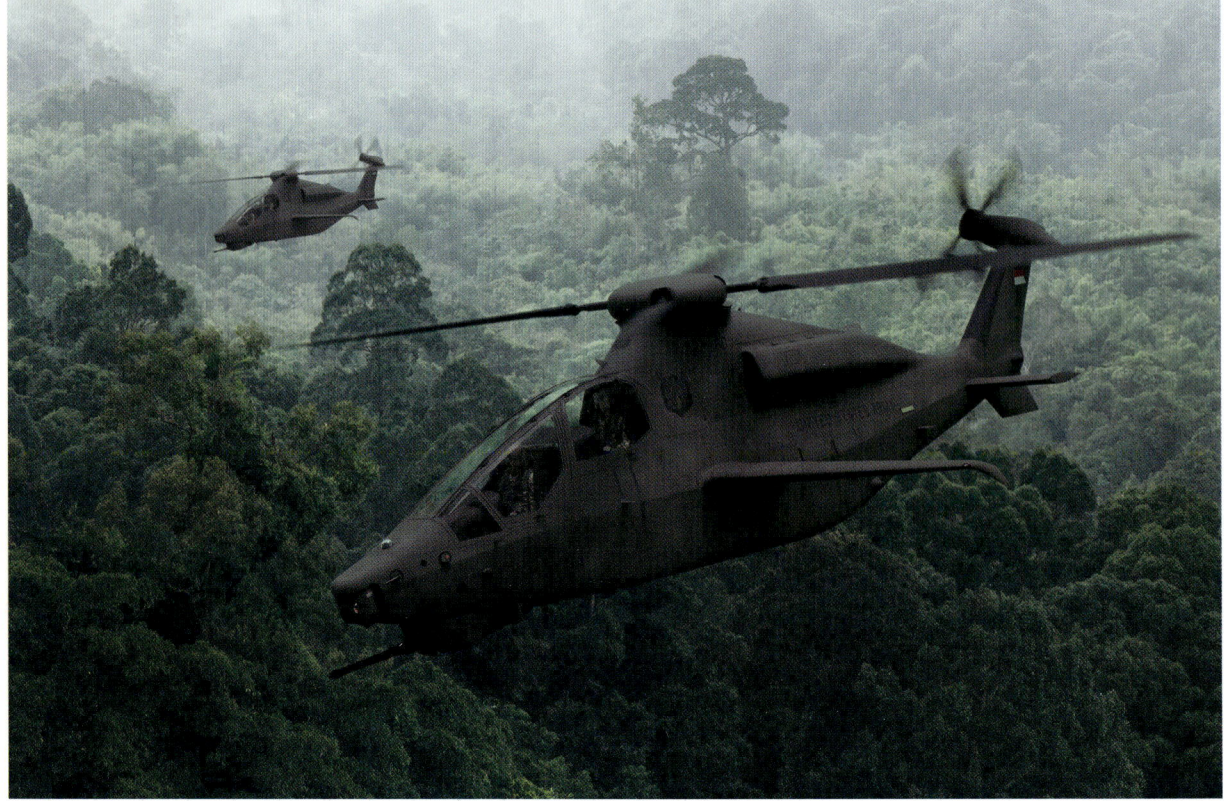